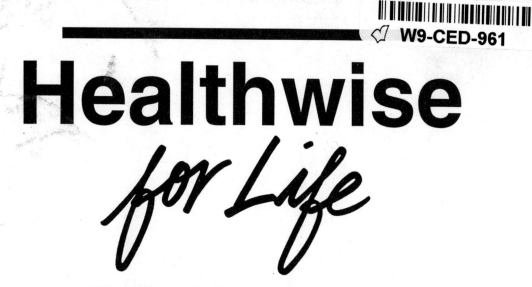

Healthwise
for Life

Medical Self-Care for Healthy Aging

Molly Mettler, MSW, and Donald W. Kemper, MPH

Diana L. Stilwell, MPH, Editor

A Healthwise® Publication
Healthwise, Inc., Boise, Idaho

Table of Contents

To Our Readers

No book can replace the need for doctors—and no doctor can replace the need for people to care for themselves. The purpose of this book is to help you and your doctors work together to manage your health problems.

Healthwise for Life includes basic guidelines on how to recognize and cope with over 190 of the most common health problems facing older adults. These guidelines are based on sound medical information from leading medical and consumer publications, with review and input from doctors, nurses, pharmacists, physical therapists, and other health professionals. We have worked to present the information in a straightforward way that is free from medical jargon. We hope you find it easy to read and easy to use.

While this book does not eliminate the need for professional medical help, it does provide a better basis for you to work with your doctors to prevent and jointly care for health problems. If you receive advice from a doctor or other health professional that conflicts with what you read in this book, look first to your health professional. Because your doctor is able to take your specific needs and history into account, his or her recommendations may prove to be the best. Likewise, if any self-care recommendations fail to provide positive results within a reasonable period of time, consult a health professional.

This book is as good as we can make it, but we cannot guarantee that it will work for you in every case. Nor will the authors or publishers accept responsibility for any problem that may develop from following its guidelines. This book is only a guide; your common sense and good judgment are also needed.

We are continually adding to and improving this book. If you have a suggestion that will make this book better, please send it to Healthwise for Life Suggestions, c/o Healthwise, P.O. Box 1989, Boise, Idaho 83701.

We wish you the best of health.

Molly Mettler and Donald W. Kemper

April 1996

Section V: Self-Care Resources

Section III: Staying Healthy and Independent

Section IV: Caregiver's Guide

About Healthwise

Healthwise is a nonprofit organization working to help people do a better job of staying healthy and taking care of their health problems. Since its founding in 1975, Healthwise has won awards of excellence and recognition from the Centers for Disease Control, the U.S. Department of Health and Human Services, the American Society on Aging, and the World Health Organization.

Healthwise works with organizations wishing to enhance the individual's role in health care. Our clients range from volunteer organizations and church groups to Fortune 500 companies, major unions, state governments, hospitals, insurers, and health maintenance organizations.

Healthwise has published six books, all with workshops and training to support them.

The *Healthwise Handbook* and the Healthwise Workshop. The use of informed medical self-care to improve the quality of care given at home and to help reduce health care costs. *La salud en casa: Guía práctica de Healthwise* is a Spanish translation of the *Healthwise Handbook*.

Healthwise for Life: Medical Self-Care for Healthy Aging and the Healthwise for Life Workshop. Medical self-care for people age 50 and better, including fitness, nutrition, caregiving, and medication management.

Pathways: A Success Guide for a Healthy Life and the Pathways to Health Workshop. A guilt-free approach to health changes in 10 areas, including stress, nutrition, fitness, smoking, alcohol and other drugs, and relationships. The book and workshop are designed to help people make the healthy changes they most want to make.

Growing Wiser: The Older Person's Guide to Mental Wellness and the Growing Wiser Workshops. Memory improvement, mental vitality, coping with loss and life change, maintaining independence, and self-esteem for older adults.

It's About Time: Better Health Care in a Minute (or two). A medical consumerism booklet, with quick, easy-to-use action steps that promote good doctor-patient relationships.

In addition to these books and workshops, Healthwise has produced videotapes and other instructional aids to support health promotion efforts. For more information contact Healthwise at P.O. Box 1989, Boise, Idaho 83701, (208) 345-1161.

Acknowledgments

Healthwise for Life is dedicated to the spirit of Betty Matzek—beloved colleague and quiet advocate for the empowerment of people of all ages. Happy trails until we meet again.

We are particularly grateful to you, the reader. Your interest in actively managing your health problems makes this book possible.

Special thanks goes to the Healthwise staff. Diana L. Stilwell, MPH, editor-in-chief, and Carrie A. Wiss, assistant editor, provided patient and precise editorial guidance. We thank them for their commitment to quality. Many thanks also go to Jean Miller, Jess Bollinger, Viki Smith, Phyllis Tomlinson, and the following individuals whose contributions were invaluable:

Associate Editor
Jane Woychick

Layout and Typesetting
Andrea Blum
Terrie Britton
Cindy Hovland
Sue Armstrong

Contributing Writers
Maria G. Essig, MS
Kattie B. Payne, RN, PhD
Ruth Schneider, RD, MPH
Terrance L. Smith, PhD, FACN
Susan Van Houten, RN, BSN, MBA

Information Specialist
Nancy Van Dinter, MLS

This book would not have been possible without the help and guidance we receive from health professionals. We depend upon them for accurate information, the latest medical developments, and spirited debate.

Primary Medical Reviewers
Steven Schneider, MD
Bradley Lauderdale, MD

Physicians
Paul H. Baehr, MD
Catherine Bannerman, MD
Lester Breslow, MD, MPH
Elizabeth Brown, MD
Randall Burr, MD
Lynn C. Chrismer, MD
Cynthia Clinkingbeard, MD

Christopher C. Colenda, III, MD, MPH
Ginger Dattilo, MD
Bruce V. Davis, MD
Chester Durnas, MD
Steven Freedman, MD
John Funai, MD
William Green, MD

Leonard W. Knapp, MD
Steve Monamat, MD
Robert B. Monroe, MD
Laura Ann Mosqueda, MD
Beverly Parker, MD
Leslie Pederson, MD
Marijo Perry, MD
James T. Pozniakas, MD
Scott Pressman, MD
Dennis E. Richling, MD
Robert Schmidt, MD, MPH, PhD
Stanford Shoor, MD
David Sobel, MD, MPH
Mary Beth Tupper, MD
Robert Vestal, MD
Michael Wasserman, MD

Nurses
Gene Drabinski, RN
Ryu Kanemoto, MN, RNC
Mary Lou Long, RNC, MSN
Jane Mayfield, RN

Health Educators
Bernice Bennett, MPH, CHES
Susan Eisendrath, MPH
David Feffer, MPH
Bob Gorsky, PhD
Joan Greathouse, MEd
Diane Katz, MPH
Joe Leutzinger, MS
Eileen Mackle-Kern, MHA

Psychologists
Karen Magee, MA
James Read, PhD

Dentist
Edwin O. Matthes, DDS

Pharmacist
Doris Denney, RPh

Physical Therapists
Nancy Casey, PT
Lynn Johnson, PT

Finally, we would like to thank the following people who helped us make this book easy to understand and easy to use:

Nancy Adrian
Loyal Barker
Joe Braun
Pris Braun
Margaret Burris
Carol Cronin
Rhonda Davis

Bonnie Mettler
Marty Shepherd
Mae States
Chuck Thompson
Dee Thompson
Grace Tucker
Ralph Tucker

Introduction

Healthwise for Life can help you improve your health and lower your health care costs. It is a book you may turn to time and again as health problems arise.

The book is divided into five sections:

Your Role in Health Care. What you need to know in order to be a wise medical consumer.

Self-Care for Health Problems. Prevention, treatment, and when to call a health professional for over 190 common illnesses and injuries.

Staying Healthy and Independent. Tips and techniques for fitness, nutrition, stress management, mental wellness, and staying independent.

Caregiver's Guide. Special advice on how to care for yourself as you care for others.

Self-Care Resources. How to manage medications and what you need to have on hand in your home to cope with health problems.

Most people will not read through the book cover to cover in one sitting. It is more of a topic-by-topic book that you can use to look up what you need when a problem or interest arises.

We do recommend that you read pages 1 and 2 and three special chapters right away.

Page 1 is the **"Healthwise Approach,"** a process to follow every time a health problem arises. Page 2, the **"Ask-the-Doctor Checklist,"** will help you get the most out of every doctor visit.

Chapter 1, **The Wise Medical Consumer,** offers important information that you can use to improve the quality and lower the cost of the health care you need.

Chapter 2, **Prevention and Early Detection,** lists the immunizations and screening tests that are important to staying healthy and detecting health problems early.

Chapter 27, **Your Home Health Center**, lists medications, supplies, and self-care equipment that you may wish to keep in stock.

The rest of the book is there when you need it. We hope it will help you succeed in better managing your own health problems.

The Healthwise Approach

Step 1. Observe the problem.
- When did it start? What are the symptoms? _____
  _____
  _____
- Where is the pain? Dull ache or stabbing pain? _____
  _____
- Measure your vital signs:
  Temperature: _____   Blood pressure: _____ / _____
  Pulse: _____ / minute   Breaths: _____ / minute
- Think back:
  Have you had this problem before?   Yes _____   No _____
  What did you do for it? _____

  Any changes in your life (stress, medications, food, exercise, etc.)?
  _____
  _____

  Does anyone else at home or work have these symptoms? _____

Step 2. Learn more about it.
- *Healthwise Handbook* (note page number): _____
- Other books or articles: _____
- Advice from others (lay or professional): _____

Step 3. Make an action plan.
- Your hunches about what's wrong (tentative diagnosis): _____
- Home care plan: _____
  _____
- When to call your doctor: _____

Step 4. Evaluate your progress.
- Are your actions working? _____

Ask-the-Doctor Checklist

Before the visit:
- Complete the Healthwise Approach on page 1 and take it with you.
- Take a list of medications and record of last visit for similar problems.
- Write down the two or three questions you want answered most.

During the visit:
- State your main problem first.
- Describe your symptoms (use page 1).
- Describe past experiences with the same problem.

Write down:
- Temperature: _____ Blood pressure: _____ / _____
- The diagnosis (what's wrong): _____
- The prognosis (what might happen next): _____
- Your self-care plan (what you can do at home): _____
  _____
  _____

For drugs, tests, and treatments, ask: (See pages 8 to 10.)
- What's its name? _____
- Why is it needed? _____
- What are the costs and risks? _____
- Are there alternatives? _____
- What if I do nothing? _____
- (For drugs) How do I take this? _____
- (For tests) How do I prepare? _____

At the end of the visit, ask:
- Am I to return for another visit? _____
- Am I to phone in for test results? _____
- What danger signs should I look for? _____
- When do I need to report back? _____
- What else do I need to know? _____
  _____
  _____

*You, the individual, can do more for your health and
well-being than any doctor, any hospital, any drug,
and any exotic medical device.*

Joseph Califano

1

The Wise Medical Consumer

Good health care begins with you.
The quality and the cost of medical
care depends as much on you as on
your doctor. By working in partnership with your doctors, you can help
them improve the care they give you.
And you can lower your own medical
costs.

You play an important role as a
partner in your care:

- At home, by managing day-to-
  day illnesses and long-term health
  problems.

- At every doctor visit, by preparing
  and asking questions.

- When you are faced with a major
  medical choice, such as surgery, by
  making informed decisions.

No matter how good your doctor is,
you can do a lot to improve the quality
of care that you receive. Your doctor

cannot practice good medicine without
your help. If you expect too much
from your doctor and too little from
yourself, you may be limiting the
quality of care you receive. The suggestions in this chapter will help you
be a good partner with your doctor.

Health Partnership at Home

Being a good partner starts at home
with your efforts to stay healthy and
take care of health problems before
they become serious.

Three Ways to Be a Good
Partner at Home

1. **Take good care of yourself**. Both
you and your doctor would prefer
that you don't get sick in the first
place. And if problems arise, you
both want a return to good health as
soon as possible.

2. At the first sign of a health problem, observe and record your symptoms. Your record of symptoms will help both you and your doctor make an accurate diagnosis. And the better job you do recording early symptoms, the better you and your doctor can manage the problem later.

- Keep written notes on the symptoms. Record when, how long, how painful, etc., for each symptom.

- Note anything unusual that might be related to the problem.

- Add regular updates and watch your progress. Note which symptoms are getting better or worse.

What Kind of Medical Consumer Are You?

The Passive Consumer

Description
You rely on the doctor's advice. You don't ask many questions or offer much information unless asked.

Message
"I'm looking for a doctor who will take charge of all my health problems. I plan to rely on the doctor's judgment in all medical decisions."

When Appropriate

- You have one main doctor whom you trust to provide or coordinate all your medical care.

- You are in an emergency situation and split-second decisions are critical.

The Active Consumer

Description
You want to actively share in making treatment decisions with your doctor. You are comfortable asking questions and expressing concerns. You strive for a working partnership with your doctor.

Message
"I'm looking for a doctor who will listen to me and involve me fully in treatment decisions. I will share responsibility for choosing among treatment alternatives."

When Appropriate

- You are confident your ideas will improve the quality of care you get.

- You believe your ideas will help keep costs down.

- For chronic problems, note any changes in symptoms or any new symptoms.

3. Practice medical self-care. You can manage many minor health problems on your own. You are also responsible for the day-to-day management of chronic health problems. Use this book, your own experience, and help from others to create a self-care plan.

- Learn all you can about the problem.

- Keep notes on your self-care plan and what you do.

- Note which home treatments seem to help.

- Set a time to call a health professional if the problem continues or if your symptoms change. See page 11 for more on calling your doctor or advice nurse.

Health Partnership With Your Doctor

Good partnerships are based on a shared effort and good communication. You can be a partner with your doctor by preparing for and playing an active role during office visits. If you are successful, you will get better care and your doctor will practice good medicine. Doctors will usually welcome your efforts to work in partnership with them to improve your care.

Two Ways to Be a Good Partner With Your Doctor

1. Prepare for office visits.

Most doctor visits are short. The better organized you are, the more value you can get from the visit.

- Prepare an Ask-the-Doctor Checklist like the one on page 2.

- Update and bring your list of symptoms and your self-care plan.

- Write down your main concern and practice describing it. Your doctor will want to hear that first.

- Write down your hunches and fears about what is wrong. These are often helpful to your doctor.

- Write down the three questions you most want answered. There may not be time to ask a long list of questions.

- Bring along a list of the medications (prescription and over-the-counter) you are taking.

2. Play an active role in the medical visit.

- Begin by stating your main concern, describing your symptoms, and sharing your hunches and fears.

- Be honest and straightforward. Don't hold anything back because of embarrassment. If you don't intend to fill a prescription, say so. If you are getting other treatments, such as chiropractic treatments or acupuncture, let your doctor know. To be a good partner, your doctor has to know what's going on.

- If your doctor prescribes a medication, test, or treatment, get more information. See pages 8 to 10.

- Take notes. The faintest ink is more accurate than the strongest memory. Write down the diagnosis, the treatment and follow-up plan, and what you can do at home.

- Take a friend along for even better understanding. A second pair of eyes, ears, and hands can be very helpful in recording the doctor's findings and suggestions.

- Review and summarize. At the end of the visit, ask if you can briefly repeat from your notes what you think the doctor said. If the doctor corrects your description, change your notes.

Health Partnership for Major Medical Decisions

Except in an emergency, you cannot be given a test or treatment without your informed consent. This means that you must be told about the risks and agree to the treatment. In a partnership, however, informed consent may not be enough. The goal of a partnership is shared decision-making, in which you actively participate in every medical decision. When you and

---

For Every Doctor Visit

1. Bring:

- The **Healthwise Approach** (page 1), including a list of your symptoms

- The **Ask-the-Doctor Checklist** (page 2)

- A list of all your medications (page 397)

2. Be honest with your doctor.

3. Ask "why?"

4. Ask about alternatives.

5. Write down important information.

6. Review and summarize.

Consumer tip: Wear clothes that you can remove easily. The time saved in undressing may allow more time with your doctor.

---

your doctor work together, the result is always better than when your doctor works alone.

Who Knows You Best?

Doctors have a tough job. They have to make treatment recommendations for lots of people whom they may not know well. Often, they recommend a treatment that will work well for the average patient. However, you may not be an average patient.

The average patient may want to have many tests to be absolutely sure what is wrong. Do you prefer to avoid tests if the results won't change your treatment?

The average patient may expect to get a prescription at every doctor visit. Do you prefer to explore other options in addition to medication?

The average patient may want to get rid of a problem regardless of the risks. Do you prefer to hear more about the side effects of treatment and decide for yourself if the benefits are worth the risks to you?

You alone are qualified to decide what is best for you. Tell your doctor your point of view about every decision.

Why should you help make decisions with your doctor? Aren't you paying him to know what to do? Well, the choices are almost never black and white. With most health problems, there is more than one option. Consider these examples:

You have an enlarged prostate. It causes some bothersome but minor urinary symptoms. Your doctor says that surgery would probably take care of the urinary symptoms, but might have other side effects, such as erection problems. Do you prefer dealing with the symptoms rather than the possible risks of the surgery?

You are just finishing menopause and are wondering about hormone therapy. Your doctor says it will reduce your risk of osteoporosis and heart disease. Do you prefer to avoid the possible risks of hormones and work on lifestyle changes such as diet and exercise to keep your bones strong and your heart healthy?

You have coronary artery disease, and your symptoms are not responding to medications and home treatment. Your doctor recommends an angiogram to measure the blockages in your coronary arteries. You ask how the test results will be used. Your doctor says that the results will determine what type of surgery would be recommended, and that you need to decide before having the test if you would want to have surgery. Would you choose to have surgery if the test indicates it would help?

Seven Ways to Share in Medical Decisions

1. Let your doctor know what you want. Tell your doctor that you want to share in making the decision about what to do for your health problem.

2. Do your own research. Sometimes you need to learn things on your own before you can fully understand what your doctor is saying. See the Resources that start on page 418 for books and other sources of information about health problems.

3. Ask about alternatives. Learn enough to understand the options your doctor thinks are feasible.

4. Consider watchful waiting. Ask your doctor if it would be risky or costly to wait a while (day, week, month) before treatment to see if symptoms improve on their own.

5. State your preferences. Tell your doctor if you prefer one option over another based on your personal desires and values.

6. Compare expectations. Tell your doctor what you are expecting from the treatment and ask if that is realistic. If appropriate, discuss side effects, pain, recovery time, long-term limitations, etc.

7. Accept responsibility. When you make shared decisions with your doctor, both of you must accept the responsibility for the outcomes.

Shared Decisions About Medical Tests

Medical tests are important tools, but they have limits. Some people think that the more tests they have, the better off they'll be. Wise consumers know medical tests have costs and risks as well as benefits. To help your doctor make good choices about tests for you, you need to:

Learn the basics.

- What is the name of the test and why do I need it?

- If the test is positive, what will the doctor do differently?

- What could happen if I don't have the test?

Consider the risks and benefits.

- How accurate is the test? How often does it indicate a problem exists when there is none (false positive)? How often does it indicate there is no problem when there is one (false negative)?

- Is the test painful? What can go wrong?

- How will I feel afterward?

- Are there less risky alternatives?

Ask about costs.

- How much does the test cost?

- Is there a less expensive test that might give the same information?

Let your doctor know:

- Your concerns about the test.

- What you expect the test will do for you. Ask if that is realistic.

- Any medications you are taking.

- Whether you have other medical conditions.

- Your decision to accept or decline the test.

If a test seems costly, risky, and not likely to change the recommended treatment, ask your doctor if you can avoid it. Try to agree on the best approach. No test can be done without your permission.

Once you agree to a test, ask what you can do to reduce the risk of errors. Should you restrict food, alcohol, exercise, or medications before the test?

After the test, ask to review the results. Take notes for your home records. If the results of the test are unexpected and the error rate of the test is high, consider redoing the test before basing further treatment on the results.

Shared Decisions About Medications

The first rule of medications is to know why you need each drug before you use it. Just as with medical tests, there are a few things you always need to know about medications.

Learn the basics.

- What is the name of the medication and why do I need it?

- How long does it take to work?

- How long will I need to take it?

- How and when do I take it (with food, on an empty stomach, etc.)?

- Are there non-drug alternatives?

Consider the risks and benefits.

- How much will this medication help?

- Are there side effects or other risks?

- Could this medication interact with other medications that I currently take?

Ask about costs.

- How much does it cost?

- Is a generic form of the medication available and appropriate for me?

- Is there a similar medication that will work almost as well and be less expensive?

- Can I start with a prescription for a few days to make sure this medication agrees with me?

Let your doctor know:

- Your concerns about the medication.

- What you expect it will do.

- All other medications you are taking (prescription and over-the-counter).

- Whether or not you plan to fill the prescription and take the medication.

See Chapter 26 for more information on how to manage medications.

Shared Decisions About Surgery

Every surgery has risks. Only you can decide if the benefits are worth the risks. Are you willing to live with the problem or do you want to have the operation? The choice is yours.

Learn the basics.

- What is the name of the surgery? Get a description of the surgery.

- Why does my doctor think I need the surgery?

- Are there other options besides surgery?

- Is this surgery the most common one for this problem? Are there other types of surgery?

Consider the risks and benefits.

- How many similar surgeries has this doctor performed? How many surgeries like this are done at this hospital?

- What is the success rate? What does success mean for the doctor? What would success mean to me?

- What can go wrong? How often does this happen?

- How will I feel afterward? How long will it be until I'm fully recovered?

- How can I best prepare for the surgery and the recovery period?

Ask about costs.

- How much does the surgery cost? How can I find out?

- Can it be done on an outpatient basis, and is that less expensive?

Let your doctor know:

- How much the problem really bothers you. Are you willing to put up with the symptoms to avoid the surgery?

- Your concerns about the surgery.

- Whether or not you want to have the surgery at this time.

- If you want a second opinion. Second opinions are helpful if you have any doubt that the proposed surgery is the best option for your problem. If you want a second opinion, ask your primary doctor or your surgeon to recommend another specialist. Ask that your test results indicating you need surgery be sent to the second doctor. Consider getting an opinion from a doctor who isn't a surgeon and who treats similar problems.

Once you understand the costs, risks, and benefits of surgery, the decision is yours.

Calling Your Doctor

Is it okay to call your doctor? Of course it is. Often a call to the doctor or advice nurse is all you need to manage a health problem at home or determine if a visit is needed. Here's how to get the most from every call:

Prepare for your call.

• Write down a short description of your symptoms and the two to three questions you want answered.

• Have your calendar handy in case you need to schedule an appointment.

Leave a clear message.

• Present your one-sentence description and ask to talk with a doctor or advice nurse.

• If no one is available, ask for a doctor or nurse to call you back. Ask when they might call (keep the line clear).

Follow through.

• When the doctor or advice nurse calls back, briefly describe your problem and your symptoms, and ask your questions.

Finding the Right Doctor

If you don't have a family doctor (primary care physician), get one. A regular doctor who knows you and your needs well can be your most valuable health care resource. A host of specialists working on separate health problems may not see the whole picture. In choosing a doctor, there are lots of questions to ask, but these three matter the most:

• Is this doctor well-trained and experienced?

• Is this doctor available when needed?

• Will this doctor work in partnership with me?

Your health plan may be able to help you find a family doctor. Some hospitals may also have a physician referral service.

Training and Experience

If you are generally in good health, a good choice for a family doctor is a board-certified family practice doctor or internist. These doctors have broad knowledge about medical problems. A geriatrician is a doctor who is board-certified in the care of older people. Geriatricians have special training to help older patients who are dealing with several chronic illnesses.

If you have a long-term chronic condition that tends to dominate your health, consider using a specialist as your primary doctor if your health plan allows you to do so. See page 17 for a brief description of medical specialists.

The Advice Nurse

Many hospitals, clinics, health plans, and health maintenance organizations (HMOs) offer an advice nurse telephone service. Advice nurses are registered nurses who have special training to help you decide what to do about symptoms, how to manage minor illnesses, and answer your questions about health problems.

A call to the advice nurse can help you decide if you need an urgent or routine appointment or may often save you a doctor visit.

Advice nurses can also help when your doctor diagnoses a health problem or recommends a test or treatment that you don't fully understand. Sometimes the advice nurse can answer your questions. Other times, he or she may help you come up with questions you can ask your doctor at your next visit.

Availability

Call or visit the office. Tell the clinic receptionist you are looking for a new doctor. Ask these questions:

- What are the office hours?

- If I called right now for a routine appointment, how soon could I be seen?

- How much time is allowed for a routine visit?

- Will the doctor discuss health problems over the phone?

- Will the doctor make home visits? What will he or she do if I am too sick to come to the office?

- Who else is around to help me when the doctor isn't available?

- Does this doctor work with nurse practitioners or physician's assistants? These health care professionals have special training for managing many common health problems. They can often see you sooner, spend more time with you, and help you just as well as a doctor can.

- Does the doctor accept Medicare assignment or participate in my health plan? (If not, your medical care may cost you more.)

- Will the office complete insurance forms for me?

Partner Potential

During your first visit, tell your doctor that you would like to share in making treatment decisions. Ask if he or she will support that. Most doctors will be happy to hear that you want to work with them to manage your health problems better. Ask how patients your age are treated differently from younger patients. You want someone who recognizes that older adults have special medical needs.

Pay attention to how you feel during the visit.

• Does the doctor listen well?

• Do you think you could build a good working partnership with this doctor?

If the answers are "no," consider looking for another doctor.

What if you don't want to be a partner with your doctor? Maybe you don't like to ask your doctor questions and you don't want to share in any decisions. Perhaps you would rather let your doctor tell you what is best for you. If that's what you prefer, tell your doctor. Most doctors have a lot of patients who choose not to be partners. Let the doctor know what you expect.

A Letter to Your Doctor

If you want your doctor to hear you, write him or her a letter. Good times to write a letter include:

• Before a visit when you will be discussing a major procedure such as surgery:

  ○ To ask questions you especially want answered.

  ○ To express concerns about a procedure or to state your preferences about treatment.

• After a visit or treatment that did not go well for you, to state your concerns and to request a different approach in the future.

• After a visit or treatment that did go well for you, to thank your doctor for what he or she did and to reinforce anything that the doctor did that made a difference to you.

Keep your letter to one page. Present your main concerns or questions clearly. Respect your doctor's expertise and appreciate what has been done well. Suggest a specific plan for dealing with any concerns.

Is It Time for a Change?

If you are unhappy with your medical care, it may be time for a change. Before you start looking for a new doctor, tell your current doctor how you would like to be treated. Your doctor would probably be pleased to work with you as a partner—if only you tell him that's what you want. Otherwise, he may think that you, like many of his patients, prefer to let him do all the work.

Managing Health Care Costs

As an active partner with your doctor, you can do a lot to reduce your health care costs. The goal is to get just the care you need, nothing more, and certainly nothing less.

Billions of dollars are spent each year on medications, tests, and treatments that patients may not need. Get the care you need when you need it, avoid unnecessary doctor visits, tests, and treatments, and use emergency services wisely to better manage your health care costs.

Nine Ways You Can Cut Health Care Costs

1. Keep immunizations current. See page 21. Ask your doctor for the screening tests on pages 25 to 26. These tests help identify serious problems early, when they are easier and less expensive to treat.

2. Don't put off needed services. If your symptoms and the guidelines in this book suggest that you should see a doctor, don't put it off. Ignoring problems often leads to complications that are more expensive to treat.

3. Reduce your medical test costs. Don't agree to medical tests until you understand how they will help you. Tests are sometimes done because "it is standard practice" or to protect doctors from possible malpractice suits. The only good reason to do a test is because the benefits to you outweigh the risks and the costs. See page 8 for more information.

4. Reduce your medication costs. Ask your doctor about every prescribed medication. Ask what would happen if you chose not to take a medication. Don't expect to get a prescription for every illness; sometimes self-care or non-drug remedies are all you need. See page 9 for more information.

5. Avoid surgery when the risks for you outweigh the benefits. Review the questions to ask about surgery on page 10. If you are not convinced that the benefits to you outweigh the risks, don't have the surgery.

6. Substitute home care for an office visit when appropriate. For some health problems, home care is all that you need. By using the information in this book, and calling your doctor or nurse for help, you can often care for a problem at home.

7. See your doctor in his or her office instead of going to the emergency room. Routine services in an emergency room cost two to three times more than in your doctor's office. Unless you have a true emergency, waiting to see your doctor can save you money. You will also be treated by your own doctor, who knows your medical history.

If you need to go to the emergency department, and there is time to prepare, do the following:

• Call your doctor first. If needed, your doctor can meet you there.

• Take your home medical records. The emergency department may not have access to your medical records. The information that you take about your medications, past test results, or treatments can be extremely important.

• Use page 1, the **Healthwise Approach**, to help you think through the problem and report symptoms to the doctor.

• Use page 2, the **Ask-the-Doctor Checklist**, to organize questions for the doctor.

Wise Use of Ambulance Services

Call 911 or your local emergency department for an ambulance if:

Someone has symptoms of a heart attack: severe chest pain, sweating, shortness of breath. See page 99.

Someone has symptoms of a stroke: loss of sight or speech, weakness or numbness in an arm or leg, severe headache. See page 108.

There is severe bleeding or blood loss. See page 276.

Someone is unconscious or is having severe difficulty breathing.

You suspect a spinal or neck injury.

Do not call an ambulance if:

The person is conscious, breathing without difficulty, and in stable condition.

It is not an emergency. Ambulance services are expensive. If it is not an emergency, it may not be covered by insurance.

- See page 8 to review the medical test checklist.

Whenever you feel you can apply home treatment safely and wait to see your regular doctor, do so. However, if you feel that it is an emergency situation, by all means go to the emergency department.

8. Substitute outpatient care for inpatient care when you can. Staying overnight in a hospital is very expensive (and not much fun). Don't check in just for tests. Hospitalization is no longer needed for most medical tests. Ask if the tests can be done on an outpatient basis. If you can control your diet and activities, outpatient tests may be appropriate for you.

For minor surgery, ask if "same-day" surgery is appropriate so that you can go home the same day and avoid a hospital stay.

If you do need inpatient care, get in and out of the hospital as quickly as possible. This will reduce costs and your risk of hospital-acquired infections.

Ask if you can avoid an additional day in the hospital by bringing in extra help at home. Ask about home health nursing services to help while you recover. With such help available, many people can shorten hospital stays.

Hospitals are not the only choice for people with a terminal illness. Many people choose to spend their remaining time at home with people they know and love. Special arrangements for the needed care can be made through hospice care programs in most communities. Try "Hospice" in the Yellow Pages or ask your doctor.

9. Save specialists for special problems. Specialists are doctors with in-depth training and experience in a particular area of medicine. For example, a cardiologist has years of special training to deal with heart problems. A visit to a specialist often costs more than a visit to your regular doctor, and the tests and treatments you receive may be more expensive. Of course, specialists often provide the information you need to decide what to do about a major health problem.

When your primary doctor refers you to a specialist, a little preparation and good communication can help you get your money's worth. Before you go see a specialist:

- Know the diagnosis or expected diagnosis.

- Learn about your basic treatment options.

- Know what your primary doctor would like the specialist to do (take over the case, confirm the diagnosis, conduct tests, etc.).

- Make sure that any test results or records on your case are sent to the specialist.

- Ask your primary doctor to remain involved in your care. Ask the specialist to send new test results or recommendations to both you and your primary doctor.

Health Fraud and Quackery

A common health fraud is bogus "cures" for chronic problems such as arthritis, cancer, impotence, and baldness. These cures often sound like the miracle answer to your problem. To avoid quackery, stay away from products that:

- Are advertised by testimonials

- Claim to have a secret ingredient

- Are not evaluated in prominent medical journals

- Claim benefits that seem too good to be true

Who Works on What?

Cardiologist (MD): heart

Dermatologist (MD): skin

Endocrinologist (MD): diabetes and hormonal problems

Family Practitioner (MD): primary care

Gastroenterologist (MD): digestive system

Geriatrician (MD): older adults

Gynecologist (MD): female reproductive system

Internist (MD): primary care

Neurologist (MD): brain and nervous system disorders

Oncologist (MD): cancer

Ophthalmologist (MD): eyes

Optometrist (OD): primary care for many eye problems*

Orthopedist (MD): surgery on bones, joints, muscles

Otolaryngologist or **Head and Neck Surgeon** (MD): ears, nose, and throat

Podiatrist (DPM): foot care

Psychiatrist (MD): mental and emotional problems

Psychologist (MA* or PhD): mental and emotional problems

Pulmonologist (MD): lungs

Rheumatologist (MD): arthritis and other connective tissue disorders

Urologist (MD): urinary and male reproductive systems

Some specialists may be MDs or Doctors of Osteopathy (DOs).

*Varies by state.

Trust Your Common Sense

Medicine is not as magical as we once thought. If someone takes the time to explain a problem or a treatment to us, we can usually make a pretty good decision about what is best for us.

The best medical tests, diagnosticians, and medical specialists are not enough. Good medical care also requires your own common sense. If you trust your common sense, you are on your way to becoming a wise medical consumer.

You Have the Right:

- To be spoken to in words that you understand.

- To be told what's wrong with you.

- To read your medical record.

- To know the benefits and risks of any treatment and its alternatives.

- To know what a treatment or test will cost you.

- To share in all treatment decisions.

- To refuse any medical procedure.

Adapted from the American Hospital Association's "Patient's Bill of Rights."

If I had known I was going to live this long,
I would have taken better care of myself.
Eubie Blake

2
Prevention and Early Detection

If you practice good prevention, you may never need most of the home treatment guidelines in this book.

Over 50 percent of all health problems are preventable. In most cases, prevention is entirely up to you. What you eat, how much exercise you get, and how well you follow safety rules will often be enough to avoid a medical problem.

Practicing good prevention does not mean giving up all pleasures. On the contrary, taking pleasure in your life is an important aspect of prevention. A happy person who enjoys a good self-image is generally a healthy person as well.

A Long Healthy Life

As much as we wish they would, good health habits do not guarantee a long life. If you start exercising, eating

right, smoking less, and relaxing more, you may extend your life by only a few years or months. However, good health habits will greatly increase your chances for a good quality of life. You will be more active, have fewer illnesses, and enjoy life more during the last five to twenty years of your life. And it's never too late to start.

Studies show that no matter how old you are, exercise, good nutrition, and a positive outlook can make a big difference in your overall quality of life. You will spend fewer days in bed, nursing homes, and hospitals. You will also have more energy to do the things you enjoy most.

If you stop smoking today, your risk of heart disease is cut in half within one year. After ten years, your risk of lung cancer drops to half that of someone who continues to smoke. And in two days, your kisses will taste much, much better. See Quitting Smoking on page 91.

If you start eating less fat, you will begin to see reductions in body fat and cholesterol in only a few weeks. Very low-fat diets can actually reverse the process of heart disease. See page 350.

Changes in levels of physical activity help, too. Beginning even a moderate exercise program can help you feel more energetic after only a few days. See Chapter 20.

Also see the information in Chapter 18 on preventing injuries.

So, don't worry that good health habits won't keep you alive forever. Instead, look forward to having all your future years be good years.

Six Keys to Healthy Aging

There is no magic to vitality and health in old age. Just develop good health habits and stick with them. You will find scores of helpful tips throughout this book. Let these six keys be your general guide.

1. Take care of your body.

- Keep physically fit. Find an exercise that you enjoy, and do something active every day. Maintain your strength, flexibility, and stamina.

- Eat well. Choose a variety of wholesome foods. Eat less fat and more beans, grains, fruits, and vegetables. Drink lots of water (eight 8-ounce glasses of water a day).

- Recharge your batteries. Get seven to eight hours of sleep per day. Try out a variety of deep breathing and relaxation techniques.

- Don't poison your body. Keep smoke out of your lungs and tobacco out of your mouth. Drink alcohol only in moderation. Avoid unneeded medications.

- Manage illnesses wisely. Use this book and other resources. Find a good doctor, and work in partnership with him or her. Maintain control of your health care decisions.

2. Stay mentally active.

If you want to keep your marbles, use them. The brain benefits from exposure to stimulating environments and activities.

Learn something new every day. Take classes or read books about new subjects. Read, write, talk, and think about what interests you.

3. Nurture the ties that bind.

Studies show that people who have many social ties, such as being married, having contact with friends and relatives, and belonging to a church or social group, are healthier than people with few social connections.

Create a support network of family and friends who will help see you through a crisis. Find a friend you can confide in. Be a confidant for someone else.

Combine physical and social health by joining a walking group or exercise class.

4. Know where your help is.

The best way to stay independent is to know when to ask for help. Become familiar with your community's support services for seniors, such as transportation, financial counseling, and Meals on Wheels. See your local senior center or Area Agency on Aging for information on available services. Also see Chapter 24.

5. Accentuate the positive.

The pictures we have in our minds and the verbal messages or self-talk we give ourselves affect both our minds and bodies.

Expect good things to happen. Count your blessings and express thanks. Add humor, laughter, and fun into every day. Also see Chapter 23.

6. Celebrate your wisdom.

Victor Hugo said, "One sees a flame in the eyes of the young, but in the eyes of the old, one sees light." More than anything else, the world needs wisdom.

Recognize your purpose for living. Think about your values and beliefs. Help others to gain wisdom, too.

Immunizations

Immunizations provide protection against many serious diseases. Chances are, you have been immunized against the major childhood illnesses, or you are immune because you had them as a child.

However, there are several immunizations that need to be updated throughout your life or given for the first time later in life. If your doctor does not suggest them to you, make a note to mention them at your next visit.

Older adults need:

- A tetanus booster every ten years.

- An annual influenza (flu) shot. (For people over age 65, and anyone who has chronic respiratory problems.)

- A one-time pneumococcal vaccine (pneumonia shot). (For anyone age 65 or older, and others at high risk.)

Tetanus Immunization

Tetanus (lockjaw) is a bacterial infection that is often fatal. The bacteria enter the body through wounds and thrive only in the absence of oxygen. Puncture wounds, such as from a rusty nail, are especially good environments for the tetanus bacteria, but any cut or scrape can become infected. The only sure protection against tetanus is immunization. Over half of tetanus cases occur in adults over age 60, because they may have forgotten to keep their immunizations up to date.

Three shots followed by a booster one year later provide immunity. Routine boosters are then recommended every 10 years throughout your life to maintain immunity. If you are age 50 or older and have not had boosters every 10 years, now is a good time to talk to your doctor about updating your tetanus boosters. If you have a wound from a dirty object, get a booster shot if you haven't had one in the past five years.

If you have never been immunized against tetanus, it is a good idea to start the series of three shots now, then have a booster every 10 years.

Influenza Immunization

Influenza (flu) is a contagious viral illness that causes fever and chills, head and muscle aches, fatigue, weakness, sneezing, and runny nose. (See page 83.)

Older people are more likely to develop complications of influenza, such as pneumonia and dehydration. To protect yourself, get a flu shot each autumn if any of the following applies to you:

- Age 65 or older and frail

- Chronic lung disease (such as asthma or emphysema)

Keep Track of Your Tests and Shots

Plan to keep home medical record files for each member of the family. Keep an immunization and routine test record in front. A list of drugs each person is taking is also important. Organize other information by problem. If the problem returns, your record of what happened the last time will be very helpful. See page 417.

- Heart disease

- Diabetes

- Sickle-cell anemia or other red blood cell disorders

- You have an illness or are receiving treatment that weakens the immune system (such as leukemia or drugs to treat cancer).

- You are in contact with someone who would be at risk of developing complications of the flu, such as a family member who has one of the high-risk conditions above, a nursing home resident, or people over age 65. If you catch the flu, he or she might catch it from you.

Side effects of the flu shot, such as a low-grade fever and minor aches, are usually mild and do not last long.

Do not get a flu shot if you are allergic to eggs. The virus in the vaccine is grown in eggs, and you may develop an allergic reaction. Medications are available for short-term protection if you are exposed to the flu. Talk with your doctor.

Pneumococcal Immunization

Most people think of pneumococci as the bacteria that cause pneumonia, but they can also cause an infection of the blood (bacteremia) or of the covering of the brain (meningitis). Older people develop pneumonia and other pneumococcal infections much more frequently than the general population.

One shot will usually give lifelong protection from pneumococcal infection. You can get the pneumococcal vaccine (pneumonia shot) at the same time as one of your yearly flu shots. Get a pneumococcal vaccine if:

- You are healthy, over 65, and have never received the shot.

- You are younger than 65, but have heart, kidney, liver, or lung disease, diabetes, Hodgkin's disease, or any immune system disorder. These conditions increase your risk of developing pneumonia. Consult with your doctor.

If you are over 65 and it has been six years or longer since you had a pneumococcal vaccine, and you have any of the conditions listed above, ask your doctor if you need another shot.

Side effects of the shot often include mild swelling and pain at the injection site.

Other Immunizations

If you are planning travel to areas where illnesses such as hepatitis, malaria, typhoid, and yellow fever are common, talk to your doctor or health department to ask about immunizations for these illnesses.

Tuberculin Test

A tuberculin test is a skin test for tuberculosis (see page 93), not an immunization. A positive result does not necessarily mean that you have active tuberculosis (TB), but it does mean that the bacteria have probably entered your body. Whether you should be tested depends on how common tuberculosis is in your area and your risk of exposure to people who have TB. If you have had a positive TB test, the test should not be repeated. Additional tests will always be positive and may cause more severe reactions.

Early Detection

If you can't prevent a health problem, the next best thing is to detect and treat it early. This section provides guidelines for what you and your doctor can do to discover disease while it is easier to treat or cure.

Annual health checkups begin to make sense for women by age 50 and for men by age 65.

The Preventive Care Schedules on pages 25 to 26 help you decide which tests are valuable for you and how often you should have them. Recommended immunizations are also listed.

The charts include recommendations for adults age 50 and older. They are based on the United States Preventive Services Task Force *Guide to Clinical Preventive Services* and other experts. This is only one possible schedule, and other organizations may make different recommendations. Experts do not agree on how often to recommend screening tests.

The most appropriate schedule of preventive exams is one you and your doctor agree upon. The schedule will depend on your health conditions, values, and risk factors.

The recommendations apply to people of average risk in each age category. You may be at higher risk for certain diseases. Family history (whether your relatives have or had the disease), other health problems, or behaviors such as smoking all increase your risk.

The risk factors for many conditions are listed in those topics in this book. Review the pages noted in the chart to see if you have any risk factors. If you do, talk with your doctor about whether you need more frequent exams.

Periodic self-exams are also an important part of staying healthy. See the breast self-exam on page 231. If you have high blood pressure, see page 103.

For more information on cholesterol screening, see page 353.

Preventive Care Schedule

(Recommended Time Intervals Between Preventive Services)
For more information about this chart, review page 24.

Preventive Service	Age 50-64	Age 65+	Comments
Blood pressure (p. 103)	1-3 years	1 year	More often if elevated.
Cholesterol (p. 353)	5 years	5 years	More often if elevated. Talk with your doctor about testing after age 65 if your cholesterol levels are normal.
Flexible sigmoidoscopy (p. 117)	3-5 years	3-5 years	More often if at risk (see page 117). Screening for colorectal cancer may also include blood in stool test. Discuss with your doctor.
Fecal occult blood test (blood in stool test) (p. 417)	1 year	1 year	Screening for colorectal cancer may also include flexible sigmoidoscopy. Discuss with your doctor.
Hearing test	Assess during regular visits for other reasons.		
Vision test	2-5 years	1-2 years	More often in people who have eye diseases.
Glaucoma test	Usually done as part of regular eye exams.		
Dental exam	6 months	6 months	

Adapted from *Guide to Clinical Preventive Services,* U.S. Preventive Services Task Force, 1996.

Preventive Care Schedule

(Recommended Time Intervals Between Preventive Services)

For more information about this chart, review page 24.

Preventive Service	Age 50-64	Age 65+	Comments
Women only			
Breast self-exam (p. 231)	Monthly	Monthly	
Clinical breast exam (p. 233)	1 year	1 year	
Mammogram (p. 233)	1-2 years	1-2 years	Discuss with your doctor whether to discontinue after age 75.
Pelvic exam (p. 235)	1 year	1 year	
Pap test (p. 235)	1-3 years	1-3 years	May discontinue after age 65 if prior exams were normal and you have no significant risk factors for cervical cancer (p. 244).
Immunizations			
Tetanus booster (p. 21)	Age 50	10 years	Update at age 50 if needed.
Influenza immunization (p. 22)		1 year	Given in the fall. Recommended before age 65 only if high-risk.
Pneumococcal immunization (p. 23)		Once	Recommended before age 65 if high-risk. Booster may be needed after 6 years or longer.

Adapted from *Guide to Clinical Preventive Services,* U.S. Preventive Services Task Force, 1996.

Stand up straight!
Mom

3
Back and Neck Pain

Few of us are lucky enough to make it through life without having back or neck pain at some time. Because it supports the weight of your body throughout your entire life, your lower back is especially prone to injury and the effects of aging. As we grow older, it is more common for back or neck pain to be caused by health problems that affect the spine or its supporting structures. These illnesses can cause chronic pain. However, most back and neck problems are the result of strain or overuse,

injuries that heal relatively quickly and can be prevented by exercising regularly and having good posture and body mechanics.

Quick Reference Guide

- First aid for back pain, page 28.

- Back pain due to arthritis, page 29.

- Neck pain, page 39.

Back Pain

Your back consists of the bones of the spine (vertebrae, which support body weight), their joints (facet joints, which allow the spine to flex and move), the discs that separate the vertebrae and absorb shock as you move, and the muscles and ligaments that hold it all together. One or more of these structures can be injured.

- You can strain or sprain ligaments or muscles during a sudden or improper movement, or by overuse.

First Aid for Back Pain

When you first feel a catch or strain in your back, try these steps to avoid or reduce expected pain. These are the most important home treatments for the first few days of back pain.

First Aid #1: Ice

As soon as possible, apply ice or a cold pack to your injured back (15 to 20 minutes every hour). Cold limits swelling, reduces pain and muscle spasms, and speeds healing.

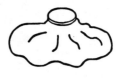

Ice

First Aid #2: Relax

Lie flat on your stomach with your arms beside your body and your head to one side. You may want to place a small pillow under your stomach. If this causes more pain, try to find the most comfortable position. Relax for one to two minutes.

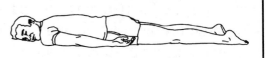

Relax

First Aid #3: Press-up

Lift yourself up on your elbows, keeping the lower half of your body relaxed. Keep hips pressed to the floor. If it's comfortable, lift your chest off the floor. Hold for two to five minutes.

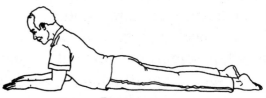

Press-up

First Aid #4: Walk

Take a short walk (three to five minutes) on a level surface (no inclines) every three hours. Walk only distances you can manage without pain, especially leg pain.

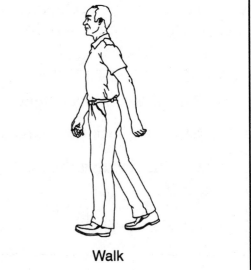

Walk

- You can damage your discs the same way so that they tear or stretch. If the tear is large enough, material may leak out of the disc and press against a nerve. A nerve may also become irritated due to swelling or inflammation in other parts of the back.

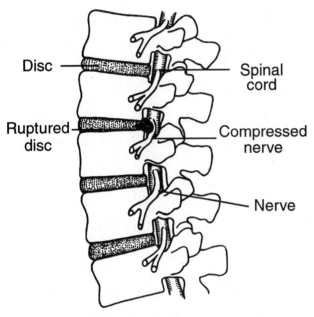

Disc	Spinal cord
Ruptured disc	Compressed nerve
	Nerve

A herniated disc can cause pressure on a nerve.

Any of these can result in two or three days of acute pain and swelling followed by slow healing and a gradual reduction in pain. Pain may be felt in the low back, the buttock, or down the leg (**sciatica**, see box at right). The goals of self-care are to relieve pain, promote healing, and avoid reinjury. Fortunately, 9 out of 10 acute back injuries will heal on their own within 8 to 12 weeks.

Sciatica

Sciatica is an irritation of the sciatic nerve, which runs from the lower back down through the buttocks and to the feet. It can result when an injured disc presses against the nerve. Its main symptom is radiating pain, numbness, or weakness that can be worse in the leg than in the back.

In addition to the home treatment for back pain on page 36, the following may help:

- Avoid sitting, unless it is more comfortable than standing.

- Alternate lying down with short walks. Increase the distance when you are able to do so without pain.

- An ice or cold pack will probably do the most good if placed in the middle of your back. See page 294.

In addition to the injuries discussed above, back pain can also be caused by conditions that affect the bones and joints of the spine. Arthritis pain may be a steady ache, unlike the sharp, acute pain of strains, sprains, or disc injuries. If you think your back pain may be caused by arthritis, combine the home treatment guidelines for back pain with those for arthritis on page 45.

Back pain can be caused by a compression fracture, which is usually the result of osteoporosis (page 55). This occurs when a thin, weak vertebra in the middle to lower part of the back breaks. Pain comes on suddenly, often without clear reason.

Prevention

The key to preventing back pain is to keep your spine in the neutral position whenever possible. When your spine is in the neutral position, the alignment of the vertebrae and discs forms an S-shaped curve (when viewed from the side) that starts at your neck and ends at your tailbone. You achieve the neutral position by aligning your ear, shoulder, hip, and ankle. The first half of this section tells you how to use proper posture and body mechanics to maintain a neutral spine when carrying out daily activities.

Maintaining a neutral spine requires muscle strength and flexibility. The exercises in the second half of this section will help you strengthen the muscles that support your spine, maintain flexibility, and improve your overall fitness. Keeping your body weight within the ideal range for the size of your frame is also important to your back's health. For tips on maintaining a healthy body weight, read Chapter 21.

Back Posture

When you have back pain, improper posture puts more stress on your back, which can lead to more discomfort. The key to good back posture is to keep the right amount of curve in your lower back. Too much curve ("swayback") or too little curve ("flat back") can result in problems.

- When you stand and walk with good posture, your ear, shoulder, hip, and ankle should be in a line. Don't lock your knees.

- When you sit, keep your shoulders back and down, chin back, and abdomen in. Slouching can stress the ligaments and muscles in your lower back. See the illustration of proper sitting posture on page 40.

Sitting

- Avoid sitting in one position for more than an hour at a time. Get up or change positions often. If you must sit a lot, see the exercises on page 33.

- If your chair doesn't give enough support, place a small pillow or rolled towel behind your lower back.

- To rise from a chair, keep your back in the neutral position and scoot forward to the edge of the seat. Use your leg muscles to stand up without leaning forward at the waist.

- When driving, pull your seat forward so the pedals and steering wheel are within comfortable reach. You may want to place a small pillow or rolled towel behind your lower back. Your forearms should be parallel to the floor. Stop often to stretch and walk around.

Sleeping

A firm bed is better than a soft mattress or waterbed. Sleep with your back in the neutral position.

- If you sleep on your back, use a towel roll to support your lower back, or put a pillow under your knees.

- If you sleep on your side, try placing a pillow between your knees.

- Sleeping on your stomach is fine if it doesn't increase back or neck pain.

- To rise from bed, lie on your side near the edge of the bed, and bend both knees. As you push yourself up to a sitting position, drop your feet over the side of the bed. Scoot to the edge of the bed and position your feet under your buttocks. Stand up, keeping your back in the neutral position.

Lifting

Follow these tips to avoid compressing the discs of the lower back:

- Keep your upper back straight and your lower back in the neutral position. Do not bend forward from the waist to lift.

- Bend your knees and let your arms and legs do the work. Tighten your buttocks and stomach muscles to further support your back.

- Keep the load as close to your body as possible, even if it is light.

- Turn with your feet, not your back.

- Never lift a heavy object above shoulder level.

- Use a hand truck, or ask someone to help with heavy or awkward objects.

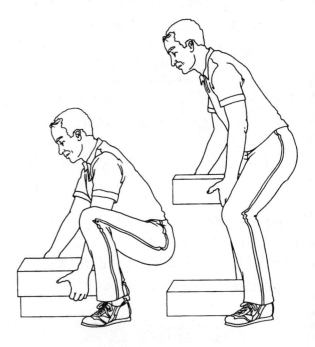

Proper lifting posture

Body Mechanics

Using good body mechanics means using the correct muscles and body alignment when you perform daily activities. Use good body mechanics all the time, not just when you have back pain.

• Keep your back in the neutral position.

• When you must stay in one position for a long time, take regular breaks to stretch and restore the neutral position of your back.

• When standing for long periods, place one foot on a small stool.

Exercises to Prevent Back Pain

Both the exercises in this chapter and general aerobic exercise (walking, swimming, cycling) will help prevent back injury and pain. They will also speed your recovery from injuries and decrease chronic pain.

Extension exercises strengthen your lower back muscles and stretch the stomach muscles and ligaments. They are particularly helpful if your pain is related to a disc problem.

Flexion exercises stretch the lower back muscles and strengthen the stomach muscles. They are most helpful if your back pain comes from muscle strain, arthritis, or inflammation of the joints where vertebrae meet.

Do not do these exercises if you have just injured your back. Instead, see "First Aid for Back Pain" on page 28.

• You do not need to do every exercise. Do the ones that help you the most.

• If any exercise causes increasing or continuing back pain, stop the exercise and try something else. Some mild strain and discomfort are okay. However, stop doing any exercise that causes pain to radiate away from your spine into your buttocks or legs, either during or after the exercise.

• Start with five repetitions three to four times a day, and gradually increase to 10 repetitions. Do all exercises slowly.

Note: You may need to hold on to a piece of furniture that will support your weight (sofa, armchair) as you lower yourself to and rise from the floor to do these exercises.

Some people become mildly lightheaded when they rise from the floor after exercising. To prevent a fall, sit up for a moment and let any lightheadedness pass before you try to rise from the floor.

Extension Exercises

1. Press-ups

Begin and end every set of exercises with a few press-ups.

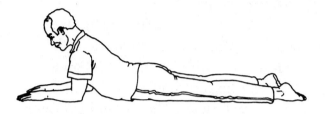

1. Press-ups

- Lie face down with arms bent, hands at shoulders, palms flat on the floor.

- Lift yourself up on your elbows, keeping the lower half of your body relaxed. If it's comfortable, lift your chest off the floor.

- Keep your hips pressed to the floor. Feel the stretch in your lower back.

- Lower your upper body to the floor.

2. Shoulder Lifts

Shoulder lifts will strengthen the back muscles that support the spine.

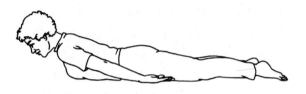

2. Shoulder lifts

- Lie face down with your arms beside your body.

- Lift your head and shoulders straight up from the floor. Keep your torso and hips pressed to the floor. Come up as high as you can without pain.

3. Backward Bend

Practice the backward bend at least once a day and whenever you work in a bent-forward position.

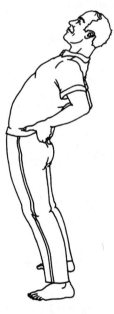

3. Backward bend

- Stand upright with your feet slightly apart. Back up to a countertop for support and greater stability.

• Place your hands in the small of your back and gently bend backward. Keep your knees straight (not locked) and bend only at the waist. See illustration. Hold the backward bend for one to two seconds.

Flexion exercises

4. Curl-ups

Curl-ups strengthen your stomach muscles, which work with your back muscles to support your spine.

• Lie on your back with knees bent (60° angle) and feet flat on the floor. Do not hook your feet under anything.

• Cross your arms over your chest.

• Slowly curl your head and shoulders up until your shoulder blades barely rise from the floor. Keep your lower back pressed to the floor. To avoid neck problems, remember to lift your shoulders, and do not force your head up or forward. Start by holding this position for two to three seconds (do not hold your breath), then curl down very slowly. As you build strength, try to remain in the curl-up position longer (5 to 10 seconds).

5. Knee-to-Chest

The knee-to-chest exercise stretches the low back and the muscles in the back of the thigh (hamstrings) and relieves pressure on the vertebral bone joints, where the vertebrae come together.

• Lie on your back with knees bent and feet close to your buttocks.

• Bring one knee to your chest, keeping the other foot flat on the floor. (You may stretch the other leg out on the floor if it feels better on your lower back). Keep your lower back pressed to the floor. Hold for 5 to 10 seconds.

• Relax and lower the knee to starting position. Repeat with the other leg.

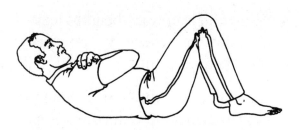

4. Curl-ups

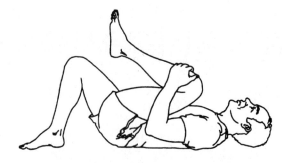

5. Knee-to-chest

Additional Stretching and Strengthening Exercises

6. Hamstring Stretch

This exercise stretches the muscles in the back of your thigh (hamstrings), which allow you to bend your legs while keeping your back in the neutral position. To stretch your right hamstring:

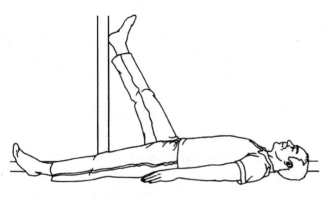

6. Hamstring stretch

• Lie on your back with your legs extended through a doorway. Your right leg should be close to the door frame.

• Raise your right leg and rest it against the door frame. Slowly straighten the leg until your heel is resting on the door frame. Flex your foot until you feel a gentle pull in the back of your thigh.

• If this causes pain, move your leg closer to or farther from the door frame until you are able to do the stretch without pain.

• Relax in this position for 30 seconds, then bend your right knee to relieve the stretch.

7. Hip Flexor Stretch

This exercise stretches the muscles in front of your hip (groin muscles or hip flexors). It will help prevent "swayback" due to tight hip muscles. To stretch your left hip flexor:

• Kneel on both knees. Bring your right leg forward, bending the knee at a 90° angle so the ankle is aligned directly under the knee. Keep your spine in the neutral position.

• Slowly shift your weight onto your front foot by dropping your hips toward the floor.

• Don't allow your right knee to move. Keep your back straight.

• You should feel a stretch in the groin of your left leg.

• Hold the stretch for 10 seconds.

8. Prone Buttocks Squeeze

This exercise strengthens the buttocks muscles, which support the back and help you lift with your legs.

• Lie flat on your stomach with your arms at your sides.

• Slowly tighten your buttocks muscles and hold for two to three seconds (do not hold your breath). Release.

• You may need to place a small pillow under your lower stomach for comfort.

9. Pelvic Tilts

This exercise gently moves the spine and stretches the lower back.

• Lie on your back with your knees bent and feet flat on the floor.

• Slowly tighten your stomach muscles and press your lower back against the floor. Hold for 10 seconds (do not hold your breath). Slowly relax.

Which Exercises for You?

• If you have no back pain, try some of the prevention exercises on pages 32 to 36.

• **Do not do the prevention exercises if you have just injured your back.**

• If you have injured your back within the last two weeks, or you have more pain in your leg than in your back or buttocks, see Home Treatment and When to Call a Health Professional on pages 36 to 38.

• Discontinue any exercise that increases pain.

• Gradually increase any exercise that helps you feel better.

Exercises to Avoid

Many common exercises actually increase the risk of low back pain. Avoid the following:

• Straight-leg sit-ups

• Leg lifts (lifting both legs while lying on your back)

• Lifting heavy weights above the waist (military press, biceps curls while standing)

• Any stretching done while sitting with the legs in a V

• Toe touches while standing

Home Treatment

Immediately after an injury and for the next few days:

• Get in a comfortable position. Apply cold packs or ice to the affected area for 15 to 20 minutes, three to four times a day, or up to once an hour for at least the first three days. Cold decreases inflammation, swelling, muscle spasms, and pain.

• Sit or lie in positions that are most comfortable and reduce your pain, especially leg pain.

• Do not sit up in bed, and avoid soft couches and twisted positions. Avoid positions that worsen your symptoms, such as sitting for long periods. Follow the posture and body mechanics guidelines on pages 30 to 32.

- Do the first aid exercises on page 28 three to four times a day.

- Bed rest can help relieve back pain but may not speed healing. Unless you have severe leg pain, it is probably best to try to continue with your usual daily activities. If any activity makes your pain worse, modify it in a way that causes less pain or avoid it altogether. If you have difficulty sleeping at night, try one of the following positions (see page 31). If it doesn't increase your pain:

  ◦ Lie on your back with your knees bent and supported by large pillows.

  ◦ Lie on your side with your knees and hips bent and a pillow between your legs.

  ◦ Lie on your stomach.

- Take aspirin, ibuprofen (Motrin), or naproxen (Aleve) regularly as directed. Call your doctor if you've been told to avoid anti-inflammatory medications. Acetaminophen (Tylenol) may also be used. Take these medications sensibly; the maximum recommended dose will reduce the pain. Masking the pain completely might allow movement that could lead to reinjury.

- As soon as you can, take short walks (three to five minutes every three hours) on level surfaces (no inclines) to keep your muscles strong. Only walk distances that you can manage without pain, especially leg pain.

- Relax your muscles. See page 368 to learn how to do progressive muscle relaxation.

After two to three days of home treatment:

- Continue with daily walks (increase to 5 to 10 minutes, three to four times a day) and the exercises above.

- Try swimming. It may be painful immediately after a back injury, but lap swimming or kicking with swim fins may help keep back pain from recurring.

Leg Weakness

Many people with low back pain say their legs feel weak. If weakness is related to back pain, you will be able to make your leg muscles work, but it will probably hurt.

True leg weakness means you are unable to use your legs, no matter how much you try to push through the pain. This may be due to a structural defect such as a herniated disc.

Significant leg weakness should be evaluated by a doctor, especially if you are unable to bend your foot upward, get up out of a chair, or climb stairs.

- When your pain has improved, begin easy exercises that do not increase your pain. One or two of the exercises on pages 32 to 36 may be helpful. Start with five repetitions twice a day and increase to 10 repetitions as you are able.

- See Resource 15 on page 419.

When to Call a Health Professional

- If new or different back pain was caused by an injury that occurred within the past 2 weeks.

- If you have evidence of nerve damage, such as:

  ◦ Loss of bowel or bladder control

  ◦ New numbness in the buttocks, genital area, or legs

  ◦ Leg weakness not due solely to pain

- If there has been a change in your pain, such as:

  ◦ Back pain that feels different than before

  ◦ A dramatic increase in your chronic back pain

  ◦ Back pain does not improve after two weeks of home treatment

- If you have new or increased back pain with unexplained fever, painful urination, or other urinary tract symptoms. See page 139.

Back Surgery

Doctors recommend back surgery much less often now than in the past. Rest, posture changes, and exercise can relieve 98 percent of back problems, even disc problems.

Surgery is often appropriate for certain conditions that do not improve with the usual treatment. If you do plan to have surgery, the posture and body mechanics guidelines and exercises in this chapter are still important. A strong, flexible back is important to a quick recovery after surgery.

Neck Pain

Neck pain and stiffness are usually caused by strain or spasm of the neck muscles or inflammation of the neck joints. However, it may also be due to arthritis or damage to the discs between the vertebrae in the neck. Pain and stiffness may limit neck movement; this usually affects one side more than the other. Neck problems often cause headaches or pain in the shoulder, upper back, or down the arm.

Neck pain and headaches are sometimes related to tension in the trapezius muscles, which run from the back of the head across the back of the shoulder. When you have neck pain, these muscles also may feel tight and painful. If neck pain occurs with headache, see Tension Headaches on page 159.

Neck muscle strain may be due to:

- Forward head posture

- Sleeping on a pillow that's too high, too flat, or doesn't support your head

- Sleeping on your stomach or with your neck twisted or bent

- Spending long periods of time in the "thinker's pose" (resting your forehead on your fist or arm)

- Watching TV or reading while lying down with the neck in an awkward position

- Stress (often people will "hold their tension" in their neck muscles)

- A poorly positioned computer monitor that causes you to hold your head in an awkward position

- Other stresses placed on the neck muscles

- Injury that causes sudden movement of the head and neck (whiplash) or a direct blow to the neck

- Strenuous activity involving the upper body and arms

Meningitis (page 158) is a serious illness that causes neck pain. If you have meningitis, you will be very sick with a severe stiff neck, headache, and fever. If all of these symptoms occur together, see a doctor promptly.

Prevention

Good posture, body mechanics, and exercise are important to preventing neck pain. Most neck pain that isn't due to arthritis or an injury is completely avoidable.

- Sit straight in your chair with your low back supported. Avoid sitting for a long time without getting up or changing positions. Take mini-breaks several times each hour to stretch your neck muscles.

- If you work at a computer, adjust the monitor so that the top of the screen is at eye level. Use a document holder that puts your work at the same level as the screen.

- If you use the telephone a lot, consider using a headset or speaker phone.

- Adjust your car seat to a more upright position that supports your head and lower back.

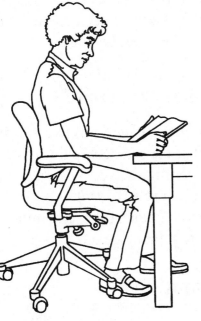

Proper sitting posture

If your neck stiffness is worse **in the morning**, check your sleeping posture (and your activities the day before).

- Improve your sleeping support. A hard mattress or special neck support pillow may solve the problem (try before buying). Or you can make a neck support at home by folding a towel lengthwise into a four-inch-wide pad and wrapping it around your neck. Pin the towel for good support.

- Use a pillow that doesn't force your head forward when you lie on your back and that allows you to align your nose with the center of your body when you lie on your side.

- If stress is a factor, practice progressive muscle relaxation exercises. See page 368.

- Strengthen and protect your neck by doing neck exercises once a day. See page 41.

Home Treatment

Much of the home treatment for back pain is also helpful for neck pain, including the guidelines on posture, body mechanics, and ice. See page 36.

- Place ice or a cold pack over painful muscles for 10 to 15 minutes at a time, as often as once an hour. This will help decrease pain, muscle spasms, and swelling. If the problem is near the back of your shoulder or upper back, it will usually help more to ice the back of the neck. If you have sharp pain in the front of your shoulder, ice the front of your neck.

- Use aspirin, ibuprofen, naproxen sodium, or acetaminophen to help relieve pain.

Neck Exercises

You do not need to do every exercise. Stick with the ones that help you the most. Stop any exercise that increases pain. Start with five repetitions twice a day. Do each exercise slowly.

1. Dorsal glide: Sit or stand tall, looking straight ahead (a "palace guard" posture). Slowly tuck your chin as you glide your head backwards. Hold for a count of five, then relax. Repeat 6 to 10 times. This stretches the back of the neck. If you feel pain, do not glide so far back. Some people find this exercise easier while lying on their back with an ice pack on the neck.

2. Chest and shoulder stretch: Sit or stand tall and glide your head backward as in exercise 1. Raise both arms so that your hands are next to your ears. Take a deep breath, and as you exhale lower your elbows down and back. Feel your shoulder blades slide down and together. Hold for a few seconds. Relax and repeat.

3. Shoulder lifts: Lie face down with your arms beside your body. Lift your head and shoulders straight up from the floor as high as you can without pain. Keep your torso and hips pressed to the floor. Repeat 6 to 10 times.

4. Hands on head: Move your head backward, forward, and side to side against gentle pressure from your hands, holding each position for several seconds. Repeat 6 to 10 times.

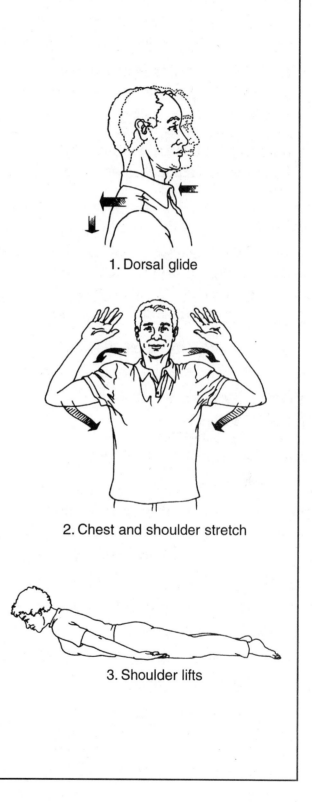

1. Dorsal glide

2. Chest and shoulder stretch

3. Shoulder lifts

- Avoid slouching or forward head posture.

- Walking is also helpful in relieving and preventing neck pain. The gentle swinging motion of your arms often relieves pain. Start with short walks of 5 to 10 minutes, three to four times a day.

- If neck pain occurs with headache, see Tension Headaches on page 159.

- Once pain subsides, do the neck exercises on page 41. Start with five repetitions twice a day. Gradually increase to 10 repetitions. Stop doing any exercise that causes pain.

- See Resource 16 on page 419.

When to Call a Health Professional

Call 911 or other emergency services:

- **If there has been a severe injury to the neck or if any of the following signs of a serious injury appear after a neck injury:**

  - **New, severe pain in the neck or back**

  - **New bruises on the head, neck, shoulders, or back**

  - **New weakness, tingling, or numbness in the arms or legs**

  - **New loss of bowel or bladder control**

  - **New bleeding or clear fluid discharge from the ears or nose**

  - **Loss of consciousness**

- **If neck pain occurs with shortness of breath or other symptoms that suggest heart problems (sweating, nausea, lightheadedness, rapid or irregular pulse), see Chest Pain on page 74.**

Call your health professional:

- If there has been a mild to moderate injury to the neck within the past two weeks, and there is pain but no evidence of injury to the spine.

- If you have new neck pain for any reason, or there has been a change in your pain, such as:

  - Neck pain that feels different than before

  - Dramatic increase in your chronic neck pain

  - Neck pain does not improve after two weeks of home treatment

- If you have evidence of nerve damage, such as:

  - Shooting pain in the arm

  - New numbness or tingling in the arms or legs

  - New weakness in the arms or any loss of function in the legs

  - Stiff neck occurs with headache and fever

*I don't deserve this award, but then I have arthritis and
I don't deserve that either.*
Jack Benny

4

Bone, Muscle, and Joint Problems

Problems with bones, muscles, and joints are the main cause of reduced activity in older people. However, you don't have to take these problems sitting down!

As your bones, muscles, and joints age, the following changes happen:

- Muscle strength declines.

- Bone mass decreases.

- Joints become less flexible and range of motion decreases.

However, you can slow these losses. Regular exercise, even as simple as walking or doing chair exercises, will help keep you strong and flexible. Exercise, a healthy diet, and good home care (and medical treatment as needed) for any problems that do develop are the best ways to keep your bones, muscles, and joints healthy, strong, and flexible.

Arthritis

Arthritis refers to a variety of joint problems that cause pain, swelling, and stiffness. Simply put, arthritis means inflammation of a joint. Arthritis can occur at any age, but it affects older people the most.

We know little about what causes most of the 100 different types of arthritis. A few types seem to run in families or are related to imbalances in body chemistry or immune system problems.

The chart on page 44 describes the three most common kinds of arthritis. Osteoarthritis is by far the most common type in people over 50 and can often be successfully managed at home. Rheumatoid arthritis and gout (page 52) will improve or can be controlled with a combination of self-care and professional care.

Joint infections, sometimes called septic arthritis, can cause joint pain and swelling and require immediate treatment.

Prevention

It may not be possible to prevent arthritis, but you can prevent a lot of pain by being kind to your joints. This is especially important if you already have arthritis.

- Protect your joints from activities that cause repeated jarring or pounding, such as high-impact aerobic activities.

- Get regular exercise.

- Control your weight.

While repeated jarring activities can increase joint pain, regular exercise can relieve or prevent it. Exercise nourishes the joint cartilage and removes waste products. It also strengthens the muscles around the

Types of Arthritis			
Type	**Cause**	**Symptoms**	**Comments**
Osteoarthritis	Breakdown of joint cartilage	Pain, stiffness, and occasionally swelling; common in fingers, hips, knees, spine.	Most common type in women and men ages 50 to 90.
Rheumatoid arthritis	Inflammation of the membrane (syno-vium) lining the joint	Pain, stiffness, and swelling in multiple joints, which may be "hot" and red; common in hands, wrists, feet.	Occurs most often around age 30 to 50; more common in women.
Gout (page 52)	Build-up of uric acid crystals in the joint fluid	Sudden onset of burning pain, stiff-ness, and swelling; common in big toe, ankle, knee, wrist, elbow.	Most common in men over 30; rare in women before menopause. May be aggravated by alcohol.

joints to support the joints and reduce injuries. Stretching exercises help maintain your range of pain-free motion. Stop any activity if you start to feel pain. Don't use pain relievers to mask pain while you continue to overuse a fatigued joint.

Controlling your weight will also reduce your chances of arthritis pain. Each extra pound adds 10 to 15 pounds to the load your hip and knee joints must carry.

Home Treatment

- Rest sore joints. Avoid activities that put weight or strain on the joint for a few days. Take short rest breaks from your regular activities throughout the day.

- A warm shower or bath may help relieve morning stiffness. Try to avoid sitting still after a warm shower or bath.

- If you have new swelling in a joint, do not apply heat. Try applying cold packs for 10 to 15 minutes every hour. Cold will help relieve pain and reduce swelling (although it may be uncomfortable for the first few minutes).

- If you have chronic joint swelling, apply either cold packs or moist heat (20 to 30 minutes, two to three times a day), whichever feels better.

- Regular exercise will help keep your muscles and joints strong and flexible. Strengthening exercises prevent the loss of muscle strength that leads to loss of function. Try low-impact activities, such as swimming, bicycling, walking, or water aerobics.

- Put each of your joints gently through its full range of motion once or twice a day. Stretching helps maintain joint mobility.

- Acetaminophen can relieve osteoarthritis pain without upsetting your stomach. Anti-inflammatory medications such as aspirin, ibuprofen, and naproxen also will relieve pain (and may relieve swelling, if present), but may cause stomach upset. Do not use different anti-inflammatory medications at the same time. See page 406.

- Try using devices that make everyday activities easier. See Resource 12 on page 419.

- Enroll in an arthritis self-management program. Participants usually have less pain and fewer limitations on their activities. See Resources 10 and 11 on page 419.

- See "Dealing With Chronic Pain" on page 61.

- Avoid fraud. There is no "miracle cure" for arthritis. Avoid products and services that promise one.

When to Call a Health Professional

- If joint pain is severe or prevents you from using a joint.

- If you have sudden onset of new and different joint pain with any of the following:

  ○ Fever of 100° or higher

  ○ Painful swelling in or around the joint

  ○ Localized pain or pain that increases when you use the joint

  ○ Redness, red streaks, or warmth

- If you experience side effects of aspirin or other arthritis medication (stomach pain, nausea, persistent heartburn, or dark tarry stools). Do not take more than the recommended dose of over-the-counter medications without your doctor's advice.

- If joint pain is not improving after two weeks of home treatment.

- If you have been diagnosed with arthritis but the pain or impaired movement is not responding to your doctor's recommended treatment or is not following the expected course.

Joint Replacement Surgery

When severe arthritis pain interferes with your quality of life and does not respond to home treatment and medications, joint replacement surgery may be appropriate. Hip and knee joints are the most commonly replaced joints. Joint replacement surgery relieves pain and may improve function, but will not restore the joint to how it was before arthritis developed.

Before having a joint replaced, consider these points (Also see page 10):

- Joint replacement surgery is seldom urgent. Get a second opinion; a few weeks or months of delay will make little difference. However, the results are often better if the joint is replaced before too much muscle and tendon strength have been lost.

- Surgery is most helpful if one joint is causing most of your problems.

- Replacement joints do not last forever. A second replacement joint may be needed in 15 to 20 years.

- The chance of success is better if you are in good shape. A regular exercise program and weight control are important both before and after the surgery.

Bunions and Hammertoes

A **bunion** is a swelling and deformity of the joint at the base of the big toe. The big toe may bend toward and overlap the other toes. A **hammertoe** is a toe that bends up permanently at the middle joint. Both conditions are irritated by wearing shoes that are too short or narrow. These problems sometimes run in families.

Morton's neuroma is a foot problem caused by pressure on the nerves in the foot. It causes pain or numbness and tingling in the ball of the foot and the toes.

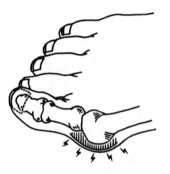

Bunion

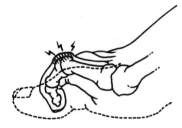

Hammertoe

Prevention

- Wear shoes with no heel (or a low heel) that give your toes plenty of room to wiggle. Tennis shoes are often best. Tight or high-heeled shoes increase the risk of bunions, hammertoes, and Morton's neuroma and irritate them if they are already present.

- Make sure that your shoes fit properly. As you age, your feet tend to get a little bigger. Have your feet measured to make sure you are buying the right size. Shop for shoes at the end of the day, because the feet tend to swell during the day.

Home Treatment

Once you have a bunion or hammertoe, there is usually no way to completely get rid of it. Home treatment will help keep it from getting worse.

- Wear low-heeled, roomy shoes that have good arch support.

- Cut out the area over the bunion or hammertoe from an old pair of shoes to wear around the house, or wear comfortable sandals that don't press on the area.

- Cushion the bunion or hammer-toe with moleskin or donut-shaped pads to prevent rubbing and irritation.

- Try aspirin, ibuprofen, or aceta-minophen to relieve pain. Ice or cold packs may also help.

When to Call a Health Professional

- If severe pain in the big toe comes on suddenly.

- If severe pain interferes with walking or daily activities.

- If the big toe begins to overlap the second toe.

- If the skin over a bunion or ham-mertoe becomes inflamed or very irritated. If you have diabetes, poor circulation, or peripheral vascular disease, be more concerned. The risk of infection is higher in people with these conditions.

- If pain does not respond to home treatment in two to three weeks.

Bursitis and Tendinitis

A bursa is a small sac of fluid that helps muscles slide easily over other muscles or bones. Injury or excessive use (overuse) of a joint or tendon may result in pain and inflammation of the bursa, a condition known as **bursitis**. Bursitis may develop quickly, over just a few days, often after a specific injury or overuse.

Tendons are tough, rope-like fibers that connect muscles to bones. Injury or overuse may cause pain, tenderness, and inflammation in the tendons or the tissues around them, a condition known as **tendinitis**.

Both bursitis and tendinitis can be related to work, sports, hobbies, or household activities that require repeated twisting or rapid joint move-ments. The same home treatment is good for both problems.

Shoulder pain is often due to bursitis or tendinitis in the tendons and mus-cles around the shoulder (the rotator cuff). This can cause pain when you move the shoulder in certain ways, such as to reach overhead or behind your back, or to comb your hair.

Prevention

- Warm up and stretch before activities to help prevent bursitis or tendinitis.

- Use good body mechanics and form when playing sports, working, or doing hobbies. Avoid repetitive, twisting movements and activities that put strain on a single joint (such as a one-handed backhand stroke in tennis).

- Prevent additional flare-ups by avoiding the activities that cause the problem.

Home Treatment

Bursitis or tendinitis will usually go away or at least subside in a few days or weeks if you avoid the activity that caused it.

The most common mistake in recovery is thinking that the problem is gone when the pain is gone. Chances are, bursitis or tendinitis will recur if you do not take steps to strengthen and stretch the muscles around the joint, and change the way you do some activities.

- As soon as you notice pain, apply ice or cold packs for 10-minute periods, once an hour or as often as you can for 72 hours. Continue applying ice (15 to 20 minutes, three times a day) as long as it relieves pain. See page 294.

Although heat may feel good, cold will relieve inflammation and speed healing.

- Rest the painful area. Avoid the activity that caused the problem, or change the way you do it so that you can do it without pain. To prevent stiffness, do not rest a joint for more than two days.

- Gently move the joint through as full a range of motion as you can without pain several times a day to prevent stiffness. As the pain subsides, continue stretching and add exercises to strengthen the muscles around the injured area.

- Aspirin, ibuprofen, or naproxen may help ease pain and inflammation, but don't use medication to relieve pain while you continue to overuse a joint.

- Warm up before and stretch after the activity that caused the pain. Apply ice to the injured area after exercise to prevent pain and swelling.

- Gradually resume the activity at an easier or slower pace. Increase slowly and only if pain does not recur.

When to Call a Health Professional

- If joint pain is severe or if you can't use a joint.

- If you have sudden onset of new and different joint pain with any of the following:

  ○ Fever of 100° or higher

  ○ Painful swelling in or around the joint

  ○ Redness, red streaks, or warmth

- If you experience side effects of aspirin or other anti-inflammatory medication (stomach pain, nausea, persistent heartburn, or dark tarry stools). Do not take more than the recommended dose of over-the-counter medications without your doctor's advice.

- If joint pain is not improving after two weeks of home treatment.

Carpal Tunnel Syndrome

The carpal tunnel is a narrow passageway of bone and ligament in your wrist. The median nerve, which controls sensation in your fingers, thumb, and some muscles in your hand, passes through this tunnel along with some of the finger tendons. Repeated motion or use of the hand or wrist may cause the wrist tendons to swell and press the nerve against the bone. This is known as carpal tunnel syndrome (CTS).

Symptoms of CTS may include numbness or tingling in one or both hands that does not affect the little finger, and wrist pain on the palm side that may affect the fingers or radiate up the arm.

Prevention

- Avoid repetitive hand motions with a bent wrist. Find ways to type, write, paint, play piano, or use tools with your wrist straight. Take 5- to 10-minute breaks every hour from repetitive hand motions.

Home Treatment

- The home treatment for bursitis and tendinitis, especially cold packs and anti-inflammatory medications, will also help carpal tunnel syndrome. See page 49.

- Consider wearing a wrist splint that keeps your wrist straight or slightly bent backward (extended). Wear the splint at night.

When to Call a Health Professional

- If pain or numbness in the hand is severe and is not relieved by rest, ice, and a normal dose of aspirin, ibuprofen, naproxen, or acetaminophen.

- If your hand grip becomes weak.

- If minor symptoms do not improve or if any numbness remains after one month of home treatment.

Fibromyalgia

Fibromyalgia (fibe-row-my-AL-ja) is a condition that causes pain in muscles and other soft tissues and occasionally in the joints. Although the joints may be sore, the condition does not cause the joints to swell or be deformed.

The cause of fibromyalgia is not known. People who have fibromyalgia have many tender spots in specific areas of their bodies. They often have trouble sleeping because of the pain. There may also be stiffness, weakness, and fatigue. Fibromyalgia is more common in women.

There is no specific treatment for fibromyalgia, although medications are sometimes prescribed to help treat the symptoms. Home treatment will help keep symptoms under control.

Home Treatment

Exercise is the cornerstone of home care for fibromyalgia. Regular exercise will strengthen your muscles and may also help you sleep better. Low-impact activities such as walking, biking, or swimming are best.

- Start slowly, with just a few minutes of exercise at a time. Increase by one minute every few days until you can exercise for 20 to 30 minutes. Try to exercise three to four times a week.

Polymyalgia Rheumatica

Polymyalgia (polly-my-AL-ja) rheumatica (roo-MAT-ik-ah) means "many aching muscles." It is a condition that causes pain and stiffness in muscles and other soft tissues, especially in the neck, shoulders, and hips. There may be inflammation and swelling in the joints, fatigue, and sometimes fever.

In contrast to fibromyalgia, the main treatment for polymyalgia rheumatica is medication. The condition is believed to be related to inflammation in small blood vessels and is related to giant cell arteritis (see page 157).

- Always stretch before and after exercise to improve flexibility, maintain good posture, and prevent injury. Stretch slowly and gently.

- When your symptoms flare, do not stop exercising, but cut back slightly.

- If pain interferes with your sleep, you may become fatigued, which may worsen the pain. See page 315 for tips on getting a good night's sleep.

- Take acetaminophen, aspirin, or ibuprofen to relieve pain.

- Apply heat to painful areas with heating pads, warm baths, or showers. Gentle muscle massage may provide some relief. A cold pack applied to the painful area may also help. Do not use for longer than 20 minutes at a time.

- If stress seems to worsen your symptoms, see page 365 for some ideas on how to manage stress.

When to Call a Health Professional

- If you have unexplained widespread muscle tenderness and pain, particularly both on the right and left sides of your body and both above and below the waist.

- If you have been diagnosed with fibromyalgia and any joints become swollen or red.

- If sleeping problems persist longer than one month despite home treatment.

Gout

Gout is a form of arthritis caused when uric acid crystallizes in the joints. Gout attacks can come on suddenly. The joint becomes tender, swollen, red, and very painful. The pain often reaches its peak in a matter of hours. A low fever of 99° to 101° is common.

Gout often attacks the big toe joint. Attacks may also involve the ankles, knees, elbows, fingers, and other joints. Gout attacks can last from several days to weeks. Between attacks, months or years can go by with no symptoms. Attacks gradually occur more often, last longer, and become more severe. Medication may be prescribed to prevent gout attacks.

Gout is far more common in men than in women. Other risk factors include a family history of gout, obesity, excessive alcohol use (particularly beer), use of aspirin, and very low-calorie starvation diets.

Prevention

Although you may not be able to prevent gout from developing, you can help reduce the frequency and severity of future attacks.

- Although you don't need to avoid specific foods, a low-fat diet that does not contain large amounts of protein is a wise choice. Avoid fasting and very low-calorie diets.

- Avoid or cut back on alcoholic beverages, especially beer. Alcohol increases uric acid production.

- Drink at least 8 to 10 glasses of water each day. This will help your kidneys flush uric acid through your system.

- Avoid aspirin.

Home Treatment

- As soon as you know you are having a gout attack, go to bed, elevate the affected joint, and stay there until the most severe symptoms have subsided. This may help prevent a second attack. Create a tent over your toe or joint to reduce pressure from bed sheets.

- Take ibuprofen to relieve pain. Do not take aspirin, because it may make it harder for your kidneys to get rid of the excess uric acid.

Caregiver's Guide for Bone, Muscle, and Joint Problems

- Encourage regular exercise, such as walking, lifting light weights (such as a can of soup), or even simple range of motion or chair exercises. People who are bedridden due to illness lose muscle strength very quickly. As soon as the person is feeling better, encourage her to start rebuilding her strength. Be patient, though. It can take several weeks to get strong again.

- Encourage the person to do for himself as much as possible. Look for devices that make daily activities, such as dressing, bathing, cooking, eating, or doing household chores, easier on sore joints. See Resource 12 on page 419.

- Look for ways to distract the person from the pain. Engage her in conversation, games, puzzles, or hobbies. Also see "Dealing With Chronic Pain" on page 61.

- Be alert for signs of depression. Pain can cause depression, and depression can worsen pain, creating a vicious cycle. See page 305.

- If your doctor has prescribed medication for use during an attack, take it as prescribed. Avoid using more than prescribed. Stop taking the drug and call your doctor if reactions such as nausea, vomiting, diarrhea, or abdominal cramping appear.

When to Call a Health Professional

- If you have sudden onset of severe joint pain, especially with swelling, tenderness, and warmth over the joint. Because gout is so painful, you'll probably need no urging to seek medical attention.

Once gout has been diagnosed, your doctor may recommend treatment for future attacks that you can start before calling for an appointment, especially if the attack is typical.

Muscle Cramps

Leg and muscle cramps are common in older adults. Nighttime leg cramps are especially common. Cramps have no clear cause, although they may occasionally be related to low levels of calcium or potassium in the blood. If you take water pills (diuretics) for high blood pressure or heart failure, you may have lower levels of these minerals in your bloodstream, or you may be slightly dehydrated. Both may contribute to muscle cramps.

Leg pain can also be due to phlebitis, an inflammation of a vein in the leg. See page 111. Atherosclerosis in the blood vessels of the leg may also cause a cramping pain called intermittent claudication that occurs during exercise. See page 107.

Pain in the front of your leg (shin) may be caused by an irritation of the tissues that hold the leg muscle to the bone. This condition is called shin-splints and may occur soon after you start an exercise program.

Prevention

- Get regular exercise during the day and do stretching exercises just before bedtime.

- Include plenty of calcium and potassium in your diet or take calcium supplements. See page 357. Potatoes, bananas, and orange juice are good sources of potassium.

- Take a warm bath before bedtime and keep your legs warm while sleeping.

- Try wearing elastic stockings during the day.

Home Treatment

- If there is heaviness and pain deep in the leg, call your doctor before applying home treatment.

- Ask someone to rub or knead a cramping muscle while you stand. Don't rub if you suspect thrombophlebitis (page 111).

- Use a heating pad or hot pack to warm the cramping muscle.

- Shinsplints are best treated with ice, anti-inflammatories (aspirin, ibuprofen, etc.), and a week or two of rest followed by a gradual return to low-impact exercise (swimming, walking, biking).

When to Call a Health Professional

Call immediately:

- If unexplained pain occurs deep in the leg or calf of one leg, especially if the leg is also swollen.

- If pain in one leg occurs with chest pain or shortness of breath.

- If you suddenly develop moderate to severe pain and cold or pale skin in the lower part of the leg.

Call a health professional:

- If pain in the leg comes on after you walk a certain distance and goes away with rest.

- If muscle cramps are not relieved with home treatment.

Osteoporosis

Osteoporosis or "brittle bones" is a condition that affects 25 percent of women over 60 years old. It is much less common and less severe in men.

Osteoporosis is caused by loss of bone mass and strength. It is more common after menopause, when estrogen levels decline. Lower estrogen levels speed up the rate of bone mass loss.

Osteoporosis is a silent disease; there may be no symptoms until a bone breaks and the condition is recognized after X-rays. Bones that are weakened by osteoporosis are easily broken, even by a minor injury. The bones that most often break are those of the spine, hip, and wrist. As the bones of the spine weaken, they often collapse, leading to stooped posture ("dowager's hump"), loss of height, and back pain.

Risk factors for osteoporosis include family history, being slender or "small-boned," white or Asian race, and inactivity. Smoking and drinking alcohol also increase the risk. To assess your risk, see "What Are Your Risks of Osteoporosis?" on page 56.

What Are Your Risks of Osteoporosis?

Risk Factors: Circle points that apply to you.

Age 35 to 64 2
Age 65 to 79 5
Age 80 or older 8
White or Asian 1
Small-boned 2
Slender 2
Mother, grandmother, or sister with osteoporosis 2
After menopause 1
Have had a hysterectomy 1
Never been pregnant 1
Have breast-fed 1
Allergic to milk 1
Smoke cigarettes 1
Drink 4 or more caffeinated drinks per day 1
Drink more than 1 ounce of alcohol per day 1
Risk Factor Score (Add risk factor points.) . . . . .____

Prevention Factors: Circle points that apply to you.
Exercise (walking or equivalent)
Walk ½ to 1 mile a day 1
Walk 1 to 2 miles a day 2
Walk 3 or more miles a day 3

Diet
Get 1000 to1500 mg of calcium per day 1
Get 1500 mg or more of calcium per day 2
Take estrogen replacement therapy .2
Get 30 minutes of sunshine or take
400 International Units of Vitamin D per day 1
Prevention Factor Score (Add prevention points.) . . . . .____

Subtract your **Prevention Factor Score** from your
Risk Factor Score to get your overall
Osteoporosis Risk Score . . . . .____

Low Risk: Less than 9   **High Risk:** 16-20
Medium Risk: 9-15   **Very High Risk:** 21 or higher

Prevention

Your bones are strongest during your twenties, but it is never too late to take steps to keep your bones strong as you get older.

- Get plenty of calcium in your diet. After menopause, women need 1,000 to 1,500 mg of calcium per day. Older men need 1,000 mg per day. Most people get only about 500 mg. The best source of calcium is low-fat dairy products:

  ○ A cup of low-fat yogurt contains about 442 mg.

  ○ A cup of skim milk contains about 313 mg.

  ○ One ounce of cheese contains about 200 mg.

  ○ Smaller amounts of calcium are also found in kidney beans, broccoli, and greens.

- If you are not able to get enough calcium in your diet, take two to three calcium carbonate tablets (TUMS) each day with meals or with milk. Don't take more than four to six tablets per day, and drink lots of water, because they can cause constipation.

- Vitamin D supplements (400 to 800 IU per day) may be helpful, especially if you do not get out in the sun much. Vitamin D is needed for strong bones.

- Hormone replacement therapy is the most effective way to prevent or reduce osteoporosis, especially when therapy is started right after menopause. Even if it has been many years since you went through menopause, starting hormone therapy may have some benefit. See page 239.

- Get regular, weight-bearing exercise, such as walking, bicycle riding, or dancing. Bones get stronger with exercise. Regular exercise will also help your coordination and strength, which will reduce your risk of falls and injuries. See the Fall Prevention Checklist on page 267.

- Don't smoke, and drink alcohol in moderation, if at all (one drink or less per day).

When to Call a Health Professional

- If a fall causes hip pain or you are unable to get up after a fall.

- If you have sudden, unexplained pain in your back that does not improve after two to three days of home treatment.

- To discuss hormone replacement therapy. See page 238.

Plantar Fasciitis and Heel Pain

Plantar fasciitis (fas-see-EYE-tis) is a condition that occurs when the thick, fibrous tissue that forms the arch of your foot (plantar fascia) becomes inflamed and painful. Athletes (especially runners), middle-aged people, and those who are overweight tend to develop plantar fasciitis. Repetitive exercises such as running and jumping sports can lead to heel pain and plantar fasciitis.

The problem may also be aggravated by poor arch support, worn-out shoes, tight calf muscles, or by running downhill or on uneven surfaces.

Achilles tendinitis can cause pain in the Achilles tendon at the back of the heel.

A **heel spur** is a calcium build-up that may occur where the plantar fascia attaches to the heel. Heel spurs are usually related to plantar fasciitis. They may cause heel pain when you walk or stand for long periods. Also, as you get older, the fatty pads that cushion your heels get thinner, which makes heel pain more likely.

Prevention

- Stretch your Achilles tendon and calf muscles several times a day (see page 336). Stretching is important even if you aren't an athlete.

- Maintain a reasonable weight for your height.

- Wear shoes with well-cushioned soles, good arch supports, and supportive heel cups. If you wear athletic shoes regularly, replace them every few months because padding wears out.

Home Treatment

Treat heel pain when it first appears to keep plantar fasciitis or other problems from becoming chronic.

- Reduce all weight-bearing activities to a pain-free level. Try low-impact activities such as cycling or swimming to speed healing.

- Apply ice to your heel. See "Ice and Cold Packs" on page 294.

- Do not go barefoot until the pain is completely gone. Wear shoes or arch-supporting sandals during all weight-bearing activities, even going to the bathroom during the night. Try an over-the-counter arch support (Spenco).

- Take aspirin, ibuprofen, or naproxen to relieve pain.

- Stretch your calf muscles. See page 336.

- For Achilles tendinitis, try putting heel lifts or heel cups in both shoes. Use them only until the pain is gone (continue other home treatment).

- Do not return to activities that cause pounding on your heels until you have been pain-free for one week. When you do return, start slowly and ice your heel afterward. If the pain recurs, start home treatment again.

When to Call a Health Professional

- If heel pain occurs with fever, redness, or heat in your heel, or if there is numbness or tingling in your heel.

- If heel pain is due to an injury or is so severe that you cannot bear weight.

- If pain continues when you are not standing or bearing any weight on your heel.

- If heel pain persists for one to two weeks despite home treatment.

Weakness and Fatigue

Weakness is a lack of physical strength that causes inability to move arms, legs, or other muscles.

Fatigue is feeling tired or exhausted, or a lack of energy.

Unexplained muscle weakness is usually more serious than fatigue. It may be due to metabolic problems such as diabetes (page 144), thyroid problems (page 152), kidney problems, or stroke (page 108). Call your doctor immediately.

Fatigue, on the other hand, can usually be treated with self-care. Most fatigue is caused by lack of exercise, stress or worry, poor sleep, depression, or boredom. Sleepiness is a common side effect of many medications. Colds and flu may sometimes cause fatigue and weakness, but the symptoms disappear as the illness runs its course.

Prevention

- Regular exercise is your best defense against fatigue. If you feel too tired to exercise, a short walk is probably the best thing you can do.

- Eat a well-balanced diet. Also consider a basic vitamin supplement as discussed on page 356.

- Make sure you are getting enough sleep. See page 315.

- Recognize and deal with any feelings of depression. See page 305.

Home Treatment

- Follow the prevention guidelines above and be patient. It may take a while to feel energetic again.

- Listen to your body. Alternate rest with exercise.

- Limit medications that might contribute to fatigue, especially tranquilizers and cold and allergy medications.

- Reduce your use of caffeine, nicotine, and alcohol. These substances can interfere with a good night's sleep, leaving you tired during the daytime.

- Take up new activities, spend time with friends, or travel to break the fatigue cycle.

When to Call a Health Professional

- If you have sudden unexplained muscle weakness in one area of your body. See Stroke on page 108.

- If severe fatigue causes you to limit your usual activities for longer than two weeks despite home treatment.

- If you have experienced sudden, unplanned weight loss.

- If you do not feel more energetic after six weeks of home treatment.

Dealing With Chronic Pain

There is no magic solution to chronic pain, whether it is caused by arthritis, osteoporosis, back problems, cancer, or any other condition. Nothing offers complete and total relief. However, the following tips may help. Also see page 375.

1. **Experiment with heat, cold, and massage.** Find out what works best for you. Touch is important, too. Ask for and give lots of hugs.

2. **Continue to exercise.** Find enjoyable exercise that does not aggravate your pain. Use the stretching exercises on pages 330 to 339 every day.

3. **Try to relax.** Severe pain makes your body tense and tight, and the tension may make the pain worse. See the relaxation techniques on page 365. It takes practice to learn any relaxation skill. Give a method a two-week trial. If it doesn't work for you, try another.

4. **Do something distracting.** Focusing all your attention on your pain makes it seem all-consuming. Refocus your attention away from the pain and onto something else. Sing a song, recite a poem, or concentrate on a visualization. See page 377.

5. **Expose yourself to humor.** A good, hearty belly laugh can provide your body with natural pain relief. Laughter *is* the best medicine.

6. **Practice positive self-talk.** Refuse to entertain negative, self-defeating thoughts or feelings of hopelessness. See page 376.

7. **Consider alternative therapies** such as biofeedback or acupuncture in addition to your regular medical care. Make sure to avoid fraud.

8. **Join a support group.** By being around others who share your problem, you and your family can learn skills for coping with pain. To find a group near you, contact the American Chronic Pain Association, P.O. Box 850, Rocklin, CA 95677, (916) 632-0922.

9. **Consider going to a pain clinic.** Be wary of those that promise complete relief from pain or that use only one method of treatment. Approved programs are registered with The Commission on Accreditation of Rehabilitative Facilities (CARF), 4891 East Grant Road, Tucson, AZ 85712, (602) 325-1044.

10. **Appeal to the Spirit.** If you believe in a higher power, ask for support and relief from the pain.

Also see Resources 48 and 49 on page 422 for books that deal with chronic pain control.

Keep breathing.
Sophie Tucker

5

Chest, Lung, and Respiratory Problems

This chapter will help you deal with the symptoms of respiratory problems. Most respiratory problems are viral infections like colds and flu that usually get better on their own. Good self-care for these minor ailments helps prevent complications.

If more serious problems develop, this chapter will help you identify them early. Prompt medical treatment from your doctor and from you will often keep even major problems from getting out of hand.

Some lung problems, like asthma and emphysema, are chronic. If you have a chronic lung disease, it's even more important to take good care of your lungs. This chapter will help.

Allergies

Allergies come in many forms. Hay fever is the most common allergy. Symptoms include itchy, watery eyes; sneezing; runny, stuffy, or itchy nose; temporary loss of smell; headache; and fatigue. Dark circles under the eyes ("allergic shiners") or postnasal drip may also accompany hay fever. Allergy symptoms are often like cold symptoms but usually last longer.

The most common causes of allergies are particles in the air, such as from pollen, house dust mites, mold or mildew, and animal dander.

You can often discover the cause of an allergy by noting when symptoms occur. Symptoms that occur at the same time each year (especially during spring, early summer, or early fall) are often due to grass, weed, or

Chest, Respiratory, Nose, and Throat Problems

Chest and Respiratory Symptoms	Possible Causes
Wheezing or difficulty breathing	See Asthma, p. 67; Bronchitis, p. 72; Pneumonia, p. 86.
Rapid, shallow, labored breathing	See Pneumonia, p. 86.
Chronic shortness of breath	See Emphysema, p. 80.
Chest-wall pain with cough that brings up yellow-green or rusty sputum; fever	See Bronchitis, p. 72; Pneumonia, p. 86.
Burning, pain, or discomfort behind the breastbone	See Heartburn, p. 125; Chest Pain, p. 74.
Chest pain with sweating, rapid pulse, lightheadedness	Possible heart attack. Call for help. See Chest Pain, p. 74.
Cough (dry or productive)	See Coughs, p. 78.
Nose and Throat Symptoms	**Possible Causes**
Stuffy or runny nose with watery eyes, sneezing	See Allergies, p. 63; Colds, p. 76.
Stuffy or runny nose, cough, with fever, headache, body aches, fatigue	See Influenza, p. 83.
Facial pain and fever with thick green, yellow, or grey nasal discharge	See Sinusitis, p. 88.
Sore throat	See Sore Throat, p. 90.
Sore throat with white spots on tonsils, swollen glands, fever of 101° or higher	See Strep Throat, p. 90.
Hoarseness, loss of voice	See Laryngitis, p. 85.

tree pollen. Allergies that persist all year long may be due to dust mites in household dust, mold spores, or animal dander. Animal allergies are often easy to detect: symptoms clear up when you stay away from the animal.

A few people have severe allergies to insect stings or certain foods or drugs, especially penicillin. For these people, the allergic reaction (**anaphylaxis**) is sudden and severe, and may cause difficulty breathing. If you have had a severe allergic reaction, carry an epinephrine syringe (Epi-pen, Anakit) that allows you to give yourself a shot that will decrease the severity of the reaction. If you are allergic to a drug, wear a medical identification bracelet that will tell health professionals about your allergy if you cannot.

Prevention

- There is no practical prevention for hay fever. However, if you have allergies, you can help prevent allergy attacks by avoiding the substances you are allergic to.

Home Treatment

If you can discover the source of your allergies, avoiding that substance is the best treatment. Keep a record of your symptoms and the plants, animals, foods, or chemicals that seem to trigger them.

If your symptoms are seasonal and seem to be related to pollen:

- Keep your house and car windows closed. Keep bedroom windows closed at night.

- Limit the time you and your pets spend outside when pollen counts are high. Pets may bring large amounts of pollen into your house.

If your symptoms are year-round and seem to be related to dust:

- Keep the bedroom as dust-free as possible, since most of your time is spent there.

- Cover your mattress and box spring with dust-proof cases and wipe them clean weekly. Avoid wool or down blankets and feather pillows. Wash all bedding weekly in hot water.

- Consider using an air conditioner or air purifier with a special HEPA filter. Rent one before buying to see if it helps.

If your symptoms are year-round and worse during damp weather, they may be related to mold or mildew:

- Keep the house well-ventilated and dry. Keep the humidity below 50 percent. Use a dehumidifier during humid weather.

- Use an air conditioner, which removes mold spores from the air. Change or clean heating and cooling system filters regularly.

- Clean bathroom and kitchen surfaces often with bleach to reduce mold growth.

If you are allergic to a pet:

- Keep the animal outside, or at least out of the bedroom. If your symptoms are severe, the best solution may be to find the pet another home.

General tips to avoid irritants and ease symptoms:

- Avoid yardwork (raking, mowing), which stirs up both pollen and mold. If you must do it, wear a mask and take an antihistamine beforehand.

- Avoid smoking or inhaling other people's smoke.

- Eliminate aerosol sprays, perfumes, room deodorizers, cleaning products, and other substances that may add to the problem.

- Antihistamines and decongestants may relieve some allergy symptoms. Use caution when taking these drugs. See pages 402 and 404.

When to Call a Health Professional

Call 911 or emergency services immediately if signs of a severe allergic reaction (anaphylaxis) develop, especially soon after taking a drug, eating a certain food, or being stung by an insect:

- **Lightheadedness or feeling like you may pass out.**

- **Swelling around the lips, tongue, or face that may interfere with breathing.**

- **Wheezing or difficulty breathing.**

Call a health professional immediately:

- If there is swelling of the lips, tongue, or face that is not interfering with breathing.

- If there is significant swelling around the site of an insect sting (e.g., the entire arm or leg is swollen).

- If there is a skin rash, itching, feeling of warmth, or hives.

Call a health professional:

- If symptoms worsen over time, and your home treatment doesn't help. Your doctor can recommend stronger medication or desensitizing shots. Allergy shots (immunotherapy) may help reduce sensitivity to some allergens.

Asthma

Asthma is a condition that causes inflammation and obstruction of the airways. The muscles surrounding the air tubes (bronchial tubes) of the lungs go into spasm, the mucous lining swells, and secretions build up. Breathing becomes quite difficult. Asthma is the Greek word for panting. Someone having an asthma attack is literally panting for breath.

Asthma usually happens in attacks or episodes. During an episode, the person may make a whistling or wheezing sound while breathing. The person usually coughs a great deal and may spit up mucus. A chronic dry cough may also be the only symptom.

Asthma may appear for the first time in adulthood, often during or following the flu or a bad cold. This type of asthma may occur throughout the year.

Infections are the most common asthma triggers. Other triggers include:

- Allergens, such as dust, pollen, mold, and animal dander

- Exercise

- Cigarette or wood smoke

- Changes in the weather

- Chemical vapors from household or workplace products

- Analgesics (especially aspirin)

- Food preservatives and dyes

- Emotional stress

Most adults can control their asthma by using medications to manage symptoms and avoiding triggers that cause attacks. Severe attacks can usually be treated with inhaled or injected medications. Asthma attacks are rarely fatal if they are treated promptly.

Prevention

No one knows for sure how to prevent asthma from developing. However, if you have asthma, you can help prevent asthma attacks by avoiding asthma triggers, by strengthening your lungs and airways, and by protecting your heart and lungs from damage.

- Review the home treatment for allergies on page 65.

- Avoid smoke of all kinds. Stop smoking and avoid second-hand smoke. Eat, work, travel, and relax in smoke-free areas.

- Avoid air pollution. Stay indoors when the air pollution is high.

- Avoid breathing cold air. In cold weather, breathe through your nose and cover your nose and mouth with a scarf or a cold weather mask (available at most drugstores).

- Aspirin, ibuprofen, and similar pain medications can cause severe reactions in some people with asthma. Use them with caution and discuss them with your doctor. If you find that these medications bother you, avoid using them.

- Do not use over-the-counter cold and cough medications unless your doctor tells you to do so.

- Reduce your risks of colds and flu by washing your hands often and getting a flu shot each year.

- If you use a humidifier, clean it thoroughly once a week.

- Get regular exercise. Swimming or water aerobics may be good choices because the moist air is less likely to trigger an attack. If vigorous exercise triggers asthma attacks, talk with your doctor. Adjusting your medication and your exercise routine may help.

- Take care of your heart (see page 98). Your lungs affect your heart, so if you have lung problems, it's important to keep your heart as healthy as possible, too.

Home Treatment

- Learn to use a peak flow meter (page 417) to monitor your ability to exhale. Used regularly, this device will give you an idea of how your lungs normally function. It also helps you tell when an attack may be coming so you can take appropriate steps sooner.

- If you have severe asthma, ask your doctor for a written care plan to guide you in adding medication as needed.

Once an asthma attack begins, good home treatment can provide relief:

- Learn to use a metered-dose inhaler. Inhalers get the right amount of medication to the airways. However, it takes some skill to use the inhaler correctly. A device called a spacer is recommended for use with an inhaler (see page 69). Ask your doctor to watch you use your inhaler and spacer to make sure you are doing it right. Ask your doctor about anti-inflammatory inhalers.

- Take control of the asthma attack. Keep a record of what triggers attacks and what helps end them. Be confident that your home treatment will control the severity of the attack.

- Practice the relaxation exercises on pages 365 to 370.

How to Use an Inhaler and Spacer

1. Shake the inhaler well for five seconds. Remove the protective cap and insert the mouthpiece of the inhaler into one end of the spacer. Hold the inhaler with your index finger on top and your thumb on the bottom.

2. Breathe out normally to empty the lungs. Tilt your head back, place the mouthpiece of the spacer tube in your mouth, and close your lips around it.

3. Press down on the top of the inhaler to release a puff of medication. Breathe in slowly and deeply, filling your lungs with as much air as possible. Some spacers make a musical sound if you are inhaling too fast. Hold your breath for at least 10 seconds, then breathe out.

4. With your lips still closed around the mouthpiece, take two or three more deep breaths, holding each one for 10 seconds. For maximum effectiveness, wait a minute or two before taking the next puff.

5. Wash the inhaler mouthpiece, spacer, and protective cap weekly with mild soapy water and allow to air dry.

- Drink extra fluids to thin the bronchial mucus. Try to drink at least two quarts of water per day.

- People with asthma usually do better in warm, moist air than in cold, dry air. If you're feeling "tight," stand or sit in a warm shower for 5 to 10 minutes.

- Follow the prevention tips on pages 67 and 68.

- Work in partnership with your doctor to increase your control over your asthma.

- If you have other chronic diseases in addition to asthma, ask your doctor how they may affect your asthma, and how your asthma may affect them. Know what symptoms to watch for, how to treat them, and when to call your doctor.

- See Resources 13 and 14 on page 419.

When to Call a Health Professional

- If you have symptoms that may indicate heart problems, such as chest pain or shortness of breath, see page 74.

- If acute asthma symptoms (wheezing, coughing, difficulty breathing) have occurred for the first time.

- If asthma symptoms fail to respond to your usual treatment or if the attack is severe (peak flow is less than 50 percent of best).

- If sputum becomes discolored, particularly green, yellow, or bloody. This may be a sign of a bacterial infection.

- If you begin to use your asthma medication more often than usual. This may be a sign that your asthma is getting worse.

- If someone with asthma or other family members have not been educated about immediate treatment, or if the medication required to treat an attack is not available.

- To discuss exactly what to do when an attack begins. Once you understand and have confidence in your asthma medication, you can often handle acute episodes without professional help.

- To discuss adjustments in medication. Your doctor needs your feedback to figure out the best medicine and the right dose for you.

- To assess allergies, which may worsen asthma attacks.

- To get a referral to a support group. Talking with others who have asthma can give you information and confidence in dealing with prevention and treatment.

Bacterial Infections

Upper respiratory infections caused by bacteria are often hard to distinguish from those caused by a virus. In particular, a bad case of the flu (page 83) may be hard to distinguish from a bacterial infection. Bacteria will sometimes attack the already weakened system of a person with a cold or flu, and bacterial infections sometimes follow viral infections.

In older adults, pneumonia or bronchitis often develops as a complication of a cold or the flu, and tends to be more serious than in younger adults.

You cannot prevent most types of bacterial infections by taking antibiotics. Antibiotics are most effective against bacterial infections once they have developed. Most doctors will not prescribe antibiotics until a bacterial infection is confirmed. For important information about antibiotics, see page 407.

When to Call a Health Professional

Call if the following symptoms of a bacterial infection develop. Bacterial infections need to be diagnosed and treated by a doctor.

- Fever of 103° or higher that does not reduce with two hours of home treatment.

- Fever of 100° or higher that lasts longer than one day in a frail or weakened person. Symptoms of a bacterial infection may be more subtle or less noticeable in people who are very old or frail. Even slight changes in temperature, breathing rate, and mental status may be signs of a serious infection.

Viral or Bacterial?

Viral Infections

- Usually involve different parts of the body: sore throat, runny nose, headaches, muscle aches. In the digestive system, viruses cause vomiting or diarrhea.

- Typical viral infections: cold, flu, stomach flu.

- Antibiotics do not help.

Bacterial Infections

- May follow a viral infection that does not improve.

- Usually are localized at a single point in the body.

- Typical bacterial infections: sinusitis, bronchitis, pneumonia, ear infection, strep throat.

- Antibiotics do help.

- Persistent fever. Many viral illnesses, especially the flu, cause fevers of 102° or higher for short periods of time (up to 12 to 24 hours). Call if a fever persists despite home treatment:

  - 102° to 103° after one full day

  - 101° to 102° after 2 full days

  - 100° to 101° after 3 full days

- New or different difficulty breathing or wheezing.

- Cough that is producing sputum from the lungs, especially with fever of 100° or higher. See Coughs, page 78.

- Ear pain (more than stuffiness) that lasts more than 24 hours. See Ear Infections, page 190.

- Localized sinus pain with fever or yellow or green nasal discharge. See Sinusitis, page 88.

- Sore throat with fever, white or yellow spots on the tonsils, or obvious swelling in the neck glands. See Sore Throat, page 90.

- If there is a change in mental status (even a minor change in a very old or frail person) or if the person seems delirious. See Delirium, page 165.

Bronchitis

Bronchitis is an inflammation and irritation of the bronchial tubes (bronchi) in the lungs. It is caused most often by bacteria or a virus but may also be caused by cigarette smoke or air pollution. Acute bronchitis often occurs after a cold or an upper respiratory infection that does not heal completely.

The inflamed bronchial tubes secrete a sticky mucus (called sputum), which is difficult for the hairs (cilia) on the bronchi to clear out of the lungs. The productive cough that comes with bronchitis is the body's attempt to get rid of the mucus. Other bronchitis symptoms include discomfort or tightness in the chest, fatigue, low fever, sore throat, runny nose, and sometimes wheezing. A severe case may lead to pneumonia.

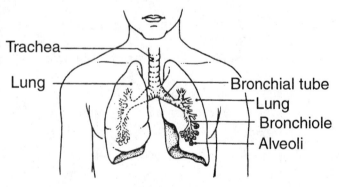

Lungs

Bronchitis is considered chronic if you have had a productive cough for more than three months per year for two years. Chronic bronchitis is caused by long-term damage to the lungs from many years of smoking or exposure to polluted air. Damage to the lungs makes it harder for the lungs to add oxygen to the blood. Symptoms such as fatigue and shortness of breath may occur.

Chronic bronchitis may occur with emphysema or chronic asthma. Any combination of these is known as chronic obstructive pulmonary disease (COPD). See page 80.

Prevention

- Give proper home care to colds and flu. See pages 76 and 83.

- Stop smoking and avoid second-hand smoke. People who smoke and those who live with them have bronchitis more often. Avoid polluted air.

If you have chronic bronchitis:

- Reduce your risk of colds and flu. Wash your hands often. Get a yearly flu shot (page 22) and a one-time pneumonia shot (page 23).

- Get regular exercise.

Home Treatment

Self-care for acute and chronic bronchitis focuses on getting rid of the mucus in your lungs.

- Drink 8 to 10 glasses of water per day (less if you have congestive heart failure). Liquids help thin the mucus in the lungs so your cough can clear it out.

- Stop smoking and avoid others' smoke.

- Breathe moist air from a humidifier, hot shower, or a sink filled with hot water. The heat and moisture will liquefy mucus and help the cough bring it up.

- Have someone massage your chest and back muscles. A massage increases blood flow to the chest and helps you relax.

- Get some extra rest. Let your energy go to healing.

- Take aspirin, ibuprofen, or acetaminophen to relieve fever and body aches.

- If you have chronic bronchitis, try roll breathing (page 365) or pursed-lip breathing (page 81) every day if it seems to help.

When to Call a Health Professional

A mild case of acute bronchitis may respond to home treatment. Watch for the following signs of a worsening lung infection or bacterial infection, and call your doctor if any of them develop:

- If you have a cough with new significant difficulty breathing or wheezing.

- If a productive cough brings up bloody sputum.

- If a cough that frequently produces yellow or green sputum from the lungs (not postnasal drainage) has lasted longer than two full days.

- If you have a productive cough with yellow or green sputum from the lungs and a fever of 100° or higher.

- If a fever of 103° or higher does not go down after two hours of home treatment, or if the fever persists after home treatment:

  ○ 102° to 103° after one full day

  ○ 101° to 102° after 2 full days

  ○ 100° to 101° after 3 full days

  ○ Fever of 100° or higher that lasts longer than one day in a frail or weakened person

- If you have significant chest-wall pain (pain in the muscles of the chest) related to coughing or breathing.

- If any cough weakens or exhausts a person who is frail.

- If a person with chronic lung problems develops symptoms of acute bronchitis.

- If the person is unable to drink enough fluids to avoid becoming dehydrated or is unable to eat.

- If any cough lasts longer than 7 to 10 days *after* other symptoms have cleared, especially if it is productive. A dry, hacking cough may last several weeks after a cold or the flu.

Get the Most Out of Your Cough

- Sit with your head bent slightly forward, feet on the floor.

- Breathe in deeply.

- Hold your breath for a few seconds.

- Cough twice, first to loosen mucus, then to bring it up.

- Breathe in by sniffing gently.

- Spit out the mucus. Swallowing it can upset your stomach.

From the American Lung Association

- If you are unable to do your normal daily activities because of fatigue or shortness of breath.

- If any cough lasts longer than four weeks.

Chest Pain

Call 911 or other emergency services immediately if chest pain is crushing (feels like someone is sitting on your chest) or squeezing, increases in intensity, or occurs with any of the symptoms of a heart attack:

- **Sweating**

- **Shortness of breath**

- **Pain that radiates to the arm, neck, or jaw**

- **Nausea or vomiting**

- **Lightheadedness**

- **Rapid and/or irregular pulse**

- **Loss of consciousness**

Chest pain is a key warning sign of a heart attack (see page 97), but it may also be caused by other problems.

If chest pain increases when you press your finger on the site, or if youcan pinpoint the spot that hurts, it is probably **chest-wall pain**, which may be caused by strained muscles or ligaments in the chest wall. An inflammation of the cartilage in the chest wall (called **costochondritis**) can also cause chest-wall pain. Chest-wall pain usually lasts only a few days. Aspirin or ibuprofen may help.

Pneumonia (page 86) may also cause chest-wall pain, especially when you cough or take a deep breath. Pain that throbs with each heartbeat may be caused by an inflammation of the outside covering of the heart (**pericarditis**).

Pleurisy is an inflammation of the outside covering of the lungs and the lining of the chest cavity (pleura). It is commonly caused by pneumonia, viral infection in the pleura, a broken rib, a blood clot in the lung, or anything that injures the chest. The pain is usually sharp and is felt along the chest wall. It will feel knifelike and stabbing after a deep breath or cough; heart pain will not. The pain from pleurisy will last until the underlying problem is treated.

Some **ulcers** (page 134) can cause chest pain, usually under the breast-bone, that is worse on an empty stomach. **Gallstones** (page 124) may cause pain in the right side of the chest or around the shoulderblade. It may be worse after a meal or in the middle of the night. **Heartburn** (page 125) can also cause chest pain.

Shingles (page 224) may cause a sharp, burning, or tingling pain that feels like a tight band around one side of the chest.

A shooting pain that lasts a few seconds or a quick pain at the end of a deep breath is not usually a cause for concern.

Home Treatment

For chest-wall pain caused by strained muscles and ligaments:

* Use pain relievers such as aspirin, acetaminophen, or ibuprofen. Ben-Gay or Vicks VapoRub may also soothe sore muscles.

* Avoid the activity that strains the chest area.

When to Call a Health Professional

Call 911 or emergency services immediately if chest pain is crushing or squeezing, increases in intensity, or occurs with any of the symptoms of a heart attack listed on page 74.

* If your chest pain has been diagnosed by a doctor and he has prescribed a home treatment plan, follow it. **Call 911 or emergency services if the pain worsens and may be due to a heart problem, or if you develop any of the heart attack symptoms on page 74.**

If minor chest pain occurs *without* symptoms of a heart attack, call a health professional:

- If you have a history of heart disease or blood clots in the lung.

- If the chest pain is constant and nagging and is not relieved by rest.

- If the chest pain lasts longer than two days without improvement.

Colds

The common cold is brought to you by any one of 200 viruses. The symptoms of a cold include runny nose, red eyes, sneezing, sore throat, dry cough, headache, and general body aches. There is a gradual, one- or two-day onset. As a cold progresses, the nasal mucus may thicken. This is the stage just before a cold dries up. A cold usually lasts about one or two weeks.

Using a mouthwash will not prevent a cold and antibiotics will not cure one. There is no cure for the common cold. If you catch one, treat the symptoms.

Sometimes a cold will lead to a bacterial infection. Frail or weakened older adults need to take extra care that their colds do not progress into pneumonia or bronchitis. Good home treatment can help prevent complications.

Prevention

- Eat well and get plenty of sleep and exercise to keep up your resistance.

- Wash your hands often, particularly when you are around people who have colds.

- Keep your hands away from your nose, eyes, and mouth.

- Humidify the bedroom or the whole house if possible.

- Don't smoke.

Home Treatment

Home treatment for a cold will help relieve symptoms and prevent complications.

- Get extra rest. Slow down just a little from your usual routine. Don't expose others.

- Drink plenty of liquids. Hot water, herbal tea, or chicken soup will help relieve congestion.

- Take aspirin, ibuprofen, or acetaminophen to relieve aches. See pages 405 and 406 for precautions.

- Humidify the bedroom and take hot showers to ease nasal stuffiness.

- Watch the back of your throat for postnasal drip. If streaks of mucus appear, gargle them away to prevent a sore throat.

- Use disposable tissues, not hand-kerchiefs, to reduce the spread of the virus to others.

- Avoid cold remedies that combine drugs such as decongestants, anti-histamines, and pain relievers to treat different symptoms. Treat each symptom separately to prevent side effects from drugs you may not need. Take a cough medicine for a cough; a decongestant for stuffiness. See pages 402 and 403 for simple remedies you can make at home. See Home Treatment for coughs on page 78.

- Avoid oral decongestants (unless approved by your doctor) if you have high blood pressure or heart disease. Some decongestants are also harmful to those with thyroid disease, glaucoma, urinary problems, enlarged prostate, or diabetes. See page 403.

- Use nasal decongestant sprays for three days or less. Continued use may lead to a "rebound effect," when the mucous membranes swell up more than before using the spray. See page 402 for nose drops you can make at home.

- Avoid antihistamines. They are not an effective treatment for colds.

When to Call a Health Professional

Call if the following symptoms of a bacterial infection develop. Bacterial infections need to be diagnosed and treated by a doctor.

- Fever of 103° or higher that does not reduce with two hours of home treatment.

- Persistent fever. Many viral ill-nesses cause fevers of 102° or higher for short periods of time (12 to 24 hours). Call if a fever persists despite home treatment:

  ○ 102° to 103° after one full day

  ○ 101° to 102° after 2 full days

  ○ 100° to 101° after 3 full days

  ○ Fever of 100° or higher that lasts longer than one day in a frail or weakened person

- New or different difficulty breath-ing or wheezing.

- Cough that is producing sputum from the lungs, especially with fever of 100° or higher. See Coughs, page 78.

- Localized sinus pain with fever or yellow or green nasal discharge. See Sinusitis, page 88.

- Sore throat with fever, white or yel-low spots on the tonsils, or obvious swelling in the neck glands. See Sore Throat, page 90.

- Ear pain (more than stuffiness) that lasts longer than 24 hours. See Ear Infections, page 190.

- If there is a change in mental status (even a minor change in a very old or frail person), or if the person seems delirious. See Delirium, page 165.

Coughs

Coughing is the body's way of removing foreign material or mucus from the lungs. Coughs have distinctive traits you can learn to recognize.

Productive coughs produce phlegm or mucus. This can be mucus that has drained down the back of the throat from the nose or sinuses (postnasal drainage) or mucus that has come up from the lungs (sputum). A cough that produces sputum from the lungs should generally not be suppressed so much that it is no longer bringing up sputum; the cough is needed to clear mucus from the lungs. A chronic productive cough in a person who smokes is often a sign of lung damage.

Nonproductive coughs are dry coughs that do not produce sputum. A dry, hacking cough may develop toward the end of a cold or after exposure to an irritant, such as dust or smoke. Dry coughs that follow viral illnesses may last up to several weeks and often get worse at night.

A chronic dry cough may be a sign of mild asthma, especially if it is hard to stop coughing. It may also be an early sign of congestive heart failure. See page 100.

Prevention

- Don't smoke. Smoking irritates the lungs and can lead to a dry, hacking "smoker's cough."

- Drink 8 to 10 glasses of water a day (less if you have congestive heart failure).

- For coughs brought on by inhaled irritants (smoke, dust, or other pollutants), avoid exposure or wear a face mask.

Home Treatment

- Drink lots of water. Water helps to loosen phlegm and soothe an irritated throat. Dry, hacking coughs respond to honey in hot water, tea, or lemon juice.

- Cough drops can soothe irritated throats, but most have no effect on the cough-producing mechanism. Inexpensive candy-flavored cough drops or hard candies work just as well as more expensive medicine-flavored cough drops.

- Elevate your head at night with extra pillows to ease a dry cough. Take an over-the-counter cough medicine if a cough is making you uncomfortable. Also see Cough Preparations on page 403.

- Use an over-the-counter cough suppressant containing dextromethorphan to help quiet a dry, hacking cough so you can sleep. Don't suppress a productive cough so much that it keeps you from clearing mucus from your lungs.

- Use an expectorant cough syrup containing guafenisin to thin mucus and make it easier for a productive cough to clear mucus from the lungs. Drink lots of water if you have a productive cough.

When to Call a Health Professional

If the following signs of a worsening lung infection or bacterial infection develop:

- If you have a cough with new significant difficulty breathing or wheezing.

- If a productive cough brings up bloody sputum.

- If a cough that frequently produces yellow or green sputum from the lungs (not postnasal drainage) has lasted longer than two full days.

- If a cough that produces yellow or green sputum from the lungs occurs with a fever of 100° or higher.

- If there is significant chest-wall pain (pain in the muscles of the chest) related to coughing or breathing.

- If a fever of 103° or higher does not go down after two hours of home treatment, or if the fever persists after home treatment:

  - 102° to 103° after one full day

  - 101° to 102° after 2 full days

  - 100° to 101° after 3 full days

  - Fever of 100° or higher that lasts longer than one day in a frail or weakened person

- If any cough weakens or exhausts a person who is frail.

- If any cough lasts longer than 7 to 10 days *after* other symptoms have cleared, especially if it is productive. A dry, hacking cough may last several weeks after a cold or the flu.

- If any cough lasts more than four weeks.

Emphysema

Emphysema is a chronic lung disease caused by repeated irritation or infection of the lung tissues. Over time, the air sacs (alveoli) in the lungs become permanently damaged and can no longer add oxygen to the blood or remove carbon dioxide. Emphysema is much more common in people who have been heavy smokers for a long time.

The primary symptom of emphysema is shortness of breath, especially on exertion, that worsens over time. Other symptoms can include fatigue, difficulty sleeping, weight loss, frequent colds and bronchitis, and wheezing. A mild productive cough may also be present. By the time symptoms develop, there has been significant lung damage.

Together with chronic bronchitis (see page 72), emphysema contributes to the condition known as **chronic obstructive pulmonary disease** (COPD).

Emphysema must be diagnosed by a health professional. There is no cure for emphysema, but early diagnosis and proper treatment will help you lead a more normal life.

Prevention

- Don't smoke and avoid second-hand smoke. The major cause of COPD and emphysema is cigarette smoking. See page 91.

- Reduce your exposure to lung irritants at home or work by using a filter mask and adequate ventilation.

Home Treatment

Self-care for emphysema and COPD focuses primarily on keeping your airways clear.

- If you smoke, quit. See page 91. Even though you cannot reverse lung damage, quitting smoking will prevent more damage.

- Drink at least 8 to 10 glasses of water a day to keep mucus thin.

- Get the most out of your cough. See page 74.

- Try pursed-lip breathing exercises (page 81) or roll breathing (page 365) if they help your breathing.

- Exercise. General fitness can help you improve your lung function.

- Avoid exposure to colds or flu. Get a yearly flu shot (page 22) and a one-time pneumonia shot (page 23).

When to Call a Health Professional

- If you have any of the following symptoms:

  ○ Increasing shortness of breath

  ○ Productive cough with green, yellow, or rust-colored sputum

  ○ Coughing up blood

  ○ Any change in the color or consistency of sputum (changes from thin to thick)

  ○ Wheezing that is not controlled by measures your doctor has recommended

- If you have symptoms such as chronic shortness of breath or a chronic cough that may be due to emphysema and have not been evaluated by a doctor.

- If you are a smoker and want help quitting. See page 91.

Pursed-Lip Breathing

Pursed-lip breathing helps release stale air trapped deep in your lungs. Practice the exercise three times a day and at the first indication that airway problems are limiting your breathing.

1. Relax your body. Let your neck and shoulders droop.

2. Breathe in slowly.

3. Purse your lips as though you were going to whistle, and blow out very slowly and evenly. Take twice as long to breathe out as you did to breathe in.

4. Check your relaxation. Repeat five times. If you get dizzy, rest for a few breaths.

Also see the roll breathing exercise on page 365.

Adapted from
American Lung Association

Fever

A fever is an abnormally high body temperature. It is a symptom, not a disease. A fever is one way your body fights illness. In healthy people, a fever up to 102° is usually beneficial, though it may be uncomfortable. The degree of the fever is not always related to the severity of the illness. This is especially true as you age, because your body loses some of its ability to produce a fever. An 80-year-old person with pneumonia who has a fever of 100° may be just as sick as a 24-year-old person with pneumonia who has a fever of 105°.

Older adults may develop symptoms that normally accompany fever even when they do not have a fever. These symptoms include headache, dizziness, restlessness, confusion, delusions, and paranoia. These symptoms may indicate an infection even if fever is not present. Fevers in older adults are more likely to cause delirium (page 165) or disorientation than fevers in younger people.

Temperatures below normal (especially below 94°) may indicate thyroid problems, hypothermia, or infection.

A high fever can place increased strain on the heart. For people who have heart disease, a high fever can sometimes trigger heart failure.

Home Treatment

Home treatment for fever depends on whether other symptoms are present with the fever. A fever up to 102° in an otherwise healthy person who has no other symptoms may just need watching. Take and record the temperature every two to four hours and whenever symptoms change.

If other symptoms are present, review the information under When to Call a Health Professional at right.

If a fever is making a person uncomfortable, the following may help:

- Take acetaminophen, aspirin, or ibuprofen to reduce the fever.

- Use a sponge bath or wet cloths with lukewarm water. Do not use ice water or rubbing alcohol.

- Drink extra water to replace fluids lost because of the fever. Watch for signs of dehydration. See page 120.

When to Call a Health Professional

- If a fever of 103° or higher does not go down after two hours of home treatment.

- If a fever of 100° or higher lasts longer than one day in someone who is frail or weak.

- If fever persists after home treatment:

  ◦ 102° to 103° after one full day

  ◦ 101° to 102° after 2 full days

  ◦ 100° to 101° after 3 full days

- If there is a change in mental status (even a minor change in a very old or frail person) or if the person seems delirious. See Delirium, page 165.

If fever occurs with any of the following symptoms, see the pages listed for more information.

- Shortness of breath and productive cough. See Bronchitis, page 72, or Pneumonia, page 86.

- Pain in the cheekbone or over the eyes. See Sinusitis, page 88.

- Painful or burning urination. See Urinary Tract Infections, page 139.

- Stomach pain, nausea, vomiting, or diarrhea. See Stomach Flu and Food Poisoning, page 132.

- Increased pain, redness, or tenderness around a skin wound, such as a cut or scrape. See page 276.

Influenza (Flu)

Influenza, or flu, is a viral illness that commonly occurs in the winter. It usually affects many people at once. (The name "influenza" comes from the Italian word for "influence.")

Influenza has symptoms similar to a cold, but they are usually much more severe and come on quite suddenly.

The flu is commonly thought of as a respiratory illness, but the whole body can be affected. Symptoms include fever (101° to 104°), chills, muscle aches, headache, pain in the muscles around the eyes, fatigue and weakness, sneezing, and runny nose. Symptoms may last five to seven days.

Older adults who are frail or who have a chronic disease, especially lung diseases like asthma or emphysema, are at higher risk of complications of influenza, such as bronchitis or pneumonia. Sinus or ear infections are other possible complications.

Prevention

- Get a flu shot each autumn if you are over 65, or if you have any of the conditions listed on page 22.

- Keep up your resistance to infection with a good diet, plenty of rest, and regular exercise.

- Avoid exposure to the virus. Wash your hands often and keep your hands away from your nose, eyes, and mouth.

Home Treatment

- Get plenty of bed rest.

- Drink extra fluids, at least 8 to 10 glasses of water every day.

- Take acetaminophen, aspirin, or ibuprofen to relieve fever, headache, and muscle aches.

When to Call a Health Professional

When trying to decide if you need to see a doctor, consider the likelihood that you have the flu versus a possible bacterial infection. If it is the flu season, and if many people in your community have similar symptoms, it is likely that you have the flu. The severity of your other symptoms (productive cough or shortness of breath) can help you decide if you need to see a doctor.

If you have any concerns, or if any of the following signs of a bacterial infection develop, call your doctor.

- New or different difficulty breathing or wheezing.

- Cough that is producing sputum from the lungs, especially with fever of 100° or higher. See Coughs, page 78.

- Localized sinus pain with fever or yellow or green nasal discharge. See Sinusitis, page 88.

- Sore throat with fever, white or yellow spots on the tonsils, or obvious swelling in the neck glands. See Sore Throat, page 90.

- Ear pain (more than stuffiness) that lasts longer than 24 hours. See Ear Infections, page 190.

- If there is a change in mental status (even a minor change in a very old or frail person), or if the person seems delirious. See Delirium, page 165.

It is common for adults who have the flu to have high fevers (up to 103°) for three to four days. However, fever may also be a symptom of a bacterial infection. If you think that you may have the flu, your fever alone will be less helpful in deciding if you need to see a doctor. Consider your other symptoms as well as the following guidelines:

- Fever of 103° or higher that does not reduce with two hours of home treatment.

- Fever that persists despite home treatment:

  ○ 102° to 103° after one full day

  ○ 101° to 102° after 2 full days

  ○ 100° to 101° after 3 full days

  ○ If a fever of 100° or higher lasts longer than one day in someone who is frail or weak.

Laryngitis and Hoarseness

Laryngitis is an infection or irritation of the voice box (larynx). The most common cause is a viral infection or a cold. It can also be caused by allergies, excessive talking, singing, or yelling, cigarette smoke, or stomach acid that backs up (refluxes) into the throat. Heavy drinking or smoking can lead to chronic laryngitis.

Symptoms of laryngitis include hoarseness or loss of voice, the urge to clear your throat, fever, tiredness, sore throat, and coughing.

Prevention

- To prevent hoarseness, stop shouting as soon as you feel minor throat pain. Give your vocal cords a rest.

Home Treatment

- Laryngitis will usually heal in 5 to 10 days. Medication does little to speed recovery.

- If the hoarseness is caused by a cold, treat the cold (see page 76). Hoarseness may last up to a week after a cold.

- Rest your voice by not shouting and by talking as little as possible. Do not whisper, and avoid clearing your throat.

- Stop smoking and avoid other people's smoke.

- Humidify the air with a humidifier, or take a hot shower.

- Drink lots of liquids.

- To soothe the throat, gargle frequently with warm salt water (one teaspoon in eight ounces of water) or drink honey in hot water, lemon juice, or weak tea.

- If you suspect stomach acid problems may be contributing to your laryngitis, see Heartburn on page 125.

Voice Changes

Some changes in the voice are normal as we age. Women's voices may get lower in pitch, while men's voices may get higher. Some people's voices may get hoarser or less clear.

Other stresses on the voice include smoking, stroke, Parkinson's disease, overuse of the vocal cords (yelling, screaming, cheering), and a low level of thyroid hormone. Leading an inactive life may also affect the voice. Keep physically active to help keep your voice strong.

When to Call a Health Professional

- If signs of a bacterial infection develop. See page 70.

- If hoarseness persists for three to four weeks.

Lung Cancer

Lung cancer is the number one cancer killer of men and women. It is most often found in long-term smokers over age 50. Lung cells can become cancerous when repeatedly damaged by smoke, chemicals, or other irritants that are inhaled.

Secondhand tobacco smoke, asbestos dust, and radon can also contribute to lung cancer. A combination of risk factors, such as a smoker who works with asbestos, greatly increases the risk of lung cancer.

If you've been diagnosed with lung cancer, see "Winning Over Serious Illness" on page 376.

Prevention

- If you smoke, quit. Ten to fifteen years after quitting, an ex-smoker's risk of cancer is about the same as a nonsmoker's. The risk of lung cancer begins to decrease almost immediately after quitting. There are other benefits as well. See page 91.

- Avoid secondhand smoke. Even if you have never smoked, inhaling other people's smoke puts you at risk.

- Test your home for radon. Call your local American Lung Association chapter for information.

When to Call a Health Professional

Symptoms of lung cancer are similar to other chest and lung problems: chronic cough, shortness of breath, wheezing, repeated lung infections or pneumonia, pain in the chest wall, or coughing up pus-filled or bloody sputum. There may be no symptoms in the early stages, making lung cancer difficult to detect. If you smoke, see your doctor about any chronic respiratory symptom.

Pneumonia

Pneumonia is an infection or inflammation of the smallest air sacs in the lungs, called alveoli. These sacs fill up with pus or mucus, preventing oxygen from reaching the blood. Pneumonia is most commonly caused by bacteria or viruses.

Pneumonia often follows or accompanies a cold, flu, or bronchitis. However, in very old or frail people, it may develop even if the person hasn't been sick.

Pneumonia can be a serious problem for older adults, especially those who have chronic diseases such as diabetes, heart disease, asthma, or emphysema. The pneumonia vaccine and good home care for colds and flu can help reduce the risk.

Someone who has bacterial pneumonia is usually very sick, and symptoms may include:

- Fever (100° to 106°) or shaking chills

- Productive cough that brings up yellow, green, rust-colored, or bloody mucus (sputum) from the lungs

- Pain in the chest wall, especially when coughing or taking a deep breath

- Labored, shallow, rapid breathing, or shortness of breath

- Fatigue that is worse than you would expect from a cold

- Sweating and flushed appearance

- Loss of appetite or upset stomach

- Mental status changes (confusion, disorientation)

Prevention

- Get a one-time pneumococcal immunization if you are over age 65, or if you have chronic heart or lung disease (asthma, emphysema) or diabetes. If it has been six years or longer since you had the shot, ask your doctor if you need a booster. See page 23.

- Keep up your resistance to infection with a good diet, rest, and regular exercise.

- Take care of minor illnesses. Don't try to "tough" your way through them. See Home Treatment for colds on page 76 and flu on page 83.

- Avoid smoke and other irritants.

Home Treatment

Call a health professional if you suspect pneumonia. If pneumonia is diagnosed, follow the home treatment below in addition to your doctor's recommended treatment.

- Drink lots of water—at least 8 to 10 glasses a day. Extra fluids are necessary to help thin the mucus.

- Get lots of rest. Don't try to rush recovery.

- Take the entire course of all prescribed medications.

- Stop smoking.

When to Call a Health Professional

- If you suspect pneumonia. See symptoms on page 87.

- If symptoms worsen after several days of antibiotic treatment.

- If there is rapid or labored breathing during any respiratory illness.

Sinusitis

Sinusitis is an inflammation or infection of the sinuses. The sinuses are cavities, or hollow spaces, in the head that are lined with mucous membranes. The sinuses usually drain easily unless there is an inflammation or infection. Sinusitis often follows a cold and may be associated with hay fever, asthma, or any air pollution that causes inflammation.

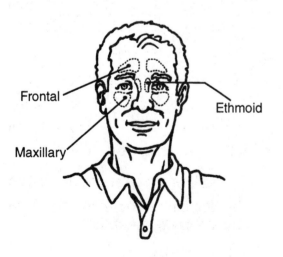

Sinus cavities

The key symptom of sinusitis is pain in the cheekbones and upper teeth, in the forehead over the eyebrows, or around and behind the eye. There may also be fever, mucus running down the back of the throat (post-nasal drip), and sore throat or cough. Sinus headaches may occur on rising and get worse in the afternoon or when bending over.

Sinusitis is usually a bacterial infection, and antibiotics are often needed. Also see page 157 for other possible causes of headache or facial pain.

Prevention

- Treat colds promptly. Blow your nose gently. Do not close one nostril when blowing your nose.

- Drink plenty of extra fluids when you have a cold to help keep mucus thin and draining.

- Stop smoking. Smokers are more prone to sinusitis.

Home Treatment

Some nasal stuffiness and facial pressure are common with a cold. Home treatment will often get your sinuses draining normally again.

- Drink extra fluids to keep mucus thin. Drink at least 8 to 10 glasses of water or juice every day.

- Breathe moist air from a humidifier, hot shower, or sink filled with hot water. Increase home humidity, especially in bedrooms.

- Use a decongestant nasal spray. See page 402 for types of decongestants. Use decongestant nasal sprays sparingly and for only three days or less.

- Salt water (saline) irrigation helps wash mucus and bacteria out of the nasal passages. Use an over-the-counter saline nasal spray or a homemade solution (see page 402):

  ○ Use a bulb syringe and gently squirt the solution into your nose, or snuff the solution from the palm of your hand one nostril at a time.

  ○ Blow your nose gently afterward. Repeat two to four times a day.

- Take aspirin, ibuprofen, or acetaminophen for headache.

- Watch the back of your throat for postnasal drip. If streaks of mucus appear, gargle with warm water to prevent a sore throat.

When to Call a Health Professional

- If you have moderate to severe pain in one or two sinus areas (such as in the cheekbone or upper teeth, forehead, or between the nose and lower eyelid).

- If you have sinus pain with a fever of 101° or higher.

- If there is swelling in the face (forehead, around the eye, side of the nose, or cheek), especially if the swollen area is red, tender, or warm.

- If you have a severe headache, different from a "typical" headache, that is not relieved by acetaminophen, aspirin, or ibuprofen.

- If moderate sinus pain or pressure persists after two days of home treatment.

- If nasal discharge has changed from clear to yellow or green, and other symptoms, such as sinus pain or fever, are worsening.

- If symptoms of sinusitis worsen after four days of antibiotic treatment or are not improving after one week.

- If yellow or green nasal discharge without other symptoms has lasted longer than two weeks.

Sore Throat and Strep Throat

Most sore throats are caused by viruses and sometimes accompany a cold. A mild sore throat is often due to low humidity, smoking, air pollution, or perhaps yelling. People who have allergies or stuffy noses may breathe through their mouths while sleeping, causing a mild sore throat.

Strep throat is a sore throat caused by streptococcal bacteria. It is much more common in children than in older adults. Symptoms of strep throat include sore throat with two of these three:

- Fever of 101° or higher (fever may be lower in adults)

- White or yellow coating on the tonsils

- Swollen glands in the neck

If a sore throat is accompanied by runny or stuffy nose and cough, it is probably due to a virus, and antibiotics will not help. Strep throat is treated with antibiotics to prevent rheumatic fever. Antibiotics are effective in preventing rheumatic fever if started within nine days of the start of the sore throat.

Another common cause of sore throat is stomach acid that backs up (refluxes) into the throat. Although this is often associated with heartburn or an "acid" taste in the mouth, sometimes a sore throat is the only symptom.

Prevention

- Try to drink at least 8 to 10 glasses of water a day (until you are urinating more often than usual).

- Identify and avoid irritants that cause sore throat (smoke, fumes, yelling, etc.). Don't smoke.

- Avoid contact with people who have strep throat.

Home Treatment

Home care is usually all that is needed for viral sore throats. If you are taking antibiotics for strep throat, these tips will also help you feel better.

- Gargle frequently with warm salt water (one teaspoon of salt in eight ounces of water) to reduce swelling, discomfort, and postnasal drip.

- Drink more fluids to soothe a sore throat. Honey and lemon in weak tea may help.

- Stop smoking and avoid other people's smoke.

- Acetaminophen, aspirin, or ibuprofen will relieve pain and reduce fever.

- Some over-the-counter throat lozenges have a local anesthetic to deaden pain. Dyclonine hydrochloride (Sucrets Maximum Strength) and benzocaine (Spec-T and Tyrobenz) are safe and effective. Regular cough drops or hard candy may also help.

- If you suspect problems with stomach acid may be contributing to your sore throat, see Heartburn on page 125.

When to Call a Health Professional

- If sore throat occurs with difficulty swallowing or difficulty breathing.

- If sore throat develops after exposure to strep throat.

- If a sore throat occurs with two of these three symptoms of strep throat:

  ○ Fever of 101° or higher (may be lower in adults)

  ○ White or yellow coating on the tonsils

  ○ Swollen glands in the neck

- If a rash occurs with sore throat. Scarlet fever is a rash that may occur when there is a strep throat infection. Like strep throat, scarlet fever is treated with antibiotics.

- If a new sore throat lasts longer than a week.

- If a chronic sore throat has not been checked out by a doctor or is getting worse.

Quitting Smoking

It's never too late to quit smoking, even if you have been smoking for 20 or 30 years. Here's the good news:

- Your risk of heart disease begins to drop almost immediately, and after 10 years it is close to that of a non-smoker.

- Your risk of lung cancer begins to decrease, and after 10 to 15 years, your risk drops to nearly that of a nonsmoker.

- Your circulation will improve, increasing the amount of blood that reaches your brain. This is important in reducing your risk of stroke.

Quitting smoking is the most important thing you can do for your own health and the health of those around you. However, it won't be easy. Chances are you have already tried once or twice. As Mark Twain once said, "Quitting smoking is the easiest thing I have ever done. I've done it a hundred times."

No one can tell you when or how to quit smoking. Only you know why you smoke and what will be most difficult as you try to stop. The important thing is that you try. Believe that you will succeed, if not the first time, then the second time, or twenty-second time.

Tips for Quitting

Preparation

- Decide how and when you will quit. About half of ex-smokers quit "cold turkey"; the other half cut down gradually.

- Figure out why you smoke. Do you smoke to pep yourself up? To relax? Do you like the ritual of smoking? Does smoking help you deal with negative feelings? Do you smoke out of habit, often without realizing you're doing it?

- Find a healthful alternative that accomplishes what smoking does for you. For example, if you like to have something to do with your hands, pick up something else: a coin, worry beads, pen or pencil. If you like to have something in your mouth, substitute sugarless gum or minted toothpicks.

- List your reasons for quitting: for your own health and your family's health, to save money, to prevent wrinkles, or whatever. Keep reminding yourself of your goal.

- Plan a healthful reward for yourself when you have stopped smoking. Take the money you save by not buying cigarettes and spend it on yourself.

- Plan things to do when you get the urge to smoke. Urges don't last long—take a walk, brush your teeth, have a mint, drink a glass of water, or chew gum.

- Choose a reliable smoking cessation program. Good programs have at least a 20 percent success rate after one year; great programs have a 50 percent success rate. Higher numbers may be too good to be true.

**Ten Good Reasons to Quit
at Age 50 or Better**

1. Your body will begin to heal itself.

2. Shortness of breath and cough will decrease.

3. Stamina and energy will improve.

4. Fewer colds and illnesses.

5. You'll smell good.

6. Taste buds and sense of smell come back to life.

7. More spending money.

8. It's good for your loved ones.

9. Be in control of your life.

10. It's a good idea.

- Think of yourself as an ex-smoker. Think positive.

Action

- Set a quit date and stick to it. Choose a time that will be busy but not stressful.

- Remember the word HALT and try to avoid becoming too Hungry, Angry, Lonely, or Tired. These are situations that make many people want to smoke. Alcohol is another trigger for many smokers; try to avoid it, too.

- Remove ashtrays and all reminders of smoking. Choose nonsmoking sections in restaurants. Do things that reduce your likelihood of smoking, like taking a walk or going to a concert.

- Ask for help and support. Choose a trusted friend, preferably another ex-smoker, to give you a helping hand over the rough spots.

- Reward yourself.

- Good books with good information can help. See Resource 52 on page 422.

Tuberculosis

Tuberculosis (TB) is a contagious disease caused by bacteria that primarily infect the lungs. TB spreads when infected people cough or sneeze the bacteria into the air and others inhale the organisms. After infection, active TB can develop immediately, many years later, or may never develop. Symptoms of active infection include a persistent cough, weight loss, fatigue, and fever.

People who are at increased risk for TB include those who are HIV-positive, IV drug users, homeless people, immigrants from countries with high rates of TB, health care workers who may be exposed to people with TB, and older adults.

Drug treatment can cure TB, but it may take up to 6 to 12 months.

To prevent TB, avoid close contact with someone who has an active TB infection, especially spending a long time together in a stuffy room. You cannot get TB by handling things an infected person has touched.

If you think you've had close contact with someone with active TB, contact your doctor or local health department about a tuberculin skin test (see page 23).

- Know what to expect. The worst will be over in just a few days, but physical withdrawal symptoms may last one to three weeks. After that, it is all psychological. Counter symptoms with relaxation. See Chapter 22.

- Keep low-calorie snacks handy for when the urge to munch hits. Your appetite may perk up, but most people gain less than 10 pounds when they quit smoking. A healthy, low-fat diet and regular exercise will help you avoid unwanted pounds and resist the urge to smoke. The health benefits of quitting outweigh a few extra pounds.

- Get out and exercise. It will distract you, help keep off unwanted pounds, and release tension.

- Don't be discouraged by slip-ups. It often takes several tries to quit smoking for good. If you do smoke, forgive yourself and learn from the experience. You will not fail as long as you keep trying.

- Good luck!

The Nicotine Patch

The nicotine patch is an adhesive patch that releases nicotine into the bloodstream through the skin. Used together with a smoking cessation program, it may help some smokers gradually withdraw from nicotine addiction by supplying smaller and smaller amounts of nicotine.

First try to stop smoking without the patch. Many people succeed without it.

The patch is most useful for people who have had serious withdrawal symptoms (headaches, anxiety, depression, difficulty concentrating, insomnia) when they try to quit smoking. Generally, it is prescribed only to those who smoke more than a pack a day.

Using the patch alone is not always successful. By combining the patch with a good smoking cessation program, your chances of success can be greatly increased.

If your heart has peace, nothing can disturb you.
The Dalai Lama

6

Heart and Circulation Problems

Your heart and blood vessels (circulatory system) supply oxygen and nutrients to every cell in your body. The heart is the key to a physically robust life at any age, but especially as you get older. To a great extent, the health of your heart and circulatory system determines how far you can walk, how late you can dance, and how long you can garden.

Your heart is a hollow muscle. When it contracts, it forces blood to surge out through the arteries to the lungs, where the blood picks up oxygen. From the lungs, the blood returns to the heart and is pumped into the circulatory system, which carries the oxygen-rich blood through the arteries to the farthest reaches of your body. Once the blood has fed its load of oxygen to your cells, it circulates through the veins back to the heart, where the whole process starts again.

Normally, your heart and circulatory system provide a constant supply of oxygen and nutrients to your body. When there is a problem in any part of the system, it may not function as well. Heart and circulatory diseases are the leading causes of death in adults. Read on for information about how to reduce your risk and manage these diseases.

Atherosclerosis

One of the most common heart and circulatory problems is atherosclerosis.

Atherosclerosis ("hardening of the arteries") is the build-up of fatty deposits called plaques (made up of cholesterol and other substances) on the inside of the arteries. As these plaques grow, the arteries are narrowed, less blood is able to flow through them, and less oxygen and nutrients reach the tissues that rely on those arteries.

Atherosclerosis is the starting point for most heart and circulation problems.

- When it affects the arteries that supply blood to the heart muscle, it is called coronary artery disease and may cause angina, heart attacks, and congestive heart failure. See below.

- When it affects the arteries in the legs or other areas, it causes a circulation problem called peripheral vascular disease. See page 107.

- When it blocks blood flow to the brain, it may cause stroke and "mini-strokes" (transient ischemic attacks). See page 109. It can also cause a type of dementia called multi-infarct dementia. See page 167.

Other types of circulatory problems include high blood pressure, blood clots or inflammation in the veins (phlebitis), irregular heartbeats, and varicose veins. These problems may be related to atherosclerosis, but in some cases they are not.

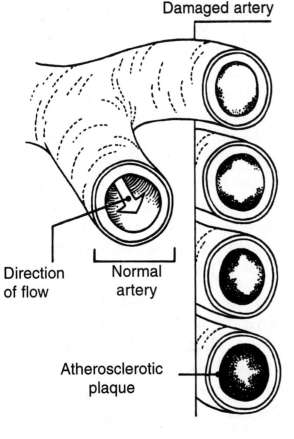

Damaged artery

Direction of flow

Normal artery

Atherosclerotic plaque

Atherosclerosis

Coronary Artery Disease

Coronary artery disease (CAD or heart disease) occurs when the blood vessels that supply blood to the heart muscle (the coronary arteries) are narrowed or blocked. This narrowing or blockage is most often caused by atherosclerosis (hardening of the arteries). When the heart muscle doesn't get enough blood, it is deprived of oxygen and nutrients. This is called ischemia (is-KEY-me-uh).

Smoking, high blood pressure, high cholesterol, diabetes, being male, and a family history of heart disease are all important risk factors for CAD. Other risk factors are stress, an inactive lifestyle, and being overweight.

Angina is the most common symptom of coronary artery disease. Angina is a pressing or squeezing chest pain (the Latin word means a choking or suffocating pain). It occurs when there is not enough oxygen to meet an increased demand on the heart muscle, such as exercise or stress. Angina pain may spread or radiate to the neck, jaws, shoulders, or arms. It is relieved by rest and use of prescribed medication (such as nitroglycerin).

Stable angina is mild to moderate chest pain that occurs predictably after a certain amount of exertion or emotion and is relieved by rest. If you have had angina for a while, you may be able to predict almost exactly how much exertion will bring on the symptoms. Angina is said to be **unstable** if it begins at rest, when you are not exercising or under stress, or is significantly different from angina that has been stable. Unstable angina requires immediate medical attention.

CAD may have no symptoms ("silent ischemia"), or it may cause symptoms in addition to angina, such as palpitations (irregular heartbeat), shortness of breath, lightheadedness, fainting, or nausea.

There are many other causes of chest pain. Most are not related to the heart (see page 74). While chest pain does not necessarily mean that you have heart disease, any chest pain that does not have a clear cause or that persists should be evaluated by a doctor.

If a coronary artery is blocked, such as by a blood clot, a portion of the heart muscle may die due to lack of oxygen. This is called a **heart attack** or myocardial (heart muscle) infarction (tissue death).

The size and location of a heart attack determine how well the heart muscle will continue to function. If only a small amount of heart muscle dies, the person may recover quickly. If there is extensive heart muscle damage, congestive heart failure (page 100) may develop, or the person may die.

Medications for CAD reduce the workload on the heart and increase the blood supply to the heart muscle. When medication and lifestyle changes do not control angina symptoms, or when blood flow to large areas of the heart muscle is impaired, surgical treatment may be necessary.

With treatment and control of risk factors, you can improve the quality of your life and, in most cases, live a long and productive life with coronary artery disease.

Prevention

A few risk factors for heart disease, such as being male or getting older, are outside your control. You can control many other risk factors, such as smoking, high blood pressure, and high cholesterol.

- Stop smoking. Smoking increases the risk of atherosclerosis. See Quitting Smoking on page 91.

- Eat a healthy, low-fat diet. This will help control your cholesterol and your weight. A very low-fat diet (less than 10 percent calories from fat) may even reduce atherosclerosis that has already started. See page 355.

- Get regular aerobic exercise. Exercise helps to control your blood pressure and your cholesterol and may make it easier for you to lose weight. Walking, swimming, cycling, jogging, hiking, and dancing are all good aerobic exercises. See your doctor before starting an exercise program if you have never been active or have not exercised for many years. Also see Chapter 20.

- Manage stress and anger wisely. These emotions may increase your blood pressure. In addition, managing stress in a healthy way will help you be successful with other lifestyle changes. See page 363.

- Review the information on page 104 about controlling blood pressure.

- If you are a woman and you have one or more risk factors for heart disease, consider taking estrogen or hormone replacement therapy after menopause. A woman's risk of heart disease goes up after menopause. Hormone therapy reduces the risk. See page 238.

- If you have diabetes, manage it as your doctor recommends to reduce your risk of heart disease. See Home Treatment for diabetes on page 146.

Home Treatment

CAD responds well to lifestyle changes and medications that reduce risk factors. If you stop smoking, maintain a healthy weight, exercise regularly, eat a healthy diet, and take your prescribed medications as directed, you can reduce your risk of heart attack. In some cases, you may even slow or reverse the process of atherosclerosis.

- Take your prescribed medications as directed. If you have been prescribed nitroglycerin for angina, be sure you understand when and how to use it and what to do if it doesn't seem to be working.

- If someone in your family has coronary artery disease, or has several risk factors for heart disease, take a cardiopulmonary resuscitation (CPR) course. CPR is a form of first aid for heart attacks, and it saves lives.

- Follow the prevention guidelines about quitting smoking, a low-fat diet, exercise, and stress management.

- Talk with your doctor about taking aspirin every day to reduce the risk of heart attack. Do not take aspirin regularly without first discussing it with your doctor.

- See Winning Over Serious Illness on page 376.

- Maintain a positive attitude. Learn all you can about heart disease and believe that you can manage it successfully. Studies show that a positive attitude helps people successfully recovery from heart attacks.

When to Call a Health Professional

Call 911 or other emergency services immediately if chest pain is crushing (feels like someone is sitting on your chest) or squeezing, increases in intensity, or occurs with any of the symptoms of a heart attack:

- **Sweating**

- **Shortness of breath**

- **Pain that radiates to the arm, neck, or jaw**

- **Nausea or vomiting**

- **Lightheadedness**

- **Rapid and/or irregular pulse**

- **Loss of consciousness**

After you call 911, begin rescue breathing and CPR if the person stops breathing or has no pulse. See page 100.

Quick action is vital when someone is having a heart attack. Medications that reduce the damage to the heart muscle are most effective when given within one hour of the onset of symptoms.

Call your doctor immediately:

- If you suspect angina and your symptoms have not been diagnosed.

- If the pattern of your angina changes (for example, symptoms begin to occur at rest).

If minor chest pain occurs without symptoms of a heart attack, call a health professional:

- If the person has a history of heart disease or blood clots in the lungs.

- If chest pain is constant, nagging, and not relieved by rest.

- If any chest pain lasts 48 hours without improvement.

Congestive Heart Failure

Heart failure occurs when your heart muscle doesn't contract hard enough to pump as much blood as the body needs. When the heart muscle has been damaged by long-term high blood pressure, coronary artery disease, a heart attack, or other conditions (such as injury or infection of the heart muscle), it is harder for the heart to pump blood effectively. "Failure" doesn't mean that the heart isn't pumping at all, just that it is failing to pump as effectively as it should.

Heart failure is most often caused by a problem with the chamber of the heart (the left ventricle) that takes in oxygen-rich blood from the lungs and pumps it out to the body.

CPR Training

Cardiopulmonary resuscitation (CPR) can save lives and improve recovery from heart attacks. Consider signing up for a CPR class or taking a refresher course. They are offered through the American Red Cross, the American Heart Association, and other community groups.

If you have never taken a CPR course and someone is unconscious and has no pulse, call 911 or emergency services.

If you have taken a CPR course, the following will refresh your memory:

1. Call 911 or other emergency services.

2. Check consciousness.

3. Open the airway and look, listen, and feel for breathing.

4. If the person is not breathing, give 2 rescue breaths.

5. Check for a pulse.

6. If no pulse, begin CPR. Give 15 chest compressions, then 2 breaths.

7. Continue until help arrives.

When you have heart failure, the left ventricle may pump out less blood with each heartbeat. As a result, there is not enough room in the left ventricle to hold all the blood that is entering from the lungs. This blood backs up in the heart and lungs. Over time, the right ventricle begins to malfunction also, causing blood to back up in the body, especially the liver and other abdominal organs.

The earliest and most common symptoms of heart failure are caused by fluid build-up in the lungs, abdomen, or legs. The symptoms may include:

- Difficulty breathing during routine activities that did not cause shortness of breath in the past

- Shortness of breath when lying down that requires the person to sit up to be able to breathe more easily

- Waking up at night with a feeling of suffocation, coughing, and rapid heart rate

- Unexplained, dry, hacking cough

- Swelling (edema) in the legs, ankles, and feet

- Rapid weight gain (due to retaining water) and increased urination at night

- Lightheadedness, fainting, fatigue, or weakness

- Swelling and discomfort in the abdomen

Prevention

The best way to prevent congestive heart failure is to keep the arteries that supply blood to your heart muscle free of atherosclerosis. See Prevention for Coronary Artery Disease on page 98.

Home Treatment

- Reduce the salt in your diet. When you have heart failure, your body retains sodium and water, which leads to fluid build-up and swelling. See page 359.

- Keep track of how much liquid you drink. Your doctor may recommend that you limit liquids to no more than 1½ to 2 quarts per day. Remember that juice, coffee, tea, milk, and soda all count toward your daily intake.

- If your doctor wants you to weigh yourself every day, do it at the same time each day (before breakfast is a good time). Call your doctor if you gain more than three to four pounds over a day or two. This may mean that fluid is building up in your body.

- If your heart failure is severe or you are having a bad episode, don't try to continue with your usual activities. Your body needs to rest. However, if you are resting in bed, avoid lying flat on your back. Prop yourself up with pillows or move to an armchair, and flex and shift your legs often. This will help keep fluid from building up in your abdomen and chest and making it hard for you to breathe. Get help with household chores if needed.

- Take your medications as directed. Not taking your pills regularly can make your symptoms worse. See page 396 for some suggestions for keeping track of your pills.

- Use care with over-the-counter medications. Some antacids and stool softeners contain sodium or ingredients that can interfere with your prescription medications.

- Get a flu shot each fall (page 22) and a one-time pneumococcal vaccine (page 23).

When to Call a Health Professional

Call 911 or other emergency services:

- **If chest pain is crushing and occurs with shortness of breath, sweating, nausea, or lightheadedness.**

- **If you have severe shortness of breath (trouble getting a breath even when resting).**

- **If you have a sudden episode of irregular heartbeat with light-headedness, nausea, or fainting.**

- **If you have a cough that produces foamy, pink mucus.**

- **If you have difficulty breathing with a sense of impending doom related to your heart or lungs not functioning well.**

Call a health professional:

- If you have difficulty breathing during previously routine activities or exercise.

- If you become short of breath when you lie down, or if you wake at night with shortness of breath or a feeling that you are suffocating.

- If you have heart failure and your symptoms get worse. In general, it's a good idea to call your doctor any time you have a sudden change in symptoms.

- If you have new and significant swelling in your feet, ankles, or legs, or if swelling that is typical for you worsens significantly.

- If you have heart failure and have had a two-day weight gain of three to four pounds or more.

Consumer Tips on Chest Pain

- Don't ignore chest pain and don't delay seeking care. If the chest pain is due to a heart attack, immediate treatment is critical.

- Stay calm. Chest pain evaluations done at the hospital often show no sign of heart attack. Practice deep breathing and relaxation. See page 365.

- At the hospital, expect some questions followed by an ECG (electrocardiogram). Practice the relaxation exercises on page 365 before the testing begins.

- Your doctor may suggest an angiogram or other test. Review "Shared Decisions About Medical Tests" on page 8.

- Always discuss other options before agreeing to angioplasty or coronary bypass surgery. Review "Shared Decisions About Surgery" on page 10.

High Blood Pressure

If a person's blood pressure readings are consistently above 140/90, he or she is said to have high blood pressure (**hypertension**).

Blood pressure is a measurement of the force of the blood against the walls of the arteries. This is most often done using a blood pressure cuff. Blood pressure readings include two numbers, for example, 130/80.

The first number in the reading is called the **systolic** pressure. It is the force of blood against the artery walls when the heart is beating or contracting to pump blood out.

The second number in the reading is the **diastolic** pressure. It is the force against the artery walls between heartbeats, when the heart is at rest.

Despite what a lot of people think, high blood pressure does not make you dizzy, tense, or nervous. It usually has no symptoms. However, high blood pressure increases the risk of heart disease and heart attacks, strokes, and kidney or eye damage. The higher the blood pressure, the higher the risk.

Risk factors for high blood pressure include:

- Black race

- Being overweight

- Family history of high blood pressure

- Inactive lifestyle

- Excess alcohol drinking

- Excess sodium (salt) intake (in some people)

- Use of certain medications, including corticosteroids, decongestants, and anti-inflammatories

Lifestyle changes (such as diet and exercise) and medications can reduce blood pressure and lower the risk of stroke, heart disease, kidney damage, and vision loss.

Prevention

Changes in your lifestyle can help prevent high blood pressure or help lower it if you have it.

- Maintain a healthy weight. This is especially important if you tend to gain weight around your waist rather than in your hips and thighs. Even losing 10 pounds can help lower blood pressure.

- Exercise regularly. Thirty to 45 minutes of brisk walking three to five times a week will help lower your blood pressure (and may also help you lose weight).

- Drink alcohol only in moderation (see page 342). Too much alcohol increases blood pressure.

- Use salt moderately. Too much salt in the diet is a problem for some people who have high blood pressure. See page 359.

Home Treatment

Even if you are taking medications to control your blood pressure, home treatment is important to keep it in control. Home treatment will also help reduce your overall risk of cardiovascular disease. In some cases, you may be able to reduce the amount of medication you need. (Don't reduce your medication without talking to your doctor.)

- Take your prescribed medications as directed. Because high blood pressure has no symptoms, it's hard to remember to take your pills every day. If you have trouble taking your medications because of bothersome side effects, talk to your doctor about alternatives.

- There is some evidence that potassium, calcium, and magnesium may be important in controlling blood pressure. A diet that includes plenty of fruits (such as bananas and oranges), vegetables, legumes, and low-fat dairy products will ensure you get enough of these minerals.

- Avoid decongestants, which can increase blood pressure.

- Follow the prevention guidelines above. Regular exercise and maintaining a healthy weight will help you control your blood pressure.

- Follow the prevention guidelines for coronary artery disease (see page 98). High blood pressure increases your risk of heart disease, so pay attention to other risk factors, such as smoking and high cholesterol.

When to Call a Health Professional

- If you have high blood pressure and your blood pressure rises suddenly, you have a sudden severe headache, or your blood pressure is 180/110 or higher.

- If your blood pressure is over 130/85 on two or more occasions (taken at home or in a community screening program). If one blood pressure reading is high, have another reading taken by a health professional to verify the reading. Some doctor's offices or clinics will take your blood pressure at no cost and without an appointment.

- If you develop significant side effects of any medication taken for high blood pressure.

Irregular Heartbeats

Normally, your heart beats in a regular rhythm and at a rate that is appropriate for the work your body is doing. Irregular heartbeats (**arrhythmias**) occur when the heart beats too fast, too slow, or with an irregular rhythm.

An arrhythmia may feel like a "skipped" beat, a palpitation, or a "flip-flop" or fluttering in your chest. Your heart may pound or race, or it may beat more slowly than usual. You may also have discomfort in the chest, shortness of breath, lightheadedness, weakness, or you may faint. When fainting occurs due to an irregular heartbeat, it is called **syncope** (sin-ko-pee).

Heavy smoking, drinking alcohol, and excess caffeine or other stimulants may cause your heart to "skip" a beat. Your heart may pound or beat rapidly when you are under stress. Your heart rate also increases when you have a fever.

Many arrhythmias are minor and do not require treatment. Others, such as a type of arrhythmia called atrial fibrillation, can be life-threatening because they increase the risk of blood clots and strokes. Arrhythmias are especially concerning in people who also have heart disease or congestive heart failure.

If treatment is needed, medications may be prescribed to help regulate the heartbeat or reduce the risk of blood clots. A device (pacemaker) may also be implanted in the chest wall to regulate the heartbeat.

Prevention

- If a rapid or irregular heartbeat seems to be related to caffeine, alcohol, or nicotine, limit your intake. Cut back on caffeine slowly to avoid headaches.

Home Treatment

- If you become lightheaded, sit down to avoid injuries that might result if you pass out and fall.

- Take deep breaths and try to relax. This may slow down a racing heartbeat.

- Keep a record of the date and time, your activities when the irregular heartbeat happened, how long the irregular beats lasted, how many "skipped" beats there were, and any other symptoms.

When to Call a Health Professional

- **Call 911 or other emergency services if a rapid and/or irregular heartbeat occurs with chest pain or other symptoms of a heart attack. See page 99.**

Call a health professional immediately:

- If an irregular heartbeat leads to fainting (a complete, brief loss of consciousness).

Call a health professional:

- If you suddenly experience a very rapid (more than 120 beats per minute) or very slow (less than 50 beats per minute) heartbeat without obvious cause.

- If you have repeated spells of lightheadedness over a few days.

- If your heart seems to beat irregularly all the time.

- If lightheadedness lasts longer than three to five days and interferes with your daily activities. Also see Vertigo and Dizziness, page 197.

Peripheral Vascular Disease

If atherosclerosis (hardening of the arteries) develops in the arteries that supply blood to the legs, abdomen, and pelvis, it is called peripheral vascular disease (PVD). The arteries in the legs are most often affected. As the artery is narrowed by atherosclerosis, the leg muscles do not get enough blood.

The main symptom of peripheral vascular disease in the leg is tight or squeezing pain in the calf, foot, thigh, or buttock that occurs during exercise (such as walking up a steep hill or a flight of stairs). This pain usually occurs after the same amount of exercise each time and is relieved by rest. As the condition worsens, leg pain may occur at rest. This pain is called intermittent claudication (claw-di-KAY-shun).

Other signs of atherosclerosis in the legs include numbness, tingling, or cold skin on the feet or legs, loss of hair on the feet or legs, and irregular toenail growth. The feet may become dusky-colored, and minor skin injuries, especially on the feet, may turn into large sores that are slow to heal or easily infected. In severe cases, foot infections may lead to gangrene, and amputation of the foot or leg may be necessary.

Atherosclerosis in the arteries of the abdomen and pelvis can also cause kidney or intestinal problems.

If you have symptoms that you think may be due to PVD, tell your doctor. These symptoms often mean that there is atherosclerosis in other arteries, such as those that supply blood to the heart.

Prevention

Risk factors for peripheral vascular disease are the same as those for coronary artery disease. Reduce your risk of peripheral vascular disease by reducing your risk of atherosclerosis and heart disease. See page 98.

Home Treatment

Once the condition has been diagnosed, the following home treatment may be useful.

- Quit smoking. People who continue to smoke have an increased risk of serious problems.

- Start a walking program (with your doctor's approval). Each day, walk until the pain starts, then rest until it goes away before continuing. Try to walk just a little farther each day before resting. Don't try to walk through the pain. The goal is to increase the amount of time you can exercise before the pain starts.

- Take good care of your feet. When your circulation is impaired, even minor injuries can lead to serious infections. See page 146.

- Avoid shoes that are too tight or that rub your feet. Avoid socks or stockings that leave elastic band marks on your legs.

When to Call a Health Professional

Call immediately:

- If unexplained pain occurs deep in the leg or calf of one leg, especially if the leg is also swollen. See Thrombophlebitis on page 111.

- If you suddenly develop moderate to severe pain and cold or pale skin in the lower part of the leg.

- If the skin of one or both legs is pale or blue-black.

Call your health professional:

- If pain in the leg comes on after you walk a certain distance and goes away with rest.

Stroke

A stroke is a medical emergency. Prompt medical treatment can reduce the amount of damage to the brain. **Call 911 or other emergency services immediately if you have the following symptoms:**

- **Progressive loss of speech or sight over a period of a few minutes to hours, or sudden onset of double vision or slurred speech**

- **Sudden weakness, numbness, or loss of sensation in an arm, leg, or the face (usually on the same side of the body)**

- **Sudden, severe headache that is new or different**

- **Sudden unexplained behavior changes, such as confusion or bizarre behavior**

- **Loss of consciousness**

A stroke occurs when an artery that supplies blood to the brain is blocked by a blood clot or bursts. Within minutes, the nerve cells in that area of the brain become damaged and die. As a result, the part of the body controlled by that part of the brain cannot function properly. The medical term for a stroke is **cerebrovascular accident (CVA)**.

A Caregiver's Guide for Heart Attack and Stroke

Someone who has had a heart attack or stroke may feel vulnerable, frightened, and depressed. Fears of never working, loving, or playing again are common. It may seem that death was close and may come again at any minute. It is hard on loved ones, too. Caregiving can be a very painful experience.

Fortunately, there are professionals who can help you and the patient. Rehabilitation and physical therapists can teach home activities that will speed healing. Occupational therapists can advise you on adaptive devices and home set-up to encourage independence.

Caregivers need support, too. Gather your friends around you. Talk with someone who has survived a stroke or heart attack. They will help you learn that much is possible in the rehabilitation process. The difficulties you see today may be much improved in the weeks and months ahead.

For more information, see Chapter 25, Caregiver Secrets. For information on support groups, contact your local chapter of the American Heart Association.

Transient ischemic attacks (TIAs) are "mini-strokes" that should be considered a warning sign of a stroke. Many people who have a stroke have had TIAs during the months before the stroke. Symptoms of a TIA are the same as those of a stroke except that they disappear completely within a few minutes to 24 hours, and there are no lingering effects.

The effects of stroke may range from mild to severe, and they may be temporary or permanent, depending on which part of the brain is damaged, how much damage there is, and how quickly blood flow is restored to the area. A stroke can affect speech, behavior, and thought processes. In addition, it can cause paralysis, coma, or death. Lingering effects may include:

- Weakness or total paralysis on one side of the body

- Difficulty speaking or making sense of words and pictures

- Loss of vision in one eye

- Changes in behavior or emotions

- Memory loss

In addition, many people who have had a stroke become depressed.

If someone has had a stroke, they will often go through a period of rehabilitation to regain their strength and mobility and to relearn how to do everyday tasks.

Prevention

Risk factors for stroke include high blood pressure, smoking, diabetes, and coronary artery disease (see page 96). Controlling these risk factors will reduce the risk of stroke.

- Control your blood pressure. High blood pressure is the most important risk factor for stroke. See page 103.

- Don't smoke. Women who smoke a pack a day are nearly four times more likely to have a stroke than women who don't smoke at all. Smoking also increases a man's risk of stroke.

- If you have diabetes, keep your blood sugar in control. See page 144.

- Ask your doctor about taking aspirin daily to reduce the risk of stroke. Do not take aspirin regularly without first discussing it with your doctor.

- Drink alcohol only in moderation. Heavy drinking increases the risk of stroke.

Home Treatment

- Know the warning signs of a stroke (see below). Seek emergency care if they occur.

- Involve family members and friends in the recovery process. Also see the box on page 109 and Chapter 25, Caregiver Secrets.

- Know the signs of depression and watch for them in the person who has had a stroke. Depression is common and very treatable. See page 305.

When to Call a Health Professional

Call 911 or other emergency services if the following signs of stroke are present:

- **Progressive loss of speech or sight over a period of a few minutes to hours, or sudden onset of double vision or slurred speech**

- **Sudden weakness, numbness, or loss of sensation in an arm, leg, or the face (usually on the same side of the body)**

- **Sudden, severe headache that is new or different**

- **Sudden unexplained behavior changes, such as confusion or bizarre behavior**

- **Loss of consciousness**

Quick action is vital when someone is having a stroke. Medications that reduce the damage to the brain are most effective when given within one hour of the onset of symptoms.

Call immediately:

• If you suspect you have had a transient ischemic attack (signs of stroke that last a short time and go away completely) within the last 12 hours. This is a warning sign of a stroke.

Call a health professional:

• If you think you have had a transient ischemic attack in the past. Your symptoms need to be evaluated.

Thrombophlebitis

When a vein becomes inflamed due to a blood clot, it is called thrombophlebitis (sometimes shortened to **phlebitis**). This can occur in any vein, but is most common in the lower leg veins. A clot may form either in a vein just under the surface of the skin (superficial thrombophlebitis) or in a vein deep in the leg.

Symptoms of superficial thrombophlebitis include pain, tenderness, warmth, and redness along a leg vein.

Clots in these veins rarely cause serious problems because they do not travel through the bloodstream.

Symptoms of thrombophlebitis in a deep leg vein include swelling and pain in one leg or a noticeable new difference in the size of one leg. There may also be pain when walking or when the foot is flexed upward. Deep vein thrombophlebitis is a serious condition, because the clot may break loose and travel through the bloodstream to the lung (pulmonary embolism). This is a life-threatening situation. Symptoms may include chest pain, shortness of breath, or coughing up blood.

The risk of thrombophlebitis is increased by:

• Long periods of inactivity, such as sitting for long plane or car rides or being bedridden following surgery, which causes blood to pool in the legs.

• Injury to the inside of the vein, such as from having intravenous medication, tests that inject dye into a vein, or an injury to the area.

• Conditions or medications that increase the chance of blood clots (such as heart disease or cancer, or estrogen).

Superficial thrombophlebitis is often treated with rest and anti-inflammatory medications. Deep vein thrombophlebitis requires hospitalization and medical treatment to avoid complications.

Prevention

- Avoid prolonged sitting or standing. If you are on a plane or in a car for long periods of time, take breaks to walk around regularly. If you cannot walk around, stretch and move your legs often. Fidgeting in your seat will help keep blood from pooling in your legs.

- Avoid stockings that leave elastic band marks on your calves or legs.

- If you frequently have superficial thrombophlebitis, ask your doctor about specially made elastic support hose.

Home Treatment

Superficial thrombophlebitis may be treated at home once it has been diagnosed. If you suspect deep vein thrombophlebitis, call your doctor immediately. Do not rub or massage the leg.

- Wear elastic support stockings to increase blood flow in your legs and prevent blood from pooling.

- Rest with your leg elevated, but be sure to continue your regular activities too. Avoid long periods of sitting or standing.

- Take aspirin or other anti-inflammatory medication as your doctor recommends.

- Apply warm moist compresses to the painful area.

When to Call a Health Professional

Call immediately:

- If unexplained pain occurs deep in the leg or calf of one leg, especially if the leg is also swollen.

- If pain in one leg occurs with chest pain, shortness of breath, or coughing up blood.

Call your health professional:

- If you suspect superficial thrombophlebitis but it has not been diagnosed by a doctor.

- If previously diagnosed thrombophlebitis does not improve after your doctor's recommended home treatment.

Cold Hands and Feet

Many older adults have cold hands and feet. Most often, this is due to reduced blood flow to the hands and feet, such as from inactivity, cold weather, or circulation problems. The following may help.

- Avoid substances that constrict your blood vessels, including caffeine (coffee, cola drinks, tea) and nicotine in cigarettes.

- Keep indoor temperatures at 65° or higher. Wear warm socks or slippers.

- If you want warm feet, wear a hat. You lose a lot of body heat from your head. Mittens are better than gloves for keeping fingers warm.

- Move around. A brisk walk or even whirling your arms around like a windmill will get your blood moving and warm you up.

A low level of thyroid hormone may cause cold intolerance (see page 152). Persistently cold hands or feet, or loss of feeling in the hands or feet, may be a sign of a more serious problem, such as nerve or blood vessel disorders. If the above home treatment doesn't warm you up, call your doctor.

Varicose Veins

Varicose veins are enlarged, twisted, or swollen veins close to the surface of the skin, most commonly in the legs. Small valves in the leg veins help blood to flow from the legs back to the heart. Varicose veins develop when these valves are weak or damaged and can no longer help move blood against the force of gravity. Blood pools in the legs, increasing pressure in the veins and causing them to swell.

Varicose veins often cause no symptoms. Some people may have aching or fatigue in the legs, especially at the end of the day, minor swelling in the feet and ankles, and itching over the vein. The blue color of the veins is often visible through the skin.

If varicose veins are more serious, there may be swelling in the leg and stretching and thinning of the skin over the veins. This can cause dry, itchy skin that breaks easily and may bleed heavily, and may cause open sores (ulcers) that are hard to heal. There may be changes in the color of the skin due to pooling blood.

Some people also have tiny red or blue veins on the surface of the skin. These are often called **spider veins**, because they may resemble a spider's web. These are not related to varicose veins, though both may occur in the same person.

Varicose veins tend to run in families and are more common in people who are overweight. In most cases, they do not require treatment. If varicose veins cause bothersome symptoms, surgery may be helpful.

You usually cannot prevent varicose veins from developing. Home treatment may help slow their progression, relieve symptoms, and prevent complications.

Home Treatment

• Wear supportive elastic stockings (full-length, not knee-highs). For mild symptoms, regular support pantyhose may work. For more bothersome symptoms, buy elastic stockings at a pharmacy.

• Avoid tight clothing that limits circulation, such as knee-high stockings that leave elastic band marks around your legs or pants that are tight in the waist and thighs. This cuts off circulation and can worsen varicose veins.

• Elevate your legs on a footstool when you are sitting. Avoid crossing your legs at the knee. Put your feet flat on the floor or cross your legs at the ankles. At the end of the day, elevate your legs above your heart for a while.

• Avoid sitting or standing for long periods of time. Get up and walk around often, or sit down and elevate your legs. Contracting the muscles in your legs helps move blood back toward the heart.

• Get regular exercise, such as walking, bicycling, dancing, or swimming. Working your leg muscles helps keep blood from pooling in the legs.

• Maintain a healthy body weight.

When to Call a Health Professional

Call immediately:

• If unexplained pain occurs deep in the leg or calf of one leg, especially if the leg is also swollen. See Thrombophlebitis, page 111.

Call a health professional:

• If a varicose vein bleeds heavily without cause or following an injury. Apply direct pressure and elevate the leg to stop the bleeding. If you are unable to slow or stop the bleeding with direct pressure, call immediately.

• If open sores develop on your legs or feet.

7
Digestive and Urinary Problems

Your digestive system absorbs useful nutrients and minerals for your body. Along with the urinary system, it eliminates waste and harmful products.

The digestive system is working all the time: 24 hours a day, 7 days a week, 52 weeks a year. Except for brief illnesses, most people have very

Abdominal pain is difficult even for a doctor to evaluate. In addition to the information in the "When to Call a Health Professional" sections of this chapter, call your doctor whenever stomach pain:

- Is severe or persistent.

- Increases over several hours.

- Localizes to one area of the abdomen (e.g., upper right, lower left).

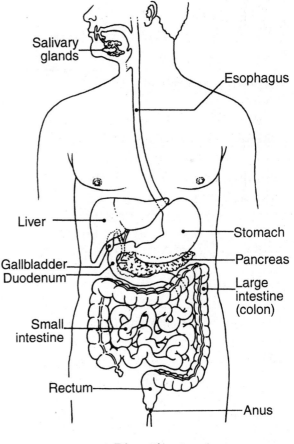

Digestive tract

Digestive and Urinary Problems

Symptoms	Possible Causes
Nausea or vomiting	See Nausea and Vomiting, p. 131; Watch for Dehydration, p. 120. Medication reaction. Call your doctor or pharmacist. See Antibiotics, p. 407.
Bowel Movements	
Frequent, watery stools	See Diarrhea, p. 122; Stomach Flu and Food Poisoning, p. 132. Watch for Dehydration, p. 120.
Stools dry and difficult to pass	See Constipation, p. 118.
Bloody or black, tarry stools	See Ulcers, p. 134.
Pain during bowel movements; bright red blood on surface of stool or on toilet paper	See Hemorrhoids, p. 127.
Abdominal Pain	
Chronic bloating with diarrhea, constipation, or both	See Irritable Bowel Syndrome, p. 129.
Pain in the abdomen, possibly with vomiting or fever	See Diverticulitis, p. 123; Gallbladder Disease, p. 124.
Burning or discomfort just below the breastbone or above the navel	See Heartburn, p. 125; Ulcers, p. 134; Chest Pain, p. 74.
Urination	
Pain or burning on urination	See Urinary Tract Infections, p. 139.
Loss of bladder control	See Urinary Incontinence, p. 137.
Difficulty urinating or weak urine stream (men)	See Prostate Problems, p. 252.
Blood in the urine	See p. 255.

few problems with their digestive tract. When you do, the guidelines in this chapter may help.

Colorectal Cancer

Cancer of the large intestine (colon) and rectum occurs in about six percent of people over age 40. Symptoms of colorectal cancer include blood in the stool, bleeding from the rectum, a persistent change in bowel movements, thin pencil-like stools, and lower abdominal pain. Fortunately, colorectal cancer can often be successfully treated if it is diagnosed at an early stage.

You are at increased risk of colon cancer if you have a family history of the disease, if you have polyps (protruding growths like skin tags) in your colon, or if you have ulcerative colitis. High-fat and low-fiber diets have also been linked to colorectal cancer.

If you have colon cancer, work with your doctor to develop a treatment plan. Also see Chapter 23.

Prevention

- Eat right. Cut down on fats and increase fiber. See Chapter 21.

Although screening tests don't prevent cancer, they can help detect it early when it may be more successfully treated. Screening for colorectal cancer may include:

- Flexible sigmoidoscopy

- Tests for blood in the stool (fecal occult blood tests)

- Digital rectal exams (controversial)

Flexible sigmoidoscopy checks for precancerous polyps and cancers of the colon and rectum. The sigmoidoscope is a flexible viewing instrument that is inserted into the rectum to examine the lower bowel. The exam takes about 10 to 15 minutes, is only mildly uncomfortable, and is very safe. The test may also be done if your doctor wants to check the cause of rectal bleeding or persistent diarrhea or constipation. See page 417 for more information about tests for blood in the stool.

See page 25 for the recommended schedule of screening tests. Increase the frequency of screening tests if you have a family history of colon cancer or if you have colon polyps or ulcerative colitis.

When to Call a Health Professional

- Call immediately if stools are dark red, black, or tarry. This usually means there is blood in the stool, which needs to be evaluated. If there is bright red blood in the stool, also see Hemorrhoids on page 127.

- If you have unexplained changes in bowel habits that persist longer than two weeks, such as:

  - Constipation or diarrhea that doesn't clear up with home treatment

  - Persistently thin, pencil-like stools

- If you have unexplained pain in the lower abdomen.

Constipation

Constipation occurs when bowel movements are difficult to pass. Some people believe that a healthy person should have a bowel movement every day. This is a misconception. Most people pass stools anywhere from three times a day to three times a week. If your stools are soft and pass easily, you are not constipated.

Constipation may be accompanied by cramping, bloating, or nausea, and pain in the rectum from the strain of trying to pass hard, dry stools. There may also be pain and small amounts of bright red blood on the stool caused by slight tearing of the skin as the stool is pushed through the anus. This should stop when the constipation is controlled. A stool may occasionally become stuck in the rectum (impacted). If this happens, mucus and fluid may leak out around the stool, or there may be leakage of stool (fecal incontinence).

Older adults are slightly more susceptible to constipation. Lack of fiber and too little water in the diet are common causes of constipation. Other causes include travel (if it disrupts your usual bowel movement schedule), lack of exercise, delaying bowel movements, medications, pain due to hemorrhoids, and laxative overuse. Some medications (antacids, antidepressants, antihistamines, diuretics, and narcotics, among others) can also cause constipation. Constipation may also be a symptom of irritable bowel syndrome (page 129).

Prevention

- Eat plenty of high-fiber foods such as fruits, vegetables, and whole grains. Other ways to add fiber include (also see page 346):

  - A bowl of bran cereal with 10 grams of bran per serving.

○ Two tablespoons of bran added to cereal or soup.

○ Two tablespoons of crushed psyllium seed (found in Metamucil and other bulk-forming agents). Start with one tablespoon or less and increase slowly to avoid bloating.

• Doctors will sometimes recommend that you take a product like Metamucil regularly. These products are not laxatives and work best if used regularly. If yours does, be sure that you drink at least two quarts of water each day, remain active, and include lots of fresh fruit and vegetables in your diet.

• Avoid foods that are high in fat and sugar.

• Drink 1½ to 2 quarts of water and other fluids every day. (However, some people find milk constipating.)

• Exercise regularly. A walking program would be a good start. See page 319.

• Pass stools when you feel the urge. Your bowels send signals when a stool needs to pass. If you ignore the signal, the urge will go away, and the stool will eventually become dry and difficult to pass.

Home Treatment

• Set aside relaxed times for bowel movements. Urges usually occur some time after meals. Establishing a daily routine (after breakfast, for example) may be helpful.

• Drink two to four extra glasses of water per day, especially in the morning.

• Add fruits, vegetables, and high-fiber foods such as bran cereal, beans, or prunes to your diet.

• If necessary, use a stool softener or very mild laxative, such as milk of magnesia. Do not use mineral oil or any other laxative for more than two weeks, as they can be habit-forming. See page 404.

When to Call a Health Professional

• If rectal pain is severe, persists longer than one-half hour after you pass stool, or prevents you from having a bowel movement.

• If you have sharp or severe pain in the abdomen.

• If rectal bleeding is heavy (more than a few bright red streaks), or if the blood is dark red or brown.

• If bleeding persists longer than two to three days after constipation has improved, or if bleeding occurs more than once.

- If constipation persists after one week of home treatment.

- If chronic constipation or other changes in bowel movement patterns persist longer than two weeks without clear reason.

- If you experience leakage of stool (fecal incontinence).

- If you are unable to have bowel movements without using laxatives.

Dehydration

Dehydration occurs when your body loses too much water. When you stop drinking water or lose large amounts of fluids through diarrhea, vomiting, or sweating, body cells and body tissues lose essential fluid. If too much fluid is lost, the blood vessels collapse, an emergency called vascular shock.

Dehydration is dangerous for everyone, but especially for people who are weak or frail. Watch closely for early signs of dehydration whenever there is an illness that causes vomiting, diarrhea, or high fever. The early symptoms of dehydration are:

- Dry mouth, dry and sticky saliva, and excessive thirst

- Little or no urine (it will be dark yellow in color)

Rehydration Drinks

When you have diarrhea or are vomiting, your body can lose large amounts of water and essential minerals called electrolytes. If you are unable to eat for a few days, you are also losing nutrients. This happens faster and is more serious in older adults who are weak or frail.

A rehydration drink (Lytren, Rehydralyte) replaces both fluids and electrolytes in amounts that are best used by your body. Sports drinks (Gatorade, All Sport) and other sugared drinks will replace fluid, but most contain too much sugar (which can make diarrhea worse) and not enough of the other essential ingredients. Plain water won't provide any necessary nutrients or electrolytes.

You can make an inexpensive homemade electrolyte solution. Measure all ingredients precisely. Even small variations can make the drink less effective or even harmful.

Mix:

- 1 quart water

- ½ teaspoon baking soda

- ½ teaspoon table salt

- 3 to 4 tablespoons sugar

- If available, add ¼ teaspoon salt substitute ("Lite Salt")

Prevention

- Prompt home treatment for illnesses that cause diarrhea, vomiting, or fever may help prevent dehydration.

  ○ Diarrhea, page 122.

  ○ Vomiting, page 131.

  ○ Fever, page 81.

- To prevent dehydration during hot weather and exercise, drink 8 to 10 glasses of fluids (water and/or rehydration drinks) each day. Drink extra water before exercise and every half hour during physical activity.

Home Treatment

Treatment of mild dehydration is simple: Stop the fluid loss and restore lost fluids as soon as possible.

- If the person is vomiting or has diarrhea, stop all foods for two to four hours to rest the stomach.

- Take frequent small sips of water or a rehydration drink.

- When vomiting is controlled, give clear liquids (water or bouillon) a sip at a time until the stomach can handle larger amounts.

- If vomiting or diarrhea lasts longer than 24 hours, sip a rehydration drink to restore lost electrolytes.

Rehydration drinks won't make the diarrhea or vomiting go away faster, but they will prevent serious dehydration from developing. See page 120.

- Watch for signs of more severe dehydration (see below).

- Continue checking to see if the dehydration is improving or getting worse.

When to Call a Health Professional

Call immediately if the following signs of severe dehydration develop:

- Little or no urine for 12 hours

- Sunken eyes

- Skin that is doughy or doesn't bounce back when pinched

- Low blood pressure and rapid heart rate

- Lethargy

Call a health professional:

- If someone cannot hold down even small amounts of liquid after 12 hours of no food or drink.

- If vomiting lasts longer than 24 hours.

- If severe diarrhea (large, loose stools every one to two hours) lasts longer than two days.

If you cannot stop the fluid loss, the person may have to be hospitalized and given fluids intravenously.

Diarrhea

Diarrhea is an increase in the frequency of bowel movements and the discharge of watery, loose stools. Someone with diarrhea may also have stomach cramps and nausea.

Diarrhea occurs when the intestines push stools through before the water in them can be reabsorbed by the body. It is your body's way of quickly clearing out any viruses or bacteria.

Most diarrhea is caused by viral stomach flu (gastroenteritis). Some medications, especially antibiotics, may also cause diarrhea. For some people, emotional stress, anxiety, or food intolerance may bring on the condition. Irritable bowel syndrome (page 129) may also cause diarrhea.

Prolonged diarrhea may lead to serious fluid loss and malnutrition, since nutrients are passed before the body can absorb them. See Dehydration, page 120.

Home Treatment

- Let your stomach rest. Stop all food for several hours or until you are feeling better. Take frequent, small sips of water or a rehydration drink to prevent dehydration. See page 120.

- Since diarrhea may sometimes speed recovery from the underlying problem, avoid antidiarrheal drugs for the first six hours. After that, use them only if the diarrhea is very bothersome and there are no other signs of illness, such as fever. See antidiarrheal preparations on page 401.

- Begin eating mild foods, such as rice, dry toast or crackers, bananas, and applesauce, the next day. Avoid spicy foods, fruit, alcohol, and coffee until 48 hours after all symptoms are gone. Avoid dairy products for three days.

When to Call a Health Professional

- Call immediately if stools are bloody or black. Pepto-Bismol or other medications containing bismuth will cause stools to look black.

- If abdominal pain or severe discomfort accompanies diarrhea and is not relieved by passing stools or gas.

- If diarrhea is accompanied by a fever of 101° or higher, chills, vomiting, or fainting.

- If signs of severe dehydration appear. See page 121.

- If severe diarrhea (large, loose stools every one to two hours) lasts longer than two days.

- If mild diarrhea continues for one to two weeks without an obvious cause.

- If diarrhea occurs after drinking untreated water.

Diverticulosis and Diverticulitis

Many older people have **diverticulosis** (diver-tick-u-LOW-sis), a condition in which small sacs, called diverticuli, form on the wall of the colon. These sacs generally cause no symptoms, although there may be occasional pain in the lower left side of the abdomen. Diverticulosis is not a serious problem. However, blood vessels inside the diverticuli can occasionally break and bleed. This can lead to blood in the stool, which requires medical treatment.

If the sacs and surrounding area become inflamed, the condition is called **diverticulitis**. Symptoms include continuous or crampy pain, usually in the lower left abdomen, constipation, and fever.

Prevention

- Keep your colon in good health by eating right and drinking 1½ to 2 quarts of water each day. Eat plenty of fruits, vegetables, and whole-grain breads and cereals. Add three to four tablespoons of wheat bran to your daily diet. See page 346 for more on fiber. When adding more fiber, drink plenty of fluids—at least two quarts every day.

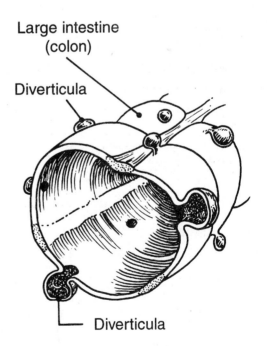

Large intestine (colon)

Diverticula

Diverticula

In diverticulosis, small sacs called diverticuli form on the wall of the colon.

- Avoid constipation and don't strain during bowel movements.

- Avoid laxatives.

- Avoid drugs that slow down bowel action, such as painkillers.

When to Call a Health Professional

Call immediately:

- If abdominal pain is severe.

- If pain that localizes to one area of the abdomen lasts longer than four hours.

Call a health professional:

- If abdominal pain occurs with fever of 100° or higher.

- If stools are dark red, black, or tarry. This usually means there is blood in the stool, which needs to be evaluated.

Gallbladder Disease

The gallbladder is a small sac located under the liver. It stores bile, a substance produced by the liver to help your body digest fats. If there are problems with the gallbladder or bile, gallstones can develop. In most cases, gallstones cause no problems and people don't even know they have them.

In some cases, however, a stone may cause the gallbladder to become inflamed. The inflammation causes pain, usually in the upper right abdomen, which can be severe. A gallstone attack often happens at night. It may waken you from sleep and last several hours. Fever and vomiting may also be present.

Gallstones can also cause problems if they start moving out of the gallbladder and become stuck in the common bile duct. This is more common in older adults. If the common bile duct is blocked, it may lead to inflammation of the pancreas (pancreatitis), jaundice, or infection.

Gallbladder disease affects twice as many women as men. Risk factors include a diet high in fat and sugar, obesity, lack of exercise, rapid weight loss, estrogen replacement therapy, diabetes, high cholesterol, and hypertension.

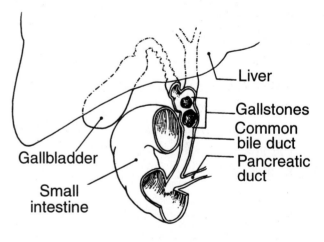

Gallstones in the common bile duct.

Gallstones that don't cause symptoms don't require treatment. If gallstones cause pain, surgery to remove the gallbladder is the most common treatment.

Prevention

- Stay close to your ideal weight based on your height and age.

- If you need to lose weight, do so slowly and sensibly (1 to 1½ pounds per week).

- Have your cholesterol checked as needed. If it is too high, try to lower it. See page 353.

Home Treatment

There is no home treatment for gallstones. If you think you have symptoms that may be due to gall-stones, call your doctor to confirm the diagnosis. If the symptoms are mild, in most cases it is safe to wait until symptoms recur several times before seeking treatment.

When to Call a Health Professional

Call immediately:

- If abdominal pain is severe.

- If pain that localizes to one area of the abdomen lasts longer than four hours.

Call a health professional:

- If abdominal pain occurs with fever of 100° or higher.

- If you have symptoms of gallstones and you have diabetes or your immune system is impaired due to other illnesses or medications.

- If there is a new yellow tint to the whites of the eyes or the skin (jaundice).

- If you have symptoms that you think are due to gallstones but there is no severe pain, fever, chills, or jaundice, call your doctor for an appointment.

Heartburn

Heartburn (indigestion) is caused by stomach acids backing up (refluxing) into the lower esophagus, the tube that leads from the mouth to the stomach. The acids produce a burning sensation and discomfort between the ribs just below the breastbone. Stomach acid may also back up into the throat or mouth, causing a bitter taste. Heartburn may occur after overeating or as a side effect of medications. The medical term for heartburn is **gastroesophageal reflux disease** (GERD).

Heartburn can also be caused by a **hiatal hernia**. This type of hernia occurs when the lower part of the esophagus and the upper part of the stomach move up into the chest cavity due to a weakness in the muscles of the diaphragm that surround the esophagus. Most people who have a hiatal hernia do not have symptoms.

Don't be concerned if you experience heartburn now and then; nearly everyone does. However, persistent heartburn can injure the esophageal lining.

Prevention

- Don't overeat. Eat smaller, more frequent meals and avoid evening and late-night snacks.

- Avoid tight-fitting clothes such as belts and girdles.

- Avoid constipation, which can increase pressure on the stomach. See page 118.

- If you use pain relievers, try acetaminophen (Tylenol) instead of aspirin, ibuprofen, or naproxen, which may cause heartburn.

- Try to figure out what causes your heartburn. Alcohol, caffeine, chocolate, peppermint, orange and tomato juices, fatty or fried foods, and carbonated drinks are common culprits. If you can make a connection between your symptoms and some food, beverage, or medication, you may be able to prevent future attacks by avoiding it.

- Stop smoking. Smoking promotes heartburn, and quitting will often relieve heartburn completely.

- If you are overweight, losing weight, even a few pounds, can reduce heartburn.

- Don't lie down too soon after eating. Try to stay upright for at least two to three hours after each meal.

- Raise the head of your bed four to six inches using wooden blocks or thick telephone books.

Home Treatment

- Try an antacid or acid controller. See page 400 for more information about these products. Follow the package instructions and your doctor's advice for their use.

  - For occasional mild heartburn, take an antacid, such as Gelusil, Maalox, Mylanta, or TUMS.

  - For more frequent or severe heartburn, take an acid controller, such as Pepcid AC, Tagamet HB, or Zantac 75.

- Whether you take an antacid or an acid controller, continue the prevention steps above to improve your chances of long-term relief.

When to Call a Health Professional

Call immediately:

- If pain occurs with shortness of breath or other symptoms that suggest heart problems: sweating, nausea or vomiting, lightheadedness, and rapid or irregular pulse. See Chest Pain on page 74.

- If stools are dark red, black, or tarry. This usually means there is blood in the stool, which needs to be evaluated.

Call a health professional:

- If heartburn is severe or is not relieved at all by antacids or acid controllers. See Ulcers, page 134.

- If you have difficulty swallowing, especially bread and meat.

- If you suspect that a prescribed medication is causing the heartburn. Antihistamines, Valium, aspirin, ibuprofen, naproxen, and other nonsteroidal anti-inflammatory drugs (NSAIDs) sometimes cause heartburn.

- If heartburn lasts for one to two weeks despite home treatment.

Hemorrhoids and Anal Itching

Hemorrhoids and piles are two terms used to describe inflammation and swelling of the veins around the anus. Hemorrhoids may be located either inside or outside the anus. Straining to pass hard, dry stools or trying to hurry a bowel movement sometimes causes these veins to become enlarged and irritated. The symptoms of hemorrhoids are tenderness or pain and sometimes bleeding. There may be a small lump at the opening to the anus. Hemorrhoids generally last several days and often recur.

Anal itching is usually caused by other conditions. The skin around the anus may become irritated by sweat or by any stool leakage that comes with diarrhea or loss of bowel control. If the skin around the anus is not kept clean, itching may result. However, trying to keep the area too clean by rubbing with dry toilet paper or using excess soap and water will injure the skin. Prolonged exposure to water is even more likely to injure the skin.

Prevention

- Keep your stools soft. Include plenty of water, fresh fruits and vegetables, whole grains, and beans in your diet. Add two tablespoons of bran or Metamucil to your diet each day. Also see Constipation on page 118.

- Try not to strain during bowel movements. Take your time and allow your body to pass the stool. Never hold your breath.

- To protect the skin around the anus, be very gentle when cleaning the area. Don't scrub or use strong soaps.

Home Treatment

- Keep the anal area clean, but even more importantly, be gentle. Warm baths are soothing and cleansing, especially after a bowel movement (though they may worsen anal itching). Sitz baths (warm baths with just enough water to cover the anal area) are helpful. Try premoistened towelettes (baby wipes) instead of toilet paper.

- Wear cotton underwear and loose clothing.

- Relieve itching by using cold compresses on the anus four times a day, ten minutes at a time.

- Ease itching and irritation with zinc oxide, petroleum jelly, hydrocortisone (0.5%), or an over-the-counter medicated cream or suppository (Anusol, Tucks, Preparation H, etc.). Avoid products with a local anesthetic, which can cause an allergic reaction. These products will have the suffix "-caine" in the name or list of ingredients.

When to Call a Health Professional

- Call immediately if bleeding is heavy (more than a few bright red streaks), or if the blood is dark red or brown.

- If any bleeding continues for longer than one week or occurs more than once.

- If bleeding occurs for no apparent reason and is not associated with straining to pass stools.

- If a lump on the anus is increasing in size or becoming more painful.

- If pain is severe or lasts longer than one week.

Irritable Bowel Syndrome

Irritable bowel syndrome (IBS) is a common digestive disorder. Symptoms of IBS often increase with stress or after eating, and include:

• Abdominal pain, gas, and bloating

• Mucus in the stool

• Feeling that a bowel movement hasn't been completed

• Irregular bowel habits with constipation, diarrhea, or both

IBS can persist for many years. An episode may be milder or more severe than the one before it, but the disorder itself does not worsen over time. It does not lead to more serious diseases such as cancer.

Prevention

There is no way to prevent IBS. However, home treatment can control or prevent future episodes. Symptoms can worsen or improve in response to stress, diet, and medications. Identifying the things that trigger your symptoms may help you avoid or minimize attacks.

Home Treatment

Good self-care for IBS is based on diet and stress management.

If **constipation** is the main symptom (also see page 118):

• Try an over-the-counter fiber supplement or bulk-forming agent that contains crushed psyllium seeds or methylcellulose. Examples include Citrucel, Fiberall, and Metamucil.

• Add fiber supplements and fiber-rich foods to your diet slowly so they do not worsen gas or cramps. See page 346.

• Use laxatives only on a doctor's recommendation.

• Drink at least two quarts of water every day.

• Get regular exercise to help maintain bowel regularity.

If **diarrhea** is the main symptom:

• Add more starchy food (bread, rice, potatoes, pasta) to your diet.

• Try an over-the-counter bulking agent. See page 404.

• Avoid smoking and avoid foods that make diarrhea worse. The following foods or drinks often worsen symptoms:

   ◦ Alcohol, caffeine

   ◦ Beans, broccoli, apples

○ Spicy foods

○ Foods high in acid, such as citrus fruits

○ Fatty foods, including bacon, sausage, butter, oils, and anything deep-fried

• Avoid dairy products that contain lactose (milk sugar) if they seem to worsen symptoms. However, get enough calcium in your diet from other sources. Yogurt may be a good choice, because it has less lactose.

• Avoid sorbitol, an artificial sweetener found in some sugarless candies and gum.

• If diarrhea persists, an over-the-counter medication such as loperamide (Imodium) may help. Check with your doctor if you are using it twice a month or more.

To reduce **stress**:

• Keep a record of the life events that occur with your symptoms. This may help you see any connection between your symptoms and stressful times.

• Get regular, vigorous exercise such as swimming, jogging, or brisk walking to help reduce tension.

• See page 365 for more tips on managing stress.

When to Call a Health Professional

Call immediately:

• If abdominal pain is severe.

• If pain that localizes to one area of the abdomen lasts longer than four hours.

Controlling Intestinal Gas

Passing intestinal gas, even as much as twenty times per day, is perfectly normal. However, if you want to reduce flatulence, there are some things you can do.

• Don't give up on beans; they are too good for you. Soak dry beans overnight and use fresh water for cooking. Cook beans thoroughly.

• If dairy products give you gas, switch to cultured milk products (yogurt and buttermilk) or add a lactase supplement (Lact-Aid) to your milk to help your digestion.

• Avoid foods that contain the sweeteners fructose and sorbitol. They may increase flatulence.

• Don't bolt your food. Large lumps of food are harder to digest.

• Avoid constipation by eating a high-fiber diet and drinking plenty of water.

Call a health professional:

- If abdominal pain occurs with fever of 100° or higher.

- If you have been diagnosed with IBS and your symptoms change significantly from their usual pattern.

- If blood appears in the stool. If there is bright red blood on the stool, also see Hemorrhoids on page 127.

Nausea and Vomiting

Nausea is a very unpleasant sensation in the pit of the stomach. A person who is nauseated may feel weak and sweaty and produce lots of saliva. Intense nausea often leads to vomiting, which forces stomach contents up the esophagus and out the mouth.

Most cases of nausea and vomiting are caused by stomach flu, stress, or medications. Nausea and vomiting can also be symptoms of other serious illnesses, such as diabetes or hepatitis. If nausea and vomiting persist, watch for signs of dehydration.

In older adults, vomiting is often a sign of a medication reaction, especially if the person has just started taking a new medication or the dose has been changed. Weakened or frail older adults can become dehydrated quickly from fluid loss due to vomiting. See Dehydration, page 120.

Home Treatment

- If vomiting is severe and persistent, stop all food for several hours or until you are feeling better. Wait an hour after vomiting, then take frequent small sips of water or a rehydration drink. See page 120.

- Drink only clear, noncarbonated liquids such as a rehydration drink, water, weak tea, diluted juice, or broth for the next 12 to 24 hours. Start one hour after the last episode of vomiting with a few sips at a time and increase gradually.

- If vomiting lasts longer than 24 hours, sip a rehydration drink to restore lost fluids and nutrients. See page 120.

- Rest in bed until you are feeling better.

- Watch for and treat early signs of dehydration. See page 120.

- When you are feeling better, begin eating clear soups, mild foods, and liquids until all symptoms are gone for 12 to 48 hours, depending on how you feel. Jell-O, dry toast, rice, crackers, and cooked cereal are good choices.

When to Call a Health Professional

Call immediately:

- If vomiting is severe or violent (continuous or shoots out in large quantities).

- If there is blood in the vomit. It may look like red or black coffee grounds.

- If vomiting occurs with severe or localized abdominal pain.

- If vomiting occurs with severe headache, sleepiness, lethargy, or stiff neck. See page 158.

- If signs of severe dehydration appear. See page 121.

- If nausea or vomiting persists longer than two hours after a head injury, or if violent vomiting lasts longer than 15 minutes. See Head Injuries on page 281.

Call a health professional:

- If vomiting lasts longer than 24 hours, or if nausea lasts longer than one week.

- If you suspect that medication is causing the problem. Antibiotics and anti-inflammatory medications (aspirin, ibuprofen, naproxen, etc.) may cause nausea or vomiting. Learn which of your medications can cause these symptoms.

- If nausea or vomiting is preventing you from taking medications you need for chronic conditions such as high blood pressure.

Stomach Flu and Food Poisoning

Stomach flu and food poisoning are different ailments with different causes. However, most people confuse the two because the symptoms are similar. Many people who get food poisoning attribute their symptoms of nausea, vomiting, diarrhea, and stomach pain to a sudden case of stomach flu. The disagreeable symptoms discourage you from eating until the problem clears up. The home treatment is the same for both problems.

Stomach flu is usually caused by a viral infection in the digestive system called viral gastroenteritis. To prevent stomach flu, you must avoid contact with the virus, which is not always easy to do.

Food poisoning is caused by bacteria that grow in food that is not handled or stored properly. Bacteria can grow rapidly when certain foods, especially meats, dairy products, and sauces, are not handled properly during preparation or are kept at temperatures between 40° and 140°. The bacteria produce a poison (toxin) that causes an acute inflammation of the intestines.

Suspect food poisoning when symptoms are shared by others who ate the same food, or after eating unrefrigerated foods, especially meat. Symptoms of food poisoning may begin 6 to 48 hours after eating. Nausea, vomiting, and diarrhea may last 12 to 48 hours.

To determine if the illness is food poisoning, ask:

- Has the sick person shared a meal with anyone who has similar symptoms?

- Has the person eaten any unrefrigerated meat recently?

Most food poisoning occurs during the summer when picnickers eat unrefrigerated meats, or on special occasions when cold cuts, turkey, dressing, sauces, and other foods are not kept under 40° or above 140°.

Botulism is a rare but often fatal type of food poisoning. It is generally caused by improper home canning methods for low-acid foods like beans and corn. Bacteria that survive the canning process may grow and produce toxin in the jar. Symptoms include blurred vision, inability to swallow, and increasing difficulty breathing. Immediate medical treatment is needed.

Prevention

To prevent food poisoning:

- Follow the 2-40-140 Rule. Don't eat meats, salads, or other foods that have been kept for more than two hours between 40° and 140°.

- Be especially careful with large cooked meats like your holiday turkey, which take a long time to cool. Thick parts of the meat may stay over 40° long enough to allow bacteria to grow.

- Use a thermometer to check your refrigerator. It should be between 34° and 40°.

- Wash your hands, cutting boards, and counter tops frequently.

- After handling raw meats, especially chicken, wash your hands and utensils before preparing other foods.

- Defrost meats in the refrigerator or by microwaving, not on the kitchen counter.

- Cover meats and poultry during microwave cooking to heat the surface of the meat.

- Cook hamburger meat until it is well done. Cook chicken until the juices run clear.

- Do not eat raw eggs or sauces made with raw eggs.

- Reheat meats to over 140° for 10 minutes to destroy bacteria. Even then, the toxin may not be destroyed.

- Put party foods on ice to keep them cool.

- Discard any cans or jars with bulging lids or leaks.

- Follow home canning and freezing instructions to the letter. Use only home canning instructions published since 1988. Call your County Agricultural Extension office for information.

- When you eat out, avoid rare and uncooked meats. Eat salad bar and deli items before they get warm.

Home Treatment

- Viral stomach flu will usually go away within 24 to 48 hours. Good home care can speed recovery. See Nausea and Vomiting on page 131 and Diarrhea on page 122.

- Watch for and treat early signs of dehydration (see page 120). Weakened or frail older adults can quickly become dehydrated from diarrhea and vomiting.

- If you suspect food poisoning, check with others who may have eaten the same food.

When to Call a Health Professional

Call immediately:

- If you suspect food poisoning from a canned product or have any of the symptoms of botulism (blurred or double vision, difficulty swallowing or breathing). If you still have a sample of the food, take it with you for testing.

- If signs of severe dehydration develop. See page 121.

Call a health professional:

- If severe diarrhea (large, loose stools every one to two hours) lasts longer than two days.

- If vomiting lasts longer than 24 hours, or if nausea lasts longer than one week.

Ulcers

An ulcer (peptic ulcer) is a sore or crater in the lining of the gastro-intestinal tract. There are two kinds of ulcers. Gastric ulcers form in the stomach. Duodenal ulcers form in the upper part of the small intestine (duodenum). It is possible to have both kinds of ulcers at the same time.

Ulcers develop when something damages the protective lining of the stomach and allows stomach acid to eat away at it. Factors that increase the risk of ulcers include:

- Regular use of aspirin, ibuprofen, naproxen, and other nonsteroidal anti-inflammatory drugs (NSAIDs)

- Smoking

- Infection with bacteria called *Helicobacter pylori*

Most people who have ulcers have *H. pylori* bacteria in their stomachs. The bacteria are not contagious. To eliminate the bacteria, treatment may include antibiotics and other medications to reduce or prevent recurrence.

Symptoms of an ulcer may include a burning or sharp pain in the abdomen between the navel and the end of the breastbone. The pain often occurs between meals and may wake you during the night. The pain can usually be relieved by eating something or taking an antacid. Ulcers may also cause heartburn, nausea or vomiting, and a bloated or full feeling during or after meals.

Ulcers can cause bleeding in the stomach, which may produce black or tarry bowel movements. Without treatment, ulcers may occasionally cause obstruction or break through (perforate) the stomach wall. Obstruction, bleeding, and perforation are serious situations that require immediate treatment.

Prevention

- Quit smoking. People who smoke are twice as likely to develop ulcers as nonsmokers.

- Discuss your use of aspirin and anti-inflammatory drugs with your doctor or pharmacist. These and other medications may increase the risk of ulcers.

- Slow down and reduce stress. For help managing your stress levels, see Chapter 22.

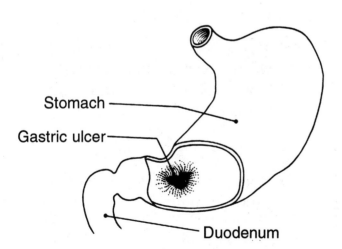

Stomach

Gastric ulcer

Duodenum

Gastric ulcers form in the stomach.

Home Treatment

When you first have symptoms that you think may be due to an ulcer, try to treat them quickly. If the symptoms are due to an irritated stomach lining, you may prevent them from worsening into an ulcer.

- Stop smoking. People who smoke are twice as likely to develop ulcers as nonsmokers. Smoking also slows healing of ulcers.

- Try an antacid or acid controller. See page 400 for more information about these products. Follow the package instructions and your doctor's advice for their use.

  ○ For occasional mild ulcer-like symptoms, take an antacid, such as Gelusil, Maalox, Mylanta, or TUMS.

  ○ For more frequent or severe ulcer-like symptoms, take an acid controller, such as Pepcid AC, Tagamet HB, or Zantac 75.

- Whether you take an antacid or an acid controller, continue the home treatment steps above to improve your chances of long-term relief.

- Avoid foods, especially alcohol, caffeine, and spicy foods, that seem to bring on symptoms. Milk and milk products slow healing and should also be avoided. It isn't necessary to eliminate any other food from your diet if it doesn't cause you problems.

- Try eating smaller, more frequent meals. If it doesn't help, return to a regular diet.

When to Call a Health Professional

Call immediately:

- If pain occurs with shortness of breath or other symptoms that suggest heart problems: sweating, nausea or vomiting, lightheadedness, and rapid or irregular pulse. See Chest Pain on page 74.

- If abdominal pain is severe.

- If pain that localizes to one area of the abdomen lasts longer than four hours.

- If stools are deep red, black, or tarry, which usually means there is blood in the stool. Ulcers are one of many possible causes of blood in the stool, which needs to be evaluated.

- If you have an ulcer and develop sudden, severe abdominal pain that is not relieved by your usual home treatment.

Call a health professional:

- If abdominal pain occurs with fever of 100° or higher.

- If you suspect an ulcer, and your symptoms have not improved after two weeks of home treatment. Your doctor can evaluate your symptoms and prescribe a treatment plan that may include antacids, acid controllers, or other medications.

Urinary Incontinence

If you suffer from loss of bladder control, called urinary incontinence, you are not alone. At least 10 to 20 percent of all older adults are coping with this problem.

Temporary incontinence can be caused by water pills (diuretics) and many other common medications. Constipation, urinary tract infections, stones in the urinary tract, or extended bed rest are other causes. Many cases of incontinence can be controlled. If the underlying problem is corrected, the incontinence can often be improved or cured.

The two most common types of persistent or chronic loss of bladder control are described here.

Stress incontinence occurs when small amounts of urine leak out during exercise or when you cough, laugh, or sneeze. It is more common in women and may affect some men after prostate surgery.

Kegel exercises often help stress incontinence. See page 138.

Urge incontinence happens when the need to urinate comes on so quickly that there is not enough time to get to the toilet. Causes include bladder infection, stroke, Parkinson's disease, and tumors.

Other types of incontinence may be caused by blockages in the bladder, injury or damage to the nerves that control bladder function, or physical or mental problems that make it hard for the person to get to the bathroom or recognize that he or she needs to urinate.

Home Treatment

- Don't let incontinence embarrass you. It is not a sign of approaching senility. Take charge and work with your doctor to treat any underlying conditions that may be causing the problem.

- Don't let incontinence keep you from doing the things you like to do. Absorbent pads or briefs, such as Attends and Depend, are available in pharmacies and supermarkets. No one will know you are wearing one.

- Avoid coffee, tea, and other drinks that contain caffeine, which over-stimulates the bladder. Do not cut down on overall fluids; you need fluids to keep the rest of your body healthy.

- Practice "double-voiding." Empty your bladder as much as possible, relax for a minute, and then try to empty it again.

- For stress incontinence, practice Kegel exercises daily. See box at right.

- Urinate on a schedule, perhaps every three to four hours during the day, whether the urge is there or not. This may help you to restore control.

- Wear clothing that can be easily removed, such as pants with elastic waistbands. If you have trouble with buttons and zippers, consider replacing them with hook-and-loop (Velcro) closures.

- Consider placing a portable commode where you can reach it easily, such as by your bed.

- Keep skin in the genital area dry to prevent rashes. Vaseline or Desitin ointment will help protect the skin from irritation due to urine.

- Incontinence is sometimes caused by a urinary tract infection. If you feel pain or burning when you urinate, see page 139.

- Pay special attention to any medications you are taking, including over-the-counter drugs, since some affect bladder control.

For more information on urinary incontinence, contact Help for Incontinent People, P.O. Box 8310, Spartanburg, SC 29305, 1-800-252-3337 (send SASE and $1.00 per request).

Kegel Exercises

Kegel exercises can help cure or improve stress incontinence. They strengthen the muscles that control the flow of urine.

- Locate the muscles by repeatedly stopping your urine in midstream and starting again. The muscles that you feel squeezing around your urethra and anus are the ones to focus on.

- Practice squeezing these muscles while you are not urinating. If your stomach or buttocks move, you are not using the right muscles.

- Hold the squeeze for three seconds—then relax for three seconds.

- Repeat the exercise 10 to 15 times per session.

- Do at least three Kegel exercise sessions per day.

Kegel exercises are simple and effective. You can do them anywhere and anytime. No one will know you are doing them except you.

When to Call a Health Professional

- If you need to wear a pad or if incontinence interferes with your life in any way.

- If your bladder feels full even after urinating.

- If you have difficulty urinating when your bladder feels full.

- If you experience burning or pain upon urination that may indicate a urinary tract infection.

Urinary Tract Infections

The urinary tract is composed of the kidneys, ureters, bladder, and urethra. The kidneys filter waste products from the blood and form urine. The ureters carry urine from the kidneys to the bladder. The bladder holds the urine until it is expelled through the urethra.

Urinary tract infections (UTIs) or bladder infections (cystitis) are generally caused by bacteria that are normally present in the digestive system. Early symptoms may include burning or pain during urination and itching or pain in the urethra. There may also be discomfort in the lower abdomen and a frequent urge to urinate without being able to pass much urine. The urine may be cloudy or reddish in color.

Chills and fever may also be present if the infection is severe, especially if it has spread to the kidneys. Men with similar symptoms may have an infection of the prostate gland. See page 254.

Men who have enlarged prostates, women who have had multiple pregnancies, and people with kidney stones or diabetes may be at higher risk for chronic urinary tract infections.

Other causes of irritation to the genital area include wearing tight pants, infrequent urination, sexual intercourse, bike riding, perfumed soaps and powders, or even spicy foods.

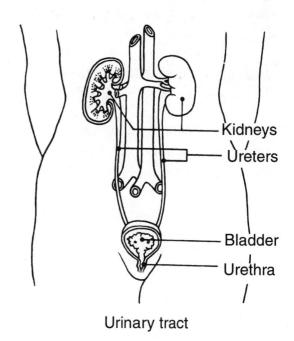

Kidneys
Ureters
Bladder
Urethra

Urinary tract

Prevention

- Drink plenty of fluids; water is best. Aim for at least two quarts a day.

- Urinate frequently.

- Women should wipe from front to back after going to the toilet. This will reduce the spread of bacteria from the anus to the urethra. Avoid frequent douching, and do not use vaginal deodorants or perfumed feminine hygiene products.

- If you are susceptible to urinary infections, drink extra water before sexual intercourse and urinate promptly afterwards.

- Wash the genital area once a day with plain water or mild soap. Rinse well and dry thoroughly.

- Wear cotton underwear, cotton-lined pantyhose, and loose clothing.

- Drinking cranberry and blueberry juice may protect against infection, especially in women.

Home Treatment

Apply home care at the first sign of irritation or painful urination. A day or so of home treatment may eliminate minor symptoms. However, if your symptoms last longer than a day or worsen despite home care, call your doctor. Because the organs of the urinary tract are connected, untreated bladder infections can spread and can lead to kidney infections and other serious problems.

- Drink as much water (think in terms of gallons) as you can in the first 24 hours after symptoms appear. This will help flush bacteria out of the bladder.

- Avoid alcohol and caffeine.

- A hot bath may help relieve pain and itching. Avoid using bubble bath and bath salts.

- Check your temperature twice daily. Fever may indicate a more serious infection is present.

- Avoid sexual intercourse until symptoms improve.

When to Call a Health Professional

- If painful urination occurs with any of the following symptoms:

  - Fever of 101° or higher and chills

  - Inability to urinate when you feel the urge

  - Low back pain just below the rib cage, usually on one side

  - Blood or pus in the urine

  - Unusual vaginal discharge

  - Nausea or vomiting

- If symptoms do not improve after 24 hours of home treatment.

- If you have diabetes and have symptoms of a urinary tract infection.

"Yes, I am an old enemy of the human race, but I am not that unbeatable once my name is said," spoke the Pale Stranger.

From an American Indian story about diabetes by John McLeod

8

Diabetes and Thyroid Problems

Your endocrine system is your body's control system. The glands that make up the endocrine system include the pituitary, thyroid and parathyroid, pancreas, adrenal glands, and the ovaries or testes. Each gland secretes special hormones, or chemical messengers, that help your body's organs do their jobs.

This chapter focuses on two common endocrine disorders: diabetes and thyroid problems. Diabetes can be successfully managed with home care and medications. Most thyroid problems respond well to medications. By following good health practices and early detection measures, you can help your endocrine system function at its best.

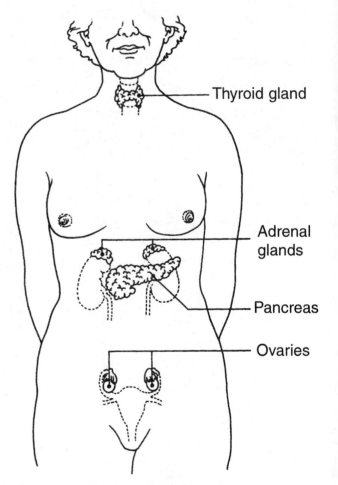

Thyroid gland

Adrenal glands

Pancreas

Ovaries

Endocrine system (women). In men, the endocrine system includes the testes.

Diabetes

When you pull up to the gas pump you have your choice of fuels: regular, super, or diesel. Your body, on the other hand, uses only one fuel to run every cell. This fuel is glucose. The starches and sugars in the food you eat are converted to glucose before your body uses it.

Insulin is a hormone released by the pancreas to control the amount of glucose (sugar) in the blood. Without insulin, the body cannot use or store glucose.

Insulin is released when blood glucose levels are high (usually after a meal). The insulin allows some glucose into cells where it is converted into energy. It helps some glucose to be stored in fat and muscle cells for later use. Excess glucose is also stored in the liver. In a healthy body, insulin keeps the amount of glucose in the blood under tight control.

Diabetes results from a breakdown in this system, which leads to a higher than normal amount of glucose (sugar) in the blood. There are two types of diabetes.

Type I, or insulin-dependent diabetes mellitus (IDDM), occurs when the pancreas fails to make insulin to keep blood glucose levels in balance. Type I diabetes generally occurs in childhood or adolescence, but it can develop at any age. People with this kind of diabetes must inject insulin every day.

Type II, or non-insulin-dependent diabetes mellitus (NIDDM), occurs when body cells become somewhat resistant to insulin. The cells require more insulin to use the same amount of glucose. Type II diabetes is the most common form among older adults, particularly those who are overweight.

Many people with type II diabetes are able to control their blood sugar through weight control, regular exercise, and a sensible diet. Others may need medications taken by mouth to lower blood sugar (oral hypoglycemic agents) or insulin injections.

Anyone with any two of the following risk factors has an increased chance of developing type II diabetes:

- Age 40 or older

- Overweight

- Family history of diabetes

- Black, Hispanic, or American Indian

- History of diabetes during pregnancy (gestational diabetes)

Symptoms of diabetes

Most of the symptoms of diabetes are vague and, by themselves, seldom lead to a doctor visit. Many people with type II diabetes think their symptoms are due to getting older. When they have a checkup, they are surprised to learn they have diabetes. These symptoms include:

- Increased thirst

- Frequent urination

- Increased appetite

- Unexplained weight loss

- Fatigue

- Frequent skin infections and slow-healing wounds

- Recurrent vaginitis

- Difficulty with erections (impotence)

- Blurred vision

- Tingling or numbness in hands or feet

Only a blood glucose test done by a health professional can accurately diagnose diabetes. Ask your doctor if you should eat or fast before the test.

Complications of diabetes

Diabetes has two types of long-term effects: damage to blood vessels and damage to nerves (called **neuropathy**). Damage to the blood vessels increases the risk of:

- Atherosclerosis (hardening of the arteries), high blood pressure, and heart disease

- Stroke

- Visual problems and blindness (See Diabetic Retinopathy on page 187.)

- Slow healing of injuries, especially on the feet, which increases the risk of serious infections that may lead to loss of a limb

- Kidney failure

Damage to the nerves increases the risk of:

- Tingling, numbness, or pain in the hands and feet

- Reduced feeling in the feet, which means that minor injuries may not be noticed

- Intestinal problems due to impaired nerve function in the digestive system

Early diagnosis and control of diabetes is important to prevent serious complications. If you are at increased risk for diabetes, have a blood glucose test once each year.

Prevention

At this time there is no known way of effectively preventing type I diabetes.

In most cases the risk of type II diabetes can be reduced by regular, daily exercise (see Chapter 20) and weight control (see Chapter 21).

Home Treatment

There are nine key points to follow for home treatment of both type I and type II diabetes.

1. Take control.

"You have diabetes." These words can be discouraging. They can make you feel shock, anger, fear, sadness, and guilt, all at the same time. You may fear that diabetes means the start of a gradual slide into poor health. You may feel overwhelmed.

It doesn't help to hear all of the things that you must do:

- Lose weight.

- Start exercising.

- Stop smoking.

- Reduce stress.

- Control your diet.

- Take your medication.

If it all feels hopeless, take heart. People with diabetes do not have to become "sick." You can take control over diabetes by making one small change at a time.

Step 1: Start with a positive vision of yourself. Read about positive thinking on page 371. If you can raise your expectations about becoming more healthy, it will be much easier to accomplish.

Step 2: Pick out one change from the list above. Choose the one that you think you can improve most easily and start there. Develop a step-by-step plan for success.

Step 3: Repeat Step 2 until you are as healthy as you want to be.

2. Take care of your feet.

Proper foot care is important for people with diabetes. Diabetes impairs nerve function and blood flow to the feet. You may lose feeling in your feet and not realize that you have a small cut or injury. Because of decreased blood flow, small cuts, sores, and even ingrown toenails take longer to heal and are more likely to become infected. If you have a sore or an injury on your foot, review the When to Call a Health Professional guidelines.

- Wash your feet daily with warm water and mild soap. Dry well.

- Avoid strong chemicals such as Epsom salts, iodine, and corn removers.

- Inspect the feet while drying. Pay special attention to any signs of cuts, cracking, or peeling between the toes or on the bottom of the foot.

- Use lanolin or other moisturizers to keep the skin soft. Do not use moisturizing lotion between the toes.

- Cut and file toenails straight across to prevent ingrown toenails.

- Break in new shoes slowly to avoid blisters.

- Don't walk barefoot, even indoors. It's easy to bruise or cut your feet.

- Stop smoking. Smoking reduces blood flow even more.

3. Get regular eye exams.

Changes in the eye caused by diabetes often have no symptoms until they are quite advanced. Early detection and treatment of diabetic retinopathy may slow its progress and save your sight. See page 187.

4. Eat a healthful diet.

People with diabetes need a healthful diet for two reasons. First, a proper diet helps keep your blood sugar levels in control. Second, a good diet helps with weight control, and being close to your ideal weight reduces your risk of type II diabetes.

See Chapter 21 for basic guidelines for healthy food choices. In general, a person with diabetes needs to:

- Eat less fat.

- Eat more high-fiber foods, such as whole-grain breads, vegetables, and fruit.

- Use less salt.

- Avoid simple sugars, such as table sugar, honey, candy, and sugary drinks. They raise blood sugar levels rapidly.

- Limit alcohol to no more than one drink per day.

- Try to avoid eating a lot of food at one meal, which could overload the blood with glucose and make it hard for the pancreas to produce enough insulin. Spread calories out over four to six meals; for example, three small meals with three snacks.

- Switching to a healthful diet may reduce your need for sugar-reducing (oral hypoglycemic) medications or insulin. Ask your doctor.

5. Exercise regularly.

Regular aerobic exercise will help you regulate your blood sugar, reduce your risk of heart disease, and control your weight—all essential ingredients to good diabetes management. However, people with diabetes also need to be aware of how exercise affects their blood glucose levels. Exercise tends to reduce blood glucose by allowing more glucose to be used by the cells.

Before beginning an exercise program, work with your doctor to identify any complications that might pose a problem, such as poor circulation or nerve damage. Your doctor can help you develop an exercise program suited to your needs. It helps to measure your blood sugar before and after exercise for several days.

Plan to check back with your doctor after any increase in regular exercise. The more you exercise, the less medication you may need.

6. Monitor your blood glucose levels.

The key to managing diabetes is careful monitoring of your blood glucose levels. Ask your doctor if you need to test your blood sugar at home. If you do, your doctor or diabetes educator can recommend a home blood sugar test. These tests measure the amount of glucose in a drop of blood, which you get from pricking your finger.

The doctor may want you to check your blood glucose several times a day, especially if you inject insulin. Using a blood sugar test to adjust the amount of insulin, you can keep your blood sugar levels within a specific range and reduce your risk for some long-term complications from diabetes. This is called "tight" or "strict" control of diabetes. Your doctor or diabetes educator can help you determine if this treatment method is best for you.

Even if you do not practice strict control of diabetes, monitoring your blood glucose for 30 days can improve your understanding and control of diabetes. This may be especially helpful if you are having trouble controlling your blood sugar levels. For example, you can learn how your diet and activities affect your blood sugar.

Keep careful records of the results of each test. Use a journal to record these items every day for 30 days:

- The time and content of each meal

- The kind and amount of exercise you get

- How tired or energetic you feel

- Your blood sugar level at least once a day at different times each day (more often if you are on insulin)

Once you understand how your body reacts to different foods and exercise, you can correct glucose imbalances before they get out of control. This is an ongoing part of managing your diabetes. Once you have learned it, you can use it as needed to help you control your blood sugar. Ask your doctor how often to keep this type of record.

7. Manage your medications.

Type II diabetes is generally managed first by weight loss and diet. However, if diet alone is not working, your doctor may prescribe an oral hypoglycemic drug for you. This medication must be taken as prescribed. Not enough medication will make your blood sugar higher than normal; too much will make it lower than normal. Consistency is important. As you improve your diet and exercise, you may need less medication. Check with your doctor.

8. Join a support group.

Diabetes support groups can add a lot to your home treatment. These groups are made up of people with diabetes and supportive health professionals. They are usually offered without cost and are excellent sources of the information you need for successful diabetes management. A local hospital may have information. Also ask about diabetes education programs available in your community.

9. Be a partner with your health professionals.

You and your doctor need to work as a team. Your team may also include a dietitian and a nurse diabetes educator. Your job is to make improvements in diet and exercise, practice good foot care, do regular glucose testing at home, keep a journal, and report all changes to your doctor.

Your health professionals' jobs are to help you understand your illness, teach you how to adjust your medications as your needs change, and treat complications before they become serious. Together, you and your health care team can control your diabetes.

For more information about diabetes management, see Resources 21 and 22 on page 420.

The National Diabetes Information Clearinghouse (Box NDIC, 9000 Rockville Pike, Bethesda, MD 20892) is a good resource for more information on diabetes management.

Diabetic Emergencies

	Hypoglycemia (Low blood sugar)	Hyperglycemia (High blood sugar)
Who	Those who take insulin or an oral hypoglycemic medication	Any person with diabetes
Onset	Rapidly, over minutes or hours	Gradually, over days
Blood test	Under 40-50 mg/% sugar	Over 300 mg/% sugar
Urine test	No sugar	High sugar
Symptoms	Fatigue, weakness, nausea	Frequent urination
	Hunger	Intense thirst
	Sweating	Dry skin
	Double or blurred vision	Dim vision
	Pounding heart, confusion, irritability, appearance of drunkenness	Rapid breathing with fruity-smelling breath (signs of ketoacidosis)
	Loss of consciousness (insulin shock)	Loss of consciousness (diabetic coma)
What to do?	If the person loses consciousness, call 911 or emergency services. For other symptoms, eat or drink something containing sugar. If symptoms recur, call your doctor immediately.	If there are signs of ketoacidosis, call your doctor immediately. If the person loses consciousness, call 911 or go to the emergency room.

If you are unsure about the cause of the diabetic emergency in a person who uses oral hypoglycemic medication, always give the person something containing sugar, such as candy, sugar under the tongue, orange juice, or a soft drink with sugar. Do not give an unconscious person anything to eat or drink.

When to Call a Health Professional

• **Call 911 or other emergency services if there are signs of insulin shock or diabetic coma (see page 150).**

Call immediately:

• If signs of ketoacidosis are present (rapid breathing and fruity-smelling breath). See page 150.

• If signs of low blood sugar (see page 150) persist after eating or drinking something containing sugar.

Call a health professional:

• If you have diabetes and there are signs of changes in your normal blood sugar levels:

  ○ Unexplained changes in home glucose tests

  ○ Continuing low blood sugar symptoms (see page 150)

  ○ A change in mental functioning (confusion, drowsiness, agitation)

• For any infection or possible infection:

  ○ Wounds that are slow to heal or are becoming infected (increased redness, warmth, pus, or fever)

  ○ Cuts, blisters, sores on the feet, ingrown toenails, athlete's foot, or a bunion or hammertoe that rubs on your shoes (call before it becomes a problem)

  ○ Genital or urinary tract infections

  ○ Complications of colds or flu such as sinus or lung infections

• If an infection is making it hard to control your diabetes.

• For a blood glucose test, if you suspect diabetes but have not been diagnosed. See symptoms on page 145.

Thyroid Problems

The thyroid is located in the front of the neck, just below the Adam's apple. This gland functions as a kind of "throttle" for the body. As the thyroid gland releases more hormones, the body runs faster. As the hormone levels decrease, the body slows down. The gland usually keeps the "throttle" fairly constant.

Thyroid problems are common among older people but often go undetected. The symptoms may develop so slowly that you do not notice them, or you may dismiss them as part of "normal aging."

The thyroid can cause problems in two ways: by producing too much hormone or by producing too little. Symptoms of too much thyroid hormone, or **hyperthyroidism**, include:

- Weight loss despite increased appetite

- Intolerance of heat

- Soft stools or diarrhea

- Itchy, irritated, and puffy eyes

- Rapid pulse and/or palpitations

- Unexplained shortness of breath, or difficulty breathing while lying down

- Night sweats

- Progressive muscle weakness, especially in the large muscles of the legs

- Anxiety, irritability, depression, forgetfulness

These symptoms are often easily confused with those of other diseases. Hyperthyroidism is easily detected with a simple blood test. **Graves' disease**, the most common cause of hyperthyroidism, occurs when the immune system makes the gland overactive. When medical (or rarely, surgery) treatment is complete, thyroid function usually returns to normal.

Symptoms of too little thyroid hormone, or **hypothyroidism,** include:

- Intolerance of cold

- Constipation

- Slowed heartbeat and reflexes

- Forgetfulness, depression, lethargy, or confusion

- Chronic fatigue

- Swelling of the face, tongue, and vocal cords. Sometimes the voice grows progressively deeper.

- An underactive thyroid can swell and form a goiter.

Treatment of a hypothyroid gland is quite simple. Your doctor can prescribe a medication that acts like natural thyroid hormone in your body. In most cases, this medication will be taken for life.

A thyroid function test can detect changes in the amount of thyroid hormone in your body, even before you have noticed symptoms. If you have a family history of thyroid problems or a history of radiation exposure (such as at work) or radiation treatment around the neck, discuss with your doctor whether you need a thyroid test.

Home Treatment

If you have a prescription for daily thyroid medications, take them every day.

When to Call a Health Professional

- If a person with hyperthyroidism develops the following symptoms:

  ○ Fever

  ○ Extreme weakness

  ○ Rapid or irregular heart rate and pulse

  ○ Heavy sweating

  ○ Restlessness, agitation, or delirium

- If the following symptoms develop, especially in a person with diagnosed hypothyroidism:

  ○ Extreme intolerance of cold

  ○ Lethargy and fatigue

- If any of the symptoms listed on page 152 cause you to suspect that you have a thyroid function problem.

I'm very brave generally,
only today I happen to have a headache.
Tweedledum in "Alice in Wonderland"

9

Headaches

Headaches are one of the most common health complaints. Some possible headache causes include muscle tension, arthritis in the neck, infection, allergy, injury, hunger, changes in the flow of blood in the vessels of the head, or exposure to chemicals.

The majority of headaches—over 90 percent—are caused by tension and respond well to prevention and home care. See page 159.

Migraines are another common cause of headaches (see page 157). Also see page 157 for information about some less common causes of pain in the head or face.

A headache that is very different from any you have had before or a change in the usual pattern of your headaches is a cause for concern. See "Headache Emergencies" in the box at right. However, if you have had similar

---

Headache Emergencies

Call your doctor now if you have:

- A very sudden "thunderclap" headache.

- A sudden, severe headache unlike any you have had before.

- Headache with stiff neck, fever, nausea, vomiting, drowsiness, confusion.

- Sudden, severe headache with stiff neck developing soon after the headache starts.

- Headache with weakness, paralysis, numbness, visual disturbances, slurred speech, confusion, or behavioral changes.

- Headaches following a recent fall or blow to the head. See page 281 for information on head injuries.

Possible Headache Causes

If headache occurs:	Possible causes
On awakening.	See Tension Headaches, p. 159; Allergies, p. 63; Sinusitis, p. 88. May also be due to low humidity.
With severe eye pain or vision disturbances.	Possible closed-angle glaucoma or temporal arteritis (pp. 185 or 157). Call a health professional immediately.
In jaw muscles or in both temples (may occur on awakening).	See Tension Headaches, p. 159; TMJ Syndrome, p. 209.
Each afternoon or evening; after hours of desk work; or following a stressful event; with sore neck and shoulders.	See Tension Headaches, p. 159.
On one side of the head.	See Migraine Headaches, p. 157; Trigeminal Neuralgia, p. 157.
After a blow to the head.	See Head Injuries, p. 281.
After exposure to chemicals (paint, varnish, insect spray, cigarette smoke).	Chemical headache. Get into fresh air. Drink water to flush poisons.
With fever, runny nose, or sore throat.	See Sinusitis, p. 88; Influenza, p. 83; Colds, p. 76.
With fever, stiff neck, nausea, and vomiting.	See "Meningitis and Encephalitis," p. 158.
With runny nose, watery eyes, and sneezing.	See Allergies, p. 63.
With fever and pain in the cheek or over the eyes.	See Sinusitis, p. 88.
On mornings when you drink less caffeine than usual.	Caffeine withdrawal headache. Cut back slowly. See p. 160.

headaches before and your doctor has recommended a treatment plan for them, emergency care may not be needed.

Other Causes of Head or Facial Pain

In addition to tension and migraine headaches, there are many causes of head and facial pain. Sinus infections (page 88), shingles (page 224), and temporomandibular joint syndrome (page 209) may cause different types of pain in the head or face. Temporal arteritis and trigeminal neuralgia are other less common conditions that can cause head or facial pain.

Temporal Arteritis

Giant cell arteritis is an inflammatory condition that affects arteries. When it affects the artery in the temple, it is called temporal arteritis and may affect the blood supply to an important nerve in the eye (the optic nerve). Temporal arteritis can cause vision problems or blindness if it is not treated.

If there is a new or different headache in one or both temples, especially with complete or partial vision loss, call your doctor immediately. Prompt medical treatment is needed to prevent permanent vision loss.

Trigeminal Neuralgia

Trigeminal neuralgia (or tic douloureux) is a painful condition caused by pressure on the trigeminal nerve. This nerve is located in front of the ear and controls sensation in certain areas of the face. Symptoms include attacks of sharp, knifelike pain, like tiny electric shocks, on one side of the face, usually around the mouth, upper jaw, and the side of the nose. The pain may occur for no apparent reason, or when the side of the face or the mouth is touched, such as when washing, shaving, chewing, talking, or brushing the teeth, or on exposure to extreme heat or cold.

Trigeminal neuralgia may be confused with a toothache, sinusitis, and temporomandibular joint (TMJ) syndrome. Medications are used to control the pain. Progressive relaxation (see page 368) may help relieve the pain and anxiety of the condition.

Migraine Headaches

Migraine headaches have very specific symptoms including throbbing pain on one or both sides of the head and sensitivity to light or noise. Because migraines may also cause nausea or vomiting, they are sometimes called "sick" headaches. Migraines are also called vascular headaches, because they are believed to be caused by changes in the flow of blood in the vessels of the head.

Although a migraine headache comes on quite suddenly, it is sometimes preceded by visual disturbances, such as zig-zagged lines, called an aura. The headaches last from a few hours to a few days and recur from several times a week to once every few years.

Migraines are more common in women and are often associated with menstrual periods. The headaches may increase or decrease at menopause, and hormone replacement therapy may make them worse.

Migraines rarely start after age 50. However, if you had migraines before age 50, they may continue. Tell your doctor about any new headache.

Prevention

Keep a diary of your headache symptoms. See "Tracking Your Headaches" on page 160. Once you know what events, foods, medications, or activities bring on a headache, you may be able to prevent or limit their recurrence.

To reduce tension, learn and practice relaxation techniques. See Chapter 22.

Home Treatment

- At the first sign of a migraine, lie down in a darkened room with a cool cloth on your forehead. Relax your entire body, starting with the forehead and eyes and working down to your toes (see page 368). Sleeping often relieves migraines.

- If a doctor has prescribed medication for your migraines, take the recommended dose at the first sign that a migraine is starting.

Meningitis and Encephalitis

Meningitis is an infection of the membranes that cover the brain and spinal cord. Encephalitis is an inflammation of the brain that may occur following a viral infection such as the flu.

Meningitis and encephalitis are serious illnesses with similar symptoms. Call a health professional immediately if the following symptoms develop:

- Fever with severe headache and stiff neck

- Vomiting

- Delirium (see page 165) or loss of consciousness

Immediate medical care is required.

- Many people find aspirin, acetaminophen, or ibuprofen helps relieve a migraine. However, if you use over-the-counter or prescription headache medications too often, they may actually make the headaches more frequent or severe. If this happens, call your doctor for advice.

- Try the home treatment advice for tension headaches. See page 160.

When to Call a Health Professional

- If you suspect that your headaches are migraine headaches. Professional diagnosis and treatment, combined with your self-care, can help decrease the impact of migraines on your life. Discuss relaxation and biofeedback techniques, which help many people prevent migraines.

- Also see "Headache Emergencies" on page 155.

Tension Headaches

More than 90 percent of headaches are tension headaches, which become more frequent and severe during times of physical or emotional stress. A tension headache may be accompanied by tightness or pain in the muscles of the neck, back, and shoulders. A previous neck injury, arthritis in the neck, or clenching the jaw muscles can also cause tension headaches.

A tension headache may cause pain all over the head, pressure, or a feeling of having a band around the head. The head may feel like it is in a vise. Some people feel a dull, pressing, burning sensation above the eyes.

The pain may also affect the jaw, neck, and shoulder muscles. You can rarely pinpoint the center or source of pain.

Prevention

- Reduce emotional stress. Take time to relax before and after you do activities that have caused a headache before. See page 365.

- Reduce physical stress. Change positions often during desk work and stretch for 30 seconds each hour. Make a conscious effort to relax your jaw, neck, shoulder, and upper back muscles.

- Evaluate your neck and shoulder posture at work or at home and make adjustments if needed. See page 39.

- Daily exercise, such as walking, helps relieve tension.

- If muscle tension seems to be related to teeth clenching, try a relaxation exercise. See page 365.

- Treat yourself to a massage. Some people find regular massages very helpful in relieving tension.

- Limit your caffeine intake to one to two cups per day. People who drink a lot of caffeinated beverages often develop a headache several hours after they have their last beverage or may wake with a headache that is relieved by drinking caffeine. Cut down slowly to avoid caffeine-withdrawal headaches.

Home Treatment

- Stop whatever you are doing and sit quietly for a moment. Close your eyes and inhale and exhale slowly. Try to relax your head and neck muscles.

- Take a stretching break or try a relaxation exercise. See page 365 or Resources 53 and 54 on page 422.

- Gently and firmly massage the neck muscles. See page 41 for neck exercises.

- Apply heat with a heating pad, hot water bottle, or a warm shower.

Tracking Your Headaches

If you have recurring headaches, keep a record of all headache symptoms. This record will help your doctor if medical evaluation is needed.

1. The date and time each headache started and stopped.

2. Any factors that seem to trigger the headache: food, smoke, bright light, stress, activity.

3. The location and nature of the pain: throbbing, aching, stabbing, dull.

4. The severity of the pain.

5. Other physical symptoms: nausea, vomiting, visual disturbances, numbness or tingling in any part of the body, sensitivity to light or noise.

6. If you are a woman, note any association between headaches and use of hormone replacement therapy or your menstrual cycle.

- If the neck muscles are tense, try applying a cold pack.

- Lie down in a dark room with a cool cloth on your forehead.

- Aspirin, acetaminophen (Tylenol), or ibuprofen (Advil) often helps relieve a tension headache. However, using over-the-counter or prescription headache medications too often may make headaches more frequent or severe. If this happens, call your doctor for advice.

When to Call a Health Professional

- If a headache is very severe and cannot be relieved with home treatment.

- If a headache occurs with fever of 103° or higher (100° in very old or frail people) and no other symptoms.

- If unexplained headaches continue to occur more than three times a week.

- If headaches become more frequent and severe.

- If headaches awaken you from a sound sleep or are worse first thing in the morning.

- If you need help discovering or eliminating the source of your tension headaches, talking with a health professional may be helpful.

- Also see "Headache Emergencies" on page 155.

If the brain was simple enough for us to understand it,
we would be too simple to understand it.
Ken Hill

10

Nervous System Problems

It's a myth that getting old means getting senile. Most people retain mental vitality as they age, though some changes do occur. (For more information on memory changes with aging, see page 312.) However, a number of conditions can affect mental functioning, including medication side effects, depression, infections, a poor diet, or heavy drinking. In many cases, treating the underlying cause will also clear up the problem.

This chapter provides some basic information about problems of the nervous system: delirium, dementia, Alzheimer's disease, Parkinson's disease, and tremor. Some of these problems respond well to treatment. Some, like dementia and Alzheimer's disease, can be managed but not cured.

This chapter will help you better understand some common nervous system problems that can occur as you get older and recognize serious symptoms if they develop so that you can seek care for yourself or someone else.

Alzheimer's Disease

Alzheimer's disease is a condition that selectively damages the brain cells that affect memory, intelligence, judgment, and speech. The destruction of brain cells eventually leads to mental impairment, dementia, and death. There is currently no cure for Alzheimer's disease.

Alzheimer's disease develops very slowly. If mental impairment has come on suddenly, the problem may be delirium, not dementia. See page 165. During the first few years, the only symptoms of Alzheimer's disease may be memory loss for recent events and occasional disorientation or confusion.

It may be difficult to distinguish the earliest symptoms from normal changes in the speed of memory recall that may occur with aging. However, the mental impairment that is associated with Alzheimer's disease is very different from normal memory changes.

Normal forgetfulness

- Forgets where the car is parked.

- Forgets to buy an item at the grocery store.

- Forgets an acquaintance's name but remembers it later.

Possible Alzheimer's disease

- Forgets how to drive the car.

- Forgets what she should be doing at the grocery store.

- Does not recognize an acquaintance or friend.

As the disease progresses, memory loss worsens and language skills and judgment become impaired. During the later stages, the person may have difficulty doing routine activities such as bathing, dressing, and eating. In the final stage of the disease, the individual may become completely dependent upon others for all activities of daily living.

Prevention

Medical science is getting closer to finding the cause of Alzheimer's disease. However, at this time, prevention guidelines are limited. Do your best to stay physically healthy and mentally active.

There have been reports linking aluminum to the brain changes that occur in Alzheimer's disease. However, at this time, there is no reason to be concerned about aluminum exposure during everyday use (cooking utensils, soda cans, deodorant).

Home Treatment

Seven out of 10 people with Alzheimer's disease are cared for at home by family and friends. The home treatment guidelines for Alzheimer's disease are the same as those for dementia on page 167. Also see "Caring for a Person With Dementia" on page 390.

Learn more about the illness by consulting Resources 8 and 9 on page 419. For more information, contact the Alzheimer's Association, 919 N. Michigan Ave., Suite 1000, Chicago, IL 60611-1676, 1-800-272-3900.

When to Call a Health Professional

- If the score on the Mental Status Exam on page 169 is 23 or lower, or if you are concerned that you may have Alzheimer's disease.

- If someone with Alzheimer's disease has a sudden worsening of symptoms or sudden significant change in the normal pattern of behavior.

- If memory loss and other symptoms begin to interfere with work, hobbies, or friendships, or result in injury or harm to the person.

- If you need help caring for a person with Alzheimer's disease.

There are no definitive tests that will identify the early stages of Alzheimer's disease. Doctors rule out other causes of dementia and are careful not to diagnose Alzheimer's without clear cause.

Delirium

Delirium is a sudden change in a person's mental status, leading to confusion and unusual behavior. It is a sign that a health problem is becoming more serious.

Unlike dementia (page 166), which comes on slowly over weeks to months, symptoms of delirium usually develop over the course of a few hours to a day or so. Symptoms may include:

- Disorganized thinking, disorientation, and confusion, which may cause rambling or incoherent speech. The person may have hallucinations (see things that aren't really there) or illusions.

- Short attention span; easily distracted or has difficulty shifting attention to something new

- Disrupted sleep-wake cycle, which may cause daytime sleepiness and nighttime wakefulness

- Fluctuations between periods when the person is very active and when he is very sleepy or hard to keep awake

- In rare cases, violent behavior

The symptoms of delirium may come and go. The person may be alert and coherent one minute, confused and drowsy the next. Delirium requires immediate medical attention so that the underlying cause can be detected and treated.

Delirium may be caused by a number of things:

- Use of many medications, a too-large dose of medication, or sudden withdrawal of certain medications

- Infection (such as pneumonia, flu, or urinary tract infection)

- Heavy drinking or sudden withdrawal of alcohol

- Added stress of hospitalization in someone who is ill

- Worsening of a chronic disease such as emphysema, heart disease, diabetes, or thyroid problems

If the patient can recover from the physical problem causing the delirium (either the acute illness or the worsening of a chronic disease), he generally does not have continuing mental impairment. Delirium is not the same as dementia. Review the information at right to understand the differences between them.

When to Call a Health Professional

If someone has had a sudden change in mental status and you suspect delirium, call a health professional immediately. Delirium is a medical emergency.

You can give the doctor information that will help uncover the cause of delirium. Tell the doctor:

- Any chronic diseases the person has (diabetes, heart disease, lung disease, anemia).

- All prescribed and over-the-counter medications the person has taken, and the doses.

- Whether the person has been ill or hospitalized recently.

- If the person has been drinking alcohol, and how much.

Dementia

The term dementia describes a condition of persistent mental deterioration. It involves memory, problem-solving, learning, and other mental functions. The mental impairment usually comes on slowly over months. Little change is noticed day to day, although many people with dementia seem better or worse at different times of the day. Over time, the mental impairment becomes severe enough to interfere with daily living activities.

The general symptoms of dementia include:

- Short-term memory loss (more than just an occasional forgetting of appointments, names, or where you put things). The person may remember events from 20 years ago but may not remember what happened two hours ago.

- Inability to complete everyday tasks (such as making soup from a can)

- Confusion

- Impaired judgment (such as walking into traffic)

- Getting lost in familiar places

- Suspicion of others (paranoia); strange behavior

The Mental Status Exam on page 169 can help to identify possible dementia. If mental impairment has come on suddenly, the problem may be delirium, not dementia. See page 165.

There are over 100 separate health conditions that can cause or mimic dementia. In some cases, if the problem can be successfully managed, the dementia is often reversible. For example, symptoms of depression are often confused with dementia. When you notice memory loss, confusion, or impaired judgment, think first of depression (page 305). Medical treatment is usually effective for depression.

For other causes of dementia, such as Alzheimer's disease, no completely effective treatment is currently available.

Alzheimer's disease (page 163) is one of the most well-known causes of dementia.

In about 25 percent of cases, dementia is caused by blockages in tiny blood vessels in the brain. This is called **multi-infarct dementia** or vascular dementia. People with untreated diabetes or high blood pressure are at increased risk. The symptoms vary depending on which area of the brain is affected. Unlike Alzheimer's disease, which develops slowly, the onset of multi-infarct dementia is usually sudden. Symptoms develop in stages, with some improvement between major declines in functioning. The prevention tips for Stroke on page 110 may also help prevent this type of dementia or slow its progress.

Other common causes of dementia include:

- Chronic infections

- Side effects of medications

- Poor nutrition

- Long-term heavy drinking

- Parkinson's disease (page 173)

- Hypothyroidism (page 152)

- Deficiency in vitamin B_1 (thiamine) or vitamin B_{12}

Home Treatment

If you suspect dementia, it is important that the person be evaluated by a doctor to rule out any possibly treatable causes. After a diagnosis is made, the following guidelines can be helpful no matter what the cause of the dementia.

- Provide visual cues to time and place such as calendars, clocks, and bulletin boards with pictures of the season, month, upcoming holidays.

- Simplify the daily routine with regular times for meals, baths, hobbies, and a limited number of activities.

- Explain what you are doing and break tasks and instructions into clear, simple steps, one step at a time. Use short, simple, familiar words and sentences.

- Use written notes or instructions. Label objects.

- Maintain eye contact and use touch to reassure and show that you are listening. Touch may be better understood than words. Holding hands or giving hugs may get through when nothing else can.

- Allow as many choices in daily activities as you can. Allow the person to select clothing, activities, foods, etc.

- Provide regular stimulation of senses: touching, singing, exercising, hugging.

- Create a safe but interesting living environment. In addition to the safety checklists on pages 266 to 268, add the following:

  ○ Keep pills and poisons locked away.

  ○ If the person may wander outside and become lost, put bells on doors and provide an ID bracelet.

- Ignore behavior that is disruptive or disturbing. Try to interest the person in another activity.

- Avoid arguing with the person about things that don't really matter. Just change the subject.

- Review with a doctor or pharmacist all medications and dosages. See the list of medications that can contribute to mental confusion on page 172.

- Provide good nutrition and plenty of fluids.

- Consider home treatment for depression (page 305), which often occurs with dementia.

- See also Chapter 25, Caregiver Secrets.

When to Call a Health Professional

- If mental impairment has come on suddenly, see Delirium on page 165.

- If someone's score on the Mental Status Exam on page 169 or other symptoms cause you to suspect dementia.

- If a person with dementia becomes uncontrollably hostile or agitated.

- For a referral to a geriatric assessment team or a specialist in geriatrics. These professionals have special training to identify causes of dementia. Some causes of dementia are reversible and many symptoms can be effectively managed.

A Checkup From the Neck Up

This three-part assessment works best if you use it to help someone who is worried about mental status problems. If you wonder whether one of these problems may be affecting you, ask someone you trust to help you with the test. You will need someone to ask the questions and write down your responses.

Step 1: Mental Status Exam

Step 2: Early Symptoms Review

Step 3: Distinguishing Between Delirium and Dementia

Step 1: Mental Status Exam

Adapted from Folstein, Folstein, and McHugh, 1975.

Orientation Questions
Read the questions out loud slowly and clearly. (Score 1 point for each correct answer.)

- What is the year?

- What is the season?

- What is the date?

- What is the day of the week?

- What is the month?

- What state are we in?

- What county are we in?

- What town are we in?

- What place are we in? (building, home, etc.)

- What room are we in?

Naming Questions
Name three objects (ball, flag, tree) one second apart. Ask the person to repeat all three. (Score 1 point for each correct answer.)

Calculation Questions
Have the person begin at 100 and count backward by 7s. Stop after 5 subtractions: 93, 86, 79, 72, 65. (Score 1 point for each correct answer.)

Or, if the person cannot or will not do the subtraction, ask him or her to spell the word "world" backwards: D L R O W. (Score 1 point for each correct letter.) Use the highest score of the subtraction and spelling questions in calculating the total score.

Recall Questions
Ask the person to name the three objects that you named earlier: ball, flag, tree. (Score 1 point for each correct answer.)

Language Questions

- Show the person a pencil and ask him or her to name it. (1 point)

- Show the person a watch and ask him or her to name it. (1 point)

- Ask the person to repeat the following phrase: "No ifs, ands, or buts." (1 point)

- Give the person the following instructions: "Take a piece of paper in your right hand. Fold it in half and place it on the floor." (1 point for completing each step.)

- Write "Close your eyes" on a piece of paper and ask the person to read it and obey the instruction. (1 point)

- Tell the person to write a sentence. (1 point)

- Ask the person to copy this design (1 point).

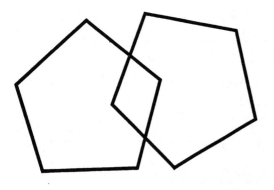

Ask the person to copy this design.

Scoring

Total all the points; there is a total of 30. Most people will score 24 or higher. A score of 23 or lower may suggest a possible problem.

If the score is below 23, don't jump to conclusions. A below-average score may be related to poor hearing, a different first language, or a low level of education. On the other hand, a high score does not guarantee there is no problem. Most doctors will use a test like this as part of a mental assessment.

If the Mental Status Exam causes you to suspect mental impairment, call your doctor to discuss the need for a more complete assessment.

Step 2: Early Symptoms Review

If the score on the Mental Status Exam was above 23 but you still have concerns, continue with Step 2 of the assessment. This step will help identify any major or persistent changes that may be early signs of dementia. Consider the following examples:

Personality changes
- A normally social person becomes withdrawn.

- A person has unusual or wild mood swings.

Memory Loss Does Not Mean Alzheimer's

Alzheimer's disease causes disability in two groups of people: those who have the disease and those who fear they have it.

Many people have heard that an early sign of Alzheimer's disease is memory loss. So when they misplace their eyeglasses or forget an acquaintance's name, they worry that it is a sign of irreversible brain damage.

The facts are:

- Some slowing of memory response time is a normal consequence of aging, although not everyone is affected. See the discussion on memory and forgetfulness on page 312.

- Many older adults express some concerns about memory. However, remember that, chances are, you've been forgetting things all your life.

- Ninety percent of all people over age 65 do not have Alzheimer's disease.

- If memory loss does not interfere with your ability to carry on normal activities, you probably don't have Alzheimer's disease.

Don't let an occasional memory lapse make you forget to pursue a full life.

Behavior changes

- A normally tidy person becomes messy.

- A person stops previous routines for no obvious reason.

- A person has become paranoid and suspicious of others.

Skill changes

- Loss of skill in balancing a checkbook.

- Loss of skill in shaving or putting on makeup.

- Loss of skill in cooking a favorite recipe.

- Inability to find previously familiar places.

- Increasing and repeated confusion about times and dates.

- Increasing forgetfulness of where items are kept.

Don't be overly concerned about minor changes in these areas. However, if the changes are major, unexplained, and causing increasing trouble, they can be clues that a more significant problem is developing. A review of the causes of dementia on page 167 may help you identify or rule out possible problems. Call a health professional if you suspect dementia.

If mental impairment has come on suddenly, the problem may be delirium, not dementia. See page 165.

Medications That Can Cause Mental Confusion

The way your body uses medications changes as you age. Taking multiple medications increases the likelihood that you will experience side effects. Confusion is just one of the side effects that medications can cause. Common medications that can cause confusion include (not a complete list):

- **Sedatives and tranquilizers** (sleeping pills and antianxiety medications):
  - chlorpromazine (Promapar, Sonazine, Thorazine)
  - haloperidol (Haldol, Halperon)
  - diazepam (Valium, Valrelease, Vazepam)
  - chlordiazepoxide (Librium, Librax, Limbitrol, Lipoxide, Menrium)

- **Parkinson's drugs**, such as levodopa (Dopar, Larodopa, Sinemet)

- **Antihistamines**, such as promethazine (K-Phen, Pentazine, Phenergan)

- **Antidepressants**:
  - fluoxetine (Prozac)
  - amitriptyline (Amitril, Elavil, Emitrip, Triavil, Endep, Limbitrol)
  - imipramine (Tofranil)
  - sertraline (Zoloft)

- **Antiseizure drugs**, such as phenytoin (Dilantin)

- **High blood pressure or heart medications**:
  - propranolol (Inderal, Inderal-LA, Inderide, Inderide-LA, Ipran)
  - digoxin (Lanoxin)

- **Painkillers**:
  - codeine (Tylenol-3)
  - propoxyphene (Darvon)

- **NSAIDs** (arthritis drugs):
  - ibuprofen (Motrin, Advil, Nuprin)
  - naproxen (Anaprox, Naprosyn)
  - indomethacin (Indocin)

- **Anticholinergic drugs** (cold medicines, chronic bronchitis medications, and drugs used to treat stomach cramps):
  - atropine (Donnatal)
  - dicyclomine (Bentyl)
  - diphenhydramine (Benadryl)

- **Antiulcer or acid reflux drugs**:
  - cimetidine (Tagamet)
  - ranitidine (Zantac)
  - famotidine (Pepcid)

Brand names are examples only; there are others. If you have questions about any drugs and their effects, ask your doctor or pharmacist.

Step 3: Distinguishing Between Delirium and Dementia

Delirium and dementia are two different problems. Delirium comes on quickly, over a few hours to days. Dementia develops gradually, often over several months. See pages 165 and 166 to help understand the differences between them. People with dementia are more likely to become delirious when they are sick. Delirium is a medical emergency. If you suspect that the problem is delirium, call a doctor immediately.

Parkinson's Disease

Parkinson's disease is caused by a degeneration of the brain cells that produce dopamine. Dopamine is a chemical needed to transmit signals that control muscle movements. Parkinson's disease seldom affects people younger than 50. Symptoms of Parkinson's disease come on slowly and gradually worsen over time. They may include:

- Shaking of the hands (tremor) when the hands are at rest. The shaking may be slight at first but gets worse over time. Eventually it starts to interfere with activities like eating or reading a newspaper. This early symptom is sometimes confused with essential tremor (page 174).

- Balance problems, stooped posture, and a shuffling walk. The person may have difficulty starting to move or have times when he seems "frozen" and unable to move.

- Loss of activity in the nerves that control the facial muscles, leading to a gradual loss of expression in the face.

- Speech changes, such as loss of volume or flat tone to the voice, or difficulty starting to speak.

- Dementia may develop in some cases.

Medication, exercise, and sometimes diet changes can slow the progression of the disease and relieve many symptoms. There is no known cure at this time.

The cause of Parkinson's disease is unknown. Parkinson-like symptoms are also a side effect of some medications.

Home Treatment

- Provide good, well-balanced nutrition, and get regular exercise.

- Review home treatment for tremor on page 174.

- Because people with Parkinson's disease may move and speak more slowly, patience is important. Meals, shopping, and other activities may take a little longer.

- See the Fall Prevention checklist on page 267 for tips on avoiding falls due to balance problems or impaired ability to walk.

- Consider home treatment guidelines for depression on page 305.

- Learn more about the illness by contacting the American Parkinson Disease Association at 1-800-223-2732 or the National Parkinson Foundation at 1-800-327-4545.

When to Call a Health Professional

- If you suspect Parkinson's disease. Medications provide effective treatment in many cases.

- If you suspect that Parkinson symptoms may be a medication side effect.

Tremor

Tremor is an involuntary shaking or twitching movement that is repeated over and over. Tremor usually affects the hands and head. Occasionally the feet or torso may also shake.

Essential tremor, which sometimes runs in families, is one of the most common types of tremor. It causes shaking that is most noticeable when the person is doing something like lifting a cup or pointing at an object.

The shaking is not present when the person is not moving. The tremor may also affect the person's voice. Medication can help reduce the shaking.

Tremors can also be caused by conditions or medications that affect the nervous system, including Parkinson's disease (page 173), liver failure, alcoholism, and mercury or arsenic poisoning. Lithium, drugs taken for arrhythmias and high blood pressure, tricyclic antidepressants, and other medications can also cause tremor.

If you notice a tremor, carefully observe its nature and record its history before calling your health professional. If a cause is discovered, the disease will be treated rather than the tremor.

Home Treatment

- Stress reduction can help to reduce tremor. See Chapter 22.

- Add a little weight to the hand (wear a heavy bracelet or watch) or hold something in your hand. This may reduce some tremors and restore more control to the hands.

- Drink beverages from half-filled cups or glasses, and use a straw.

- Get enough rest and sleep. Fatigue often makes a tremor worse.

- Convince yourself and those around you that although your hands may shake, your mind is steady.

When to Call a Health Professional

- If you suddenly develop a tremor or it suddenly becomes much worse.

- If shaking interferes with your ability to do daily activities or keeps you from taking part in social events.

- If you suspect that tremor may be a side effect of a medication.

You can observe a lot just by watching.
Yogi Berra (naturally)

11
Eyes and Seeing

By age fifty, most people have become aware of vision changes. Typical changes include:

- A gradual decline in the ability to see small print or focus on close objects (presbyopia)

- A decrease in the sharpness of vision

- The need for more light for reading, driving, sewing, and other activities

- Some trouble distinguishing subtle color differences; blue may appear gray, for example

---

Eye Emergencies

If you have any of the following symptoms, call your eye doctor immediately:

- Severe, aching pain in the eye

- Sudden onset of vision disturbances, such as flashes of light, partial blindness, or dark spots in your field of vision

These symptoms may indicate a serious eye problem that could lead to blindness if not treated. Immediate medical care may help save your sight.

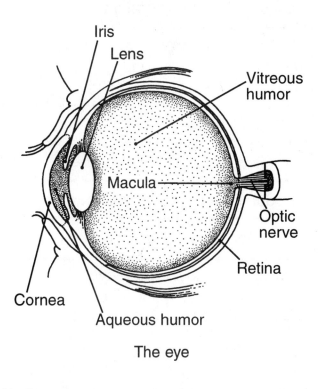

The eye

Eye Problems

Symptoms	Possible Causes
Severe, aching pain in the eye	Call a health professional immediately! Possible closed-angle glaucoma, p. 185.
Sudden onset of vision changes such as flashes of light, partial blindness, or dark spots in the visual field	Call a health professional immediately. Possible retinal detachment, p. 186.
Gradual onset of blurry or fuzzy vision	See Presbyopia, p. 186; Cataracts, p. 180.
Tunnel vision (gradual loss of side or peripheral vision)	See Glaucoma, p. 185.
Halos around lights	See Cataracts, p. 180; Glaucoma, p. 185.
Distorted vision, dark spot in the center of vision; straight lines appear wavy	See Macular Degeneration, p. 186.
Blood in the white of the eye	See Blood in the Eye, p. 179.
Excessive discharge from the eye; red swollen eyelids, sandy feeling in eyes	See Conjunctivitis, p. 182.
Dry, scratchy eyes	See Dry Eyes, p. 184.
Red, irritated, scaly eyelids	See Eyelid Problems, p. 184.
Drooping eyelids; excess tearing	See Drooping Eyelids, p. 183.
Pimple or swelling on eyelid	See Styes, p. 188.
Object or chemical in the eye	See Objects in the Eye, p. 290; Chemical burns to the eye, p. 270.

The information in this chapter will help you adjust to normal vision changes and know what symptoms may indicate a serious problem.

This chapter includes eye problems that are more common with aging and that can impair your vision, such as cataracts, glaucoma, and retinal disorders. These conditions usually require medical treatment. The chapter also includes minor irritations like eyelid problems, dry eyes, excessive tearing, and floaters, which often respond well to self-care and usually do not affect vision.

Vision Protection Tips

Keep an eye on your sight throughout your life by following these general guidelines:

- Avoid overexposure to sunlight to reduce the risk of cataracts (page 180). Wear sunglasses that screen out ultraviolet (UV) rays.

- Wear goggles or protective glasses when you are handling chemicals, operating power tools, or playing racquet sports.

- Get periodic vision checkups: every two years if you wear glasses; every five years if you don't. If you have a family history of eye disorders, diabetes, or a diagnosed vision disorder, such as glaucoma, cataracts, or macular degeneration, have your vision checked according to the schedule your eye doctor recommends.

- Keep your blood pressure under control. High blood pressure can damage the blood vessels that supply blood to the eye. See page 103.

- If you have diabetes, follow the home treatment guidelines on page 146. People with diabetes are at risk of a vision problem called diabetic retinopathy. See page 187.

Blood in the Eye

Sometimes, blood vessels in the whites of the eyes break and cause a red spot or speck on the eye. This is called a subconjunctival hemorrhage. The blood in the eye may look alarming, especially if the spot is large. It is usually not a cause for concern and will clear up in two to three weeks.

When to Call a Health Professional

- If there is blood in the colored part of the eye.

- If blood that covers more than one-quarter of the white of your eye does not clear after five days.

- If the bleeding followed a blow to the eye.

- If blood in the eye appears while you are taking blood thinners (anti-coagulants).

Cataracts

Cataracts are thickened, hardened, and cloudy parts of the eye lens. The cloudy lens blocks or distorts light coming into the eye and blurs vision. Cataracts usually affect both eyes and develop at different rates. Some remain quite small and do not impair vision. When they become large enough to cause visual problems, the only effective treatment is surgery.

Symptoms include painless blurring or fuzziness of vision, decreased night vision, and problems with glare. Double vision may occur, spots may be seen, and lights may have a halo around them. If left untreated, the lens will become milky, and vision will be greatly reduced.

Cataracts are very common; 70 percent of people over age 75 have some type of cataract. Cataracts may also be caused by a direct injury or blow to the eye, chemical burns, and

electrical shocks. Smokers, American Indians, people with diabetes, and those who have taken steroids are at risk for cataracts at an early age.

In the past, surgery was delayed until the cataract became "ripe" or very cloudy. Now, cataract surgery is recommended as soon as visual impairment becomes a problem. The surgery is very successful at restoring clear vision.

Prevention

- Avoid overexposure to sunlight. Use sunglasses that block ultraviolet (UV) light. Wearing a brimmed hat while outdoors helps too.

- Wear protective glasses or goggles to avoid eye injury when using strong chemicals or power tools and when playing racquet sports.

- Eat foods high in beta carotene and vitamin C (cantaloupes, oranges, carrots, etc.) These foods seem to help prevent or delay cataracts.

- If you have diabetes, keep it under control. See page 146.

Home Treatment

Although you cannot stop or slow the progress of cataracts once they have developed, there are many things you can do to make the gradual changes in your vision easier to live with.

• Make sure you have plenty of light indoors. Standard 60- to 100-watt light bulbs seem to work best for most people; fluorescent lights are less helpful. Use table or floor lamps for reading or other close work.

• When outdoors, wear sunglasses with yellow-tinted lenses, which will help to reduce glare. A large-brimmed hat or visor will help also. However, sunglasses do not help everyone, so experiment before you buy an expensive pair.

• When you watch television, don't have a light on between you and the screen. It will produce glare.

• Try large-print books and newspapers. Magnifying glasses may help you read some things, but only if the type is very clear. Magnified blurry print will be larger but will still be blurry.

• For more information on cataracts and other vision problems, contact The Lighthouse, 800 Second Avenue, New York, NY 10017, (800) 334-5497.

When to Call a Health Professional

• If you are bothered by blurred or fuzzy vision.

• If your night vision is impaired.

• To schedule periodic eye exams. See page 179 for recommended frequency.

Light Up Your Life

Improve the lighting in your home to compensate for any vision loss you may have. Good lighting will make your home safer and your activities more enjoyable.

• Increase lighting on steps and stairways.

• Use more than one light source in a room. It will help your eyes feel less tired.

• Use concentrated light for tasks that require near vision, such as reading or sewing.

• Cut down on glare. Use blinds or shades to cut down on direct sunlight. When you watch television, position the set so it doesn't reflect glare.

Conjunctivitis

Conjunctivitis, or "pinkeye," is an inflammation of the delicate membrane (conjunctiva) that lines the inside of the eyelid and the surface of the eye. It can be caused by bacteria, viruses, allergies, pollution, or other irritants.

The symptoms are redness in the whites of the eyes, red and swollen eyelids, lots of tears, and a sandy feeling in the eyes. There may be a discharge that causes the eyelids to stick together during sleep and occasional sensitivity to light.

Prevention

• Wash your hands thoroughly after treating a person with pinkeye.

• Avoid eye-rubbing as it can transfer the condition from one eye to the other.

• Do not share towels, handkerchiefs, or washcloths with an infected person.

• If a chemical or object gets into your eye, immediately flush it with water. See page 271 or 290.

Home Treatment

Although most cases of conjunctivitis will clear up in five to seven days on their own, viral pinkeye can last many weeks. Conjunctivitis due to allergies or pollution will last as long as you are exposed to the irritating substance. Good home care will speed healing and ease the discomfort.

• Apply moist compresses several times a day to relieve discomfort.

• Gently wipe the edge of the eyelid with moist cotton or a clean wet washcloth to remove encrusted matter.

• Don't wear contact lenses or eye makeup until the infection is gone. Throw out eye makeup after an eye infection.

• If eyedrops are prescribed, insert as follows: Pull the lower lid down with two fingers to create a little pouch. Put the drops there. Close the eye for several minutes.

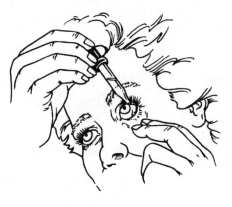

Inserting eyedrops

- Be sure the dropper is clean and does not touch any surface. Eyedrops are washed out by normal tearing, so they will need to be replaced frequently.

- Make sure any over-the-counter medicine you use is *ophthalmic* (for eyes), not *otic* (for ears).

When to Call a Health Professional

- If the eye is very red with either a thick, greenish-yellow discharge or swollen, red eyelids.

- If there is severe, aching pain in the eye.

- If the problem continues for more than a week.

Drooping Eyelids

As we get older, the lower eyelids sometimes start to droop away from the eyeball. This is called **ectropion** (eck-TRO-pea-un). If the lid droops far enough, it may no longer be able to protect the eye, and the eye may become dry and irritated. The upper lid may also droop and interfere with vision. Both are due to reduced muscle tone in the muscles that control the eyelids.

Floaters

Floaters are spots, specks, and lines that "float" across the field of vision. They are caused by stray cells or strands of tissue that float in the vitreous humor, the gel-like substance that fills the eyeball.

Floaters can be annoying but are not usually serious. However, if you notice persistent loss of vision in one spot, a sudden increase in the number of floaters, or if floaters occur with flashes of light, call a health professional. This may be a sign of retinal detachment. See page 186.

Drooping eyelids can prevent tears from draining normally, and they may run down the cheek. **Excessive tearing** can also be a sign of increased sensitivity to light or wind. Tearing may also be a symptom of an eye infection or a blocked tear duct. If your eyes tear in bright light or wind, wear protective glasses.

When to Call a Health Professional

- If drooping eyelids came on suddenly.

- If drooping eyelids interfere with vision.

- If the eye is dry and irritated, or if the eyelids do not close completely during sleep.

- If the lashes of the lower lid begin to rub on the eyeball.

Dry Eyes

Dry eyes occur when the tear glands are not producing enough tears. Your eyes will feel itchy, scratchy, and irritated. This may be associated with certain medications (diuretics, antihistamines, decongestants, and antidepressants).

Home Treatment

Try an over-the-counter artificial tear solution, such as Akwa-Tears, Duratears, or Hypotears. Do not use eye drops that reduce eye redness (such as Visine) to treat dry eyes.

When to Call a Health Professional

- If dry eyes are persistent and artificial tears do not help. Excessive dryness can damage your eyes.

Eyelid Problems

One of the most common eye problems in older adults is a skin condition called **blepharitis** (blef-air-EYE-tis). Symptoms include redness, irritation, and scaly skin at the edges of the eyelids. The scales may be dry or greasy, and the eyelashes may fall out. The cause is not clear, although it is more common in people who have dandruff, skin allergies, or eczema, and those who often have styes. The problem is often chronic.

The Eye Specialists

Ophthalmologists are medical doctors (MD) or osteopathic doctors (DO) who are trained and licensed to provide total eye care. They can prescribe corrective lenses, diagnose and treat eye disorders, and perform eye surgery.

Optometrists (OD) perform eye examinations and prescribe corrective lenses. In some states, they are also licensed to diagnose and treat some types of eye problems.

Opticians make eyeglasses and fill prescriptions for corrective lenses.

Home Treatment

- Wash your eyelids, eyebrows, and hair daily with baby shampoo. Use a few drops of shampoo in a cup of water and a cotton ball or soft washcloth to wash the eyelids. Rinse well with clear water.

When to Call a Health Professional

Blepharitis often requires antibiotic ointment. Call a health professional:

- If your eye is painful.

- If the eyelids are bleeding.

- If the problem is not improving after a week of home care.

Glaucoma

Glaucoma is an eye disorder caused by too much pressure within the eyeball. This pressure (ocular hypertension) builds up when the fluid (aqueous humor) in the chamber between the lens and the cornea is unable to drain normally. If the pressure is not relieved, it may eventually damage the retina and optic nerve and result in blindness. Untreated glaucoma is a leading cause of blindness in older adults.

Glaucoma is normally painless and can develop slowly over several years without being detected. By the time symptoms such as reduced side vision (tunnel vision) and halos around lights appear, the disease has progressed enough to permanently affect vision.

An uncommon form of the disorder called closed-angle glaucoma comes on quite suddenly and can lead to permanent eye damage in a matter of 24 hours. Symptoms include severe aching pain in the eye and blurred vision. Call a health professional immediately if these symptoms occur.

Blacks and those with a family history of glaucoma are at increased risk for developing the disorder.

Prevention

Regular eye exams, including glaucoma tests, will help detect glaucoma before it affects your vision. People aged 50 to 64 are advised to have a glaucoma test every five years. If you are at high risk for glaucoma, schedule an exam every year after age 50.

Home Treatment

If you have been diagnosed with glaucoma, use your prescribed medications exactly as directed.

When to Call a Health Professional

- Call immediately if there is severe aching pain in the eye.

- If vision is blurred or if you see halos around lights.

Presbyopia

Presbyopia (prez-bee-OH-pea-ah) is a condition that affects everyone sometime after age 40. As the eye ages, the lens becomes less flexible and can no longer easily focus on near objects or small print. You may find that you hold objects at arm's length to see them clearly. (People with presbyopia sometimes say that they don't need glasses, they just need longer arms.)

Home Treatment

Glasses or contact lenses will give you clear vision again. If you already wear glasses, you may need bifocals. Over-the-counter reading glasses may be appropriate for some people.

When to Call a Health Professional

Presbyopia usually develops gradually, over months to years. If your vision changes more quickly, over just a few weeks, call your doctor. This may be an early symptom of another condition, such as diabetes.

Retinal Disorders

The retina is a light-sensitive membrane that covers the inside of the eyeball. It transmits images from your eye to your brain. Problems with the retina can lead to impaired vision or blindness.

Detached or Torn Retina

Most retinal detachments are caused by small tears or holes in the retina. Although it may occur at any age, older people, those who are nearsighted, and those with a family history of retinal detachments are at higher risk. A blow to the head or eye may also cause the retina to detach. Symptoms of a retinal detachment or tear may include a sudden onset of flashes of light, partial blindness, or seeing dark spots.

Most retinal tears or detachments can be treated if they are detected early, although perfect vision may not always return after treatment.

Macular Degeneration

Macular degeneration is caused by damage or breakdown of the part of the retina that provides clear, sharp central vision (the macula). It may occur in one or both eyes. The signs may range from blurry or distorted vision to a blind spot in the center of the visual field. Straight lines (such as in the Amsler grid, below) may appear wavy, and colors may appear faded or dim.

As the condition progresses, central vision in the eye is lost. Peripheral (side) vision is not affected, and many people function well despite the

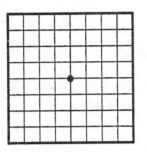

Amsler grid: Cover one eye and look at the grid above. Repeat with the other eye covered. If the lines around the center dot look wavy or distorted, you may have a macular problem.

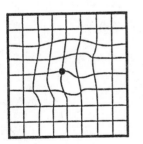

The lines around the center dot are distorted as they would appear to someone with macular degeneration.

loss of central vision, although walking and other activities that require central vision are more difficult.

There is some evidence that a diet that contains plenty of dark, leafy green vegetables (spinach and collard greens) may reduce the risk of macular degeneration.

Laser treatment may be effective for one type of macular degeneration if it is detected early, but it doesn't help everyone.

Diabetic Retinopathy

This retinal problem affects people who have diabetes. It occurs when the blood vessels that supply blood to the retina are damaged. It often has no symptoms until it is quite advanced. If untreated, it can lead to blindness. Keeping your blood sugar in control is important to help reduce your risk of retinal changes. See page 146. Regular eye exams can detect this problem early when it can be more successfully treated.

When to Call a Health Professional

- Call immediately if you have a sudden onset of vision disturbances such as flashes of light, partial blindness, or dark spots in your field of vision.

- If you have vision changes that may be due to a macular problem, such as loss of sharp vision, a dark spot in your center of vision, or if the lines on the Amsler grid appear wavy or distorted.

- For regular eye exams if you have diabetes or macular degeneration.

Styes

A sty is a noncontagious infection of an eyelash root (follicle). It appears as a small, red bump, much like a pimple, either in the eyelid or on the edge of the lid. It comes to a head and breaks open after a few days.

Styes are very common and are not a serious problem. Most will respond to home treatment and don't require removal.

Home Treatment

- Do not rub the eye, and do not squeeze the sty.

- Apply warm, moist compresses for 10 minutes, five to six times a day until the sty comes to a point and drains.

When to Call a Health Professional

- If the sty interferes with vision.

- If the sty gets worse despite home treatment.

- If redness centered on the sty spreads to involve most of the eyelid.

Help for Vision Problems

The National Eye Care Project is a public service program sponsored by the Foundation of the American Academy of Ophthalmology and volunteer ophthalmologists. It provides medical and surgical eye care for disadvantaged older adults who are:

- 65 or older

- US citizens or legal residents

- Without access to an ophthalmologist

Call toll-free for help:

- **1-800-222-EYES**

To get a free catalog of low-vision aid devices, write to: American Foundation for the Blind, Consumer Products Division, 15 West 16th Street, New York, NY 10011, 1-800-232-5463 or (212) 620-2147 for NY residents.

The older I grow,
the more I listen to people who don't say much.
Germain Glidden

12
Ears and Hearing

The human ear is designed to channel and modify sound waves. Sound waves enter the ear and cause the eardrum to vibrate, setting in motion the tiny bones of the middle ear: the hammer, anvil, and stirrup. These bones transfer sounds to the structures of the inner ear: the cochlea and auditory nerve. The cochlea contains tiny hairs that convert sounds to nerve impulses that are transmitted to the brain by the auditory nerve.

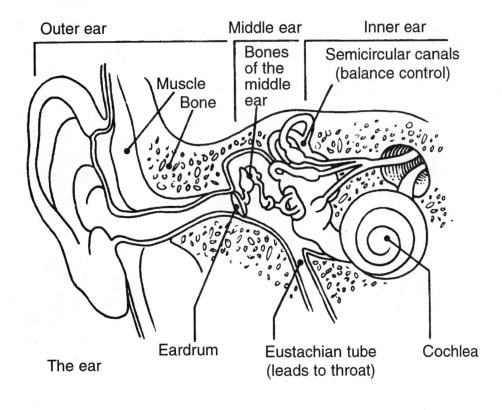

Outer ear   Middle ear   Inner ear

Bones of the middle ear

Semicircular canals (balance control)

Muscle
Bone

Eardrum

Eustachian tube (leads to throat)

Cochlea

The ear

Ear Problems

Ear Symptoms	Possible Causes
Earache and fever	See Ear Infections, below.
Ear pain while chewing; headache	See TMJ Syndrome, p. 209.
Feeling of fullness in the ear; with runny or stuffy nose, cough, fever	See Colds, p. 76; Ear Infections, below.
Hearing loss	See Hearing Loss, p. 192; Earwax, p. 191.
Dizziness or lightheadedness; sensation that room is spinning around you; problems with balance	See Vertigo and Dizziness, p. 197; "Meniere's Disease," p. 198.
Ringing or noise in the ears	See Tinnitus, p. 196.

As we get older, a number of changes within the ear can affect how well we hear. For example, the tiny hairs in the cochlea begin to deteriorate and do not conduct the sound vibrations as well. This breakdown is probably due to lifelong exposure to noise.

It is impossible to go back in time and undo noise damage, but there is still plenty you can do to get the most out of your hearing.

This chapter will tell you how to protect your hearing and what you can do to cope with hearing losses and other ear problems.

Ear Infections

Middle ear infections (otitis media) are much more common in children but do occur in adults. They usually start when a cold causes the eustachian tube between the ear and throat to swell and close. When the tube closes, fluid seeps into the ear and bacteria start to grow. As the body fights the infection, pressure builds up, causing pain.

Symptoms of a bacterial ear infection may include earache, dizziness, ringing or fullness in the ear, hearing loss, fever, headache, and runny nose.

Antibiotic treatment stops bacterial growth, which will help relieve pressure and pain.

Prevention

- Treat a cold rapidly, especially if you have frequent ear infections. See page 76.

- Blow your nose gently to avoid forcing fluid into the eustachian tubes.

Home Treatment

- Use a warm washcloth or heating pad to apply heat to the ear. This will ease pain.

- Drink plenty of clear liquids.

- Take aspirin, ibuprofen, or acetaminophen to help relieve pain.

- If dizziness occurs, see page 197.

- Take the full course of antibiotics, if prescribed. Call your doctor if you have any reaction to the medication.

When to Call a Health Professional

- If a severe earache lasts over two hours or any earache lasts longer than 12 to 24 hours. If hearing loss or a significant feeling of fullness in the ear persists after the pain is gone, call your doctor.

- If you suspect an eardrum rupture. Look for a white, yellow, or bloody discharge from the ear.

- If there is no improvement after three to four days of antibiotics.

Earwax

Earwax is a protective secretion, similar to mucus or tears, that filters dust and keeps the ears clean. Normally, earwax is semi-liquid, self-draining, and does not cause problems. Occasionally, the wax will build up, harden, and cause some hearing loss.

Poking at the wax with cotton swabs, fingers, or other objects will only pack the wax more tightly against the eardrum. The same old advice still applies: Never stick anything smaller than your elbow in your ear. You can handle most earwax problems by avoiding cotton swabs and following the home treatment tips below. Professional help is needed to remove tightly packed wax.

Home Treatment

- Warm mineral oil helps loosen wax. Wash the wax out with an ear syringe and warm mineral oil. (Cold oil may make you dizzy.) Use very gentle force. Do not do this if there is discharge from the ear or if you suspect an ear infection or a ruptured eardrum.

- If the warm mineral oil does not work, use an over-the-counter wax softener, followed by gentle flushing with an ear syringe, each night for a week or two. Do not use it if you suspect infection or eardrum rupture.

When to Call a Health Professional

- If the above home treatment does not work and the wax build-up is hard, dry, and compacted.

- If you suspect that earwax is causing a hearing problem.

- If the ear is sore or bleeding.

Hearing Loss

Hearing loss is one of the most common conditions affecting people over 50. There are three types of hearing loss: sensorineural, conductive, and central deafness.

Most hearing loss is caused by problems in the inner ear or acoustic nerve. This is called **sensorineural** hearing loss. The damage to the inner ear can be the result of changes that come with age, exposure to loud noise, and some medications, especially aspirin. People with this type of hearing loss are usually not totally deaf. They may have trouble understanding the speech of others yet be very sensitive to loud sounds. They may also hear ringing, hissing, or clicking noises.

Hearing loss that is caused by something that blocks or interferes with sound reaching the inner ear is called **conductive** hearing loss. The most common cause is packed earwax in the ear canal, which is easily treated (see page 191). Infection, abnormal bone growth, and excess fluid in the ear are other causes.

Help for Hearing Problems

- SHHH (Self Help for Hard of Hearing People, Inc.), 7910 Woodmont Ave., Suite 1200, Bethesda, MD 20814

  - (301) 657-2248 (Voice)

  - (301) 657-2249 (TDD)

- American Speech-Language-Hearing Association

  - 1-800-638-8255

- For free booklets on hearing problems or a free over-the-phone hearing test, call

  - 1-800-222-EARS

- The Better Hearing Institute provides information on hearing protection and deafness prevention.

  - 1-800-EAR-WELL

People with conductive hearing loss often say that their own voice sounds loud while other voices sound muffled. There may be a low level of tinnitus, or ringing in the ear. Depending on the underlying problem, conductive hearing loss is usually treated by ear-flushing, medication, or surgery.

A rare form of hearing loss is caused by damage to the hearing centers in the brain. This is called **central deafness** and can occur after a head injury or stroke. The person's ear works normally, but the brain has difficulty understanding what is heard.

Prevention

- Wear ear plugs when exposed to loud noise, or avoid it if possible.

- Keep your ears clean and periodically check for wax build-up. Do not use cotton swabs or other objects to clean your ears. See page 191.

- Keep circulatory problems, such as heart disease, high blood pressure, and diabetes, under control. Some hearing loss may be the result of decreased blood flow to the inner ear.

- Be aware of medication side effects on hearing. For example, antibiotics (gentamicin), blood pressure medicines (diuretics such as Lasix), ibuprofen, and large doses of aspirin (8 to 12 pills per day) are linked to hearing impairment.

Home Assessment

To check your hearing, you can do a few simple tests:

The Clock Test

- Have a friend hold a ticking clock out of sight some distance from one side of your head.

- Have the friend move slowly closer. Tell him when you first hear the ticking.

- Repeat for the other ear. You should hear the sound about the same distance away from each ear.

- Test your friend's hearing in the same way to see if he can hear the clock from much farther away than you can. (Be sure to ask a friend whose hearing is good!)

The Radio Test

- Have someone adjust the volume on a radio or television so it is pleasing to that person. Can you hear it well or do you have to strain?

The Telephone Test

- When you talk on the telephone, switch the phone from ear to ear to hear if the sound is the same. Although the hearing loss of aging usually affects both ears, it is possible that only one ear is affected.

Facts About Hearing Aids

Elements

- Microphone to pick up the sound and an amplifier to make it louder. Some models have digital electronics that can be custom-programmed to amplify certain frequencies of sound differently.
- Speaker to transmit the sound to the ear
- Battery for power
- Volume control to regulate sound level
- Ear mold to keep the aid in place

Models

- In-the-ear or in-the-canal styles
- Behind-the-ear styles

Questions to Ask Before You Buy

- What kind of hearing aid will best suit my needs?
- How much does each hearing aid cost? The price will depend on the style of hearing aid, the amount of power needed, the manufacturer, and where you buy the aid.
- Will Medicare, Medicaid, or private health insurance pick up any of the costs? Medicare may pay for some of the fitting costs. Your insurance or health plan coverage may also pay some of the costs.
- What does the cost of the hearing aid cover? Check to see if special services, follow-up visits, and adjustments are covered. Also ask about warranties.
- Is there a 30- to 60-day trial period before the purchase becomes final?

Considerations

- Not all hearing loss can be corrected with a hearing aid; it depends on the underlying cause of the loss.
- Hearing aids work by making all sounds, both soft and loud, louder. They do not restore normal hearing. Digitally programmable aids may allow you to choose different settings depending on whether you are in a noisy or quiet place.
- It takes time and practice to get used to a hearing aid; you may need to try more than one type to get the best results. Wear your hearing aid every day and gradually accustom yourself to the way it works.

Caregiver Tips: Living With a Hearing-Impaired Person

- Speak to the person at a distance of three to six feet. Make sure that your face, mouth, and gestures can be seen clearly. Arrange furniture so everyone is completely visible.

- Avoid speaking directly into the person's ear. Visual clues will be missed.

- Speak slightly louder than normal, but do not shout. Speak slowly.

- Cut down on background noise. Turn down the television or radio. Ask for quiet sections in restaurants.

- If a particular phrase or word is misunderstood, find another way of saying it. Avoid repeating the same words over and over.

- If the subject is changed, tell the person, "We are talking about _____ now."

- Treat the hearing-impaired person with respect and consideration. Involve the person in discussions, especially about him or her. Do what you can to ease feelings of isolation.

When to Call a Health Professional

- If hearing loss develops suddenly (within a matter of days or weeks).

- If you have hearing loss in one ear only.

- After age 50, hearing assessments are recommended periodically during regular doctor visits. Have exams more frequently if hearing problems exist.

- To consider a hearing aid. Make an appointment with a hearing specialist if you find:

  ○ You often ask people to repeat themselves.

  ○ You cannot hear soft sounds, such as a dripping faucet, or high-pitched sounds.

  ○ You continuously hear a ringing or hissing background noise.

  ○ You have difficulty understanding words.

  ○ You have difficulty hearing when someone speaks in a whisper.

  ○ A hearing problem is interfering with your personal and social life.

The Hearing Specialists

Otologists or otolaryngologists (MD or DO) are medical doctors who have extensive training in ear and hearing disorders. They can diagnose and treat hearing disorders and perform surgery. Many have audiologists on staff.

Audiologists are hearing specialists who usually have a graduate degree. They identify, diagnose, and measure hearing problems and recommend the most appropriate type of hearing aid or other method to treat hearing loss. Look for an audiologist who is licensed by the state or who is certified by the American Speech-Language-Hearing Association (they will have CCC-A after their name).

Hearing aid specialists or **dispensers** are licensed in nearly all states and may be certified by the National Board for Certification in Hearing Instrument Sciences (BC-HIS). They can fit you with a hearing aid and adjust it to meet your hearing needs.

If you are considering buying a hearing aid, first have an evaluation by a medical doctor or an audiologist to help determine what type of hearing loss you have and whether it may be treated in other ways. The FDA recommends that you have a hearing evaluation by a doctor within six months before you buy a hearing aid (unless you sign a waiver).

Tinnitus

Almost everyone has experienced an occasional ringing (or hissing, buzzing, or tinkling) sound in their ears, which usually lasts only a few minutes. It is often more noticeable in quiet places. If it becomes persistent, you may have tinnitus.

Tinnitus is usually caused by damage to the nerves in the inner ear from prolonged exposure to loud noise. Other, more treatable causes include excess earwax, ear infections, and medications, especially antibiotics and large amounts of aspirin. Heavy drinking can also cause tinnitus.

Home Treatment

- Limit or avoid exposure to loud noises, such as power tools, loud music, gunshots, jet engines, or industrial machinery. If you can't avoid loud noises, wear ear plugs or a headset to protect your ears.

- Limit your use of aspirin and products containing aspirin.

- Tinnitus is often worse in quiet places. A radio played at low volume or a white noise machine may help make it less noticeable.

- Cut back on or eliminate alcohol, caffeine, and nicotine.

- Try to relax. Stress and fatigue seem to aggravate tinnitus. See pages 365 to 370 for some simple relaxation techniques.

- Find emotional support. Tinnitus can be difficult to deal with. The American Tinnitus Association is a helpful support group. Write P.O. Box 5, Portland, OR 97207 (enclose a self-addressed stamped envelope) or call 503-248-9985.

When to Call a Health Professional

- If tinnitus becomes persistent and interferes with your daily activities or sleep.

- If ringing occurs with dizziness, loss of balance, vertigo, nausea, or vomiting.

- If tinnitus persistently affects only one ear.

Vertigo and Dizziness

Dizziness or **lightheadedness** is usually not due to a serious problem; in fact, it is common to feel lightheaded occasionally. (Dizziness or lightheadedness is not the same as vertigo. Vertigo involves a sensation of spinning or movement.)

Lightheadedness is often due to a momentary drop in blood pressure and blood flow to the head that occurs when you get up too quickly from a seated or lying position. This is called **orthostatic hypotension**. It is most commonly caused by dehydration or medications, such as water pills (diuretics).

When you sit up or stand up, the blood flow in your body changes to keep blood moving to the brain. With aging, these changes may occur more slowly, which can lead to lightheadedness when you stand up quickly. Other things that can affect your balance include stress, anxiety, problems with vision or hearing, and poor circulation to the legs. Other causes of lightheadedness or vertigo include drinking alcohol or side effects of medications (such as blood pressure medications and antidepressants).

An uncommon cause of lightheadedness is an abnormality in your heart rhythm (see page 105). This can cause recurrent spells of lightheadedness for a short period of time when the irregular heartbeat is present. This can lead to a fainting spell, called **syncope** (SIN-ko-pee). Unexplained fainting spells need to be checked out by your doctor.

Vertigo is a sensation that your body or the world around you is spinning or moving. Vertigo is usually related to inner ear problems. It may occur with nausea and vomiting. It may be impossible to walk when you have severe vertigo.

The most common form of vertigo is triggered by changes in the position of the head, such as when you move your head from side to side or bend your head back to look up. This is called **benign positional vertigo**. Vertigo may also be caused by inflammation (called labyrinthitis) in the part of the inner ear that controls balance. Labyrinthitis is usually caused by a viral infection and sometimes occurs following a cold or the flu.

Other underlying problems that can contribute to vertigo are Meniere's disease (see box at right) and multiple sclerosis.

Home Treatment

Lightheadedness is usually not a cause for concern unless it is severe, persistent, or occurs with other symptoms such as irregular heartbeat or fainting. The biggest danger of lightheadedness is the injuries that might result if you keel over.

- When you feel lightheaded, sit down for a minute or two and take some deep breaths. Stand up again slowly.

Meniere's Disease

Meniere's disease is a balance problem believed to be caused by a build-up of fluid in the inner ear. The symptoms include attacks of vertigo and unsteadiness, tinnitus, hearing loss in one ear, nausea, and vomiting. The person may also have a feeling of fullness in the ear and be very sensitive to loud noises. The attacks can last for hours and occur as frequently as once a week or as seldom as once every few years.

If you have been diagnosed with Meniere's disease, these measures may help ease symptoms:

- Restrict salt, caffeine, and alcohol.

- Stop smoking.

- Ease stress with relaxation techniques. Attacks often come during periods of emotional upset. See Chapter 22.

In some cases, diuretics or medications like those used to treat motion sickness may help.

- Get up from bed or from a chair slowly. Sit on the edge of the bed for a few minutes before standing. Sit up or stand up slowly to avoid sudden changes in blood flow to the head that can make you feel lightheaded.

If you have vertigo (sense of spinning and world moving around you):

- Avoid head positions or changes in position that bring on vertigo. However, some experts suggest that practicing these positions may help you overcome the problem. If you have vertigo, ask your doctor about this approach.

- If you have vertigo, avoid lying flat on your back. Prop yourself up slightly to relieve the spinning sensation.

When to Call a Health Professional

Call 911 or emergency services immediately:

- **If vertigo (dizziness) is accompanied by headache, confusion, loss of speech or sight, weakness in the arms or legs, or numbness in any part of the body.**

- **If someone who says he is dizzy loses consciousness.**

Call a health professional immediately:

- If a sensation that you may faint persists.

- If you experience vertigo (sensation that the room is spinning around you) that is severe (usually with vomiting) or occurs with hearing loss.

Call a health professional:

- If you suspect dizziness may be a side effect of a medication.

- If dizziness lasts more than three to five days and interferes with your daily activities.

- If you experience vertigo that:

  o Has not been diagnosed.

  o Persists for more than five days.

  o Is significantly different from previous episodes.

- If you have repeated spells of lightheadedness over a few days.

- If your pulse is less than 50 or more than 130 beats per minute when you are feeling lightheaded.

Be true to your teeth or your teeth will be false to you.
Dental Proverb

13

Mouth and Dental Problems

Your teeth will last a lifetime if you care for them properly. Understanding how your mouth and teeth change as you age will help you keep an attractive smile. Typical changes include:

- A dryer mouth, which can alter your sense of taste and also increases the risk of tooth decay.

- Receding gums, which expose the roots of the teeth, making them more vulnerable to cavities. Decay may also develop around the edges of fillings.

- Loss of teeth, which can affect your ability to eat a healthy diet. Dentures and bridgework are more common and require special care. See page 206.

This chapter also covers irritations to your mouth that know no age limits, such as canker sores and cold sores.

Canker Sores

Canker sores are painful little blisters on the inner membranes of the mouth and cheek that break and leave open sores. There are many possible causes of canker sores. Injury to the inside of the mouth, genetic predisposition, female hormones, and stress all seem to play a role. The sores usually heal by themselves in about ten days. Ulcer-like mouth sores may also be a side effect of some medications.

Prevention

Avoid injury to the inside of your mouth:

- Chew food slowly and carefully.

- Use a soft-bristle toothbrush and brush your teeth thoroughly but gently.

Mouth and Dental Problems

Problem	Possible Causes
White spots, sores, or bleeding in mouth	See Canker Sores, p. 201; Oral Cancer, p. 208. If unexplained sores last longer than 14 days, call a health professional.
Bleeding gums	Gum disease. See Dental Problems, p. 204.
Toothache	See p. 206.
Sores on the lips	See Cold Sores, p. 203.
Bad breath	May be a sign of dental problems, indigestion, or upper respiratory infection.
Pain and stiffness in jaw, with headache	See TMJ Syndrome, p. 209; Tension Headaches, p. 159.
Hoarseness or voice changes	See Laryngitis and Hoarseness, p. 85.
Dry mouth	See p. 207.

Home Treatment

- Avoid coffee, spicy and salty foods, and citrus fruits.

- Try one of the following several times a day:

  - Apply an oral paste, like Orabase, to the canker sore. It will protect the sore, ease pain, and speed healing.

  - Rinse your mouth with a mixture of one tablespoon of hydrogen peroxide in eight ounces of water.

  - Apply a thin paste of baking soda and water to the sore.

When to Call a Health Professional

- If mouth sores develop after starting a medication.

- If a canker sore, or any sore, does not heal after 14 days.

- If a sore is very painful or comes back frequently.

- If white spots that are unlike canker sores appear in the mouth and do not heal within one to two weeks.

Cold Sores

Cold sores (fever blisters) are small red blisters that usually appear on the lip and outer edge of the mouth. They often weep a clear fluid and form scabs after a few days.

Cold sores are caused by a herpes virus. Herpes viruses (chickenpox is one kind) stay in the body after the first infection. Later, something triggers the virus and causes it to become active again. Cold sores may appear after colds, fevers, exposure to the sun, or stressful times. Sometimes they appear for no apparent reason.

Prevention

- Cold sores are contagious, so avoid direct contact with the sores. Avoid kissing someone who has a cold sore, and avoid direct skin contact with genital herpes sores. Both types of herpes can affect either the mouth or genitals. If you have a cold sore, do not share drinking glasses and eating utensils.

- Use a sunscreen on your lips and wear a hat if exposure to the sun seems to trigger cold sores.

- Reducing stress may help in some cases. Practice relaxation exercises often. See page 365.

Home Treatment

- At the first sign of a cold sore (tingling or prickling at the site where the sore will appear), apply ice to the area. This may help reduce the severity of the sore.

- Blistex or Campho-Phenique may ease the pain. Don't share them with others.

- Apply petroleum jelly (Vaseline) to ease cracking and dryness.

- Cornstarch may be soothing. Apply several times a day in a paste made with a little water.

- Be patient. Cold sores usually go away within 7 to 10 days.

When to Call a Health Professional

- If cold sores last longer than two weeks or occur frequently.

Dental Problems

Dental disease is preventable. You can keep all of your teeth by practicing good home care and having regular professional checkups. Be on the lookout for tooth decay and gum disease — both can appear as the result of bacterial plaque.

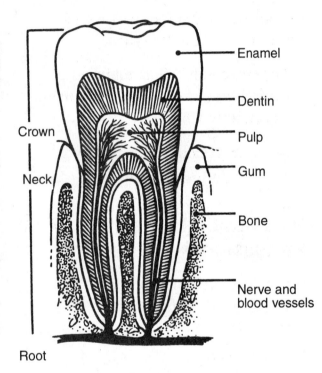

Crown

Neck

Root

— Enamel

— Dentin

— Pulp

— Gum

— Bone

— Nerve and blood vessels

The tooth

Plaque and Tooth Decay

Bacteria are always present in the mouth. When they are not removed by brushing and flossing, bacteria stick to the teeth and multiply into larger and larger colonies called plaque. Plaque appears as a sticky, colorless film on your teeth.

This sticky plaque damages teeth in two ways. First, food particles, especially refined sugars, stick to it. The plaque uses that food to grow more bacteria and to produce acid. Second, the plaque holds the acid against the tooth surface. If not removed, the acid will eventually eat through the tooth enamel, causing tooth decay.

If you eat only at meal times, it takes about 24 hours for bacteria and acid to harm your teeth. This is enough time for you to brush the plaque off and to wash away the acid. If you eat a lot of between-meal snacks, plaque builds up faster and you need to brush more often.

Plaque and Gum (Periodontal) Disease

Periodontal (perry-oh-DON-tal) disease is an inflammation around the gums and in the bone supporting the gums. It is the primary cause of tooth loss in older adults. It is caused by bacterial plaque that builds up and sticks to the teeth.

The first stage of the disease, called **gingivitis**, is marked by swollen, bleeding gums and bad breath. This stage is painless and, unfortunately, many people do not seek treatment.

As the disease progresses, the supporting bones and ligaments are affected. The gums recede, creating gaps between the teeth, which eventually fall out.

People with diabetes and those who smoke or chew tobacco are at increased risk. However, everyone is at risk; an estimated 75 to 80 percent of Americans have some form of periodontal disease.

Occasional bleeding when you brush or floss your teeth is an early sign of gum disease. However, with good care, it won't take long to get your gums back to normal. Brush and floss your teeth every day, and follow the prevention guidelines. Faithful home care and regular visits to the dentist can prevent tooth decay and periodontal disease.

Prevention

- Brush and floss every day to remove plaque. A thorough job once a day (three to five minutes each time) is better than two or three quick brushings. Clean every part of every tooth.

- Use fluoride toothpaste or mouth rinses. Fluoride is a mineral that strengthens tooth enamel and reduces the harmful effects of plaque.

- Eat crunchy foods that naturally clean the teeth (apples, carrots, and other raw vegetables), and foods with lots of vitamin C, like citrus fruits and broccoli.

- Have your teeth checked and cleaned at least twice a year by a dentist or dental hygienist.

Get Hold of Your Toothbrush

If you have difficulty brushing your teeth because your hands are stiff, painful, or weak, consider these simple solutions:

- Enlarge the brush handle by wrapping a sponge, elastic bandage, or adhesive tape around it. You might also push the handle through a rubber ball.

- Lengthen the handle by taping popsicle sticks or tongue depressors to it.

- Use an electric toothbrush.

There are also specially designed toothbrushes, toothpaste dispensers, and floss holders. See Resource 12 on page 419.

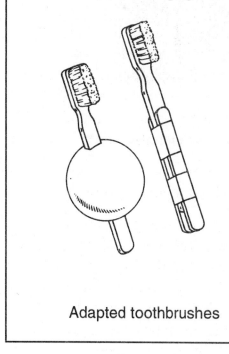

Adapted toothbrushes

When to Call a Health Professional

- For regular cleanings and exams. Every six months is the recommended schedule.

- If your gums bleed when you press on them or bleed often when you brush your teeth.

- If teeth are loose or moving apart.

- If there are changes in the way your teeth fit together when you bite or in the way partial dentures or removable bridgework fits.

- If gums are very red, swollen, or tender, or if pus is present.

- If you have a toothache. Toothaches are caused when the inside of the tooth (the dentin) is exposed. The pain may go away temporarily, but the problem will not. Take aspirin, ibuprofen, or acetaminophen (Tylenol) for pain relief until you can get an appointment. A cold pack on the jaw may also help. Oil of clove may help, too, although there is no scientific proof.

Denture Care

- Clean your dentures every day with a brush and a denture cleaner such as Polident.

- For cleaning fixed bridges, use a floss threader or special floss with a stiff threader section.

- Store dentures in lukewarm water or denture-cleansing liquid overnight. Don't let them dry out.

- Examine your gums daily before putting in your dentures. Let red, swollen gums heal before wearing your dentures again. If the redness does not go away in a few days, call your dentist. White patches on the inside of the cheeks could also indicate poorly fitting dentures.

- Give your mouth at least six hours of rest from your dentures every day. Your mouth heals more slowly as you age and needs time to recover from the friction of wearing dentures.

- Don't put up with dentures that are too big, click when you eat, or feel uncomfortable. Dentures take some time to get used to, but if they are still giving you trouble after the first few weeks, consult your dentist about a refitting.

- Have your dentures replaced about every five years. Dentures suffer from daily wear and tear and need to be replaced regularly.

Dry Mouth

Many older adults experience dry mouth (xerostomia, pronounced zero-STOW-me-ah). It can be caused by:

- Breathing through the mouth in dry environments

- Diabetes

- Many common medications, particularly diuretics, antihistamines, and antidepressants

- Not drinking enough water throughout the day

- Gum disease

- Radiation therapy to the head or neck

- Autoimmune diseases such as rheumatoid arthritis

Sjogren's (show-gruns) **syndrome** is a condition that affects some older women. It causes dry mouth, itchy burning eyes, and vaginal dryness. Sjogren's syndrome often accompanies rheumatoid arthritis or lupus.

Chronic lack of saliva can cause mouth problems such as tooth decay and bacterial infections.

Prevention

- Drink two quarts of water a day.

- Humidify your home, especially the bedroom.

- Breathe through your nose rather than through your mouth.

- Avoid antihistamines, which dry the mucous membranes.

Taste Changes

As you age, you lose some of your sense of taste. Some of this loss may be linked to a decline in the sense of smell. However, there's no need to put up with poor taste! There are many preventable and reversible causes for taste loss:

- Smoking

- Not thoroughly brushing both teeth and tongue

- Gum disease

- Dry mouth

- Medications. If you notice a marked decrease in taste while you are taking any medication, report it to your doctor.

- Viral infection

Home Treatment

- Follow the prevention guidelines.

- Practice good dental care. Lack of saliva increases your risk of tooth decay. Regular brushing and flossing are very important to protect your teeth.

- Suck on sugarless candies or chew sugarless gum to increase saliva production.

- Add extra liquid to foods to make them easier to chew and swallow. Drink water with meals.

- Avoid caffeinated beverages, tobacco, and alcohol, all of which increase dryness in the mouth.

- Try saliva substitutes, such as Xerolube, which are available over-the-counter.

When to Call a Health Professional

- If dry mouth is causing difficulty in swallowing food.

- If dry mouth is accompanied by persistent sore throat.

- If dry mouth causes denture discomfort.

- If dry mouth may be linked to medications that you are taking.

Oral Cancer

Oral cancer may develop in any part of the oral cavity. It is most commonly found on the lips, the tongue, the lining of the cheeks, the gums, the floor of the mouth, and the area behind the wisdom teeth. Risk factors for oral cancer include smoking or chewing tobacco and excessive use of alcohol.

It is important to check regularly for symptoms of oral cancer. Symptoms include:

- A sore in the mouth that bleeds easily and does not heal within two to three weeks

- A lump or thickening in the cheek that can be felt with the tongue

- A persistent white or red patch on the gums, tongue, or lining of the mouth

- Soreness or a feeling that something is caught in the throat

- Unexplained difficulty chewing or swallowing or moving the jaw or tongue

- Persistent numbness of the tongue or other areas of the mouth

- Persistent swelling of the jaw that causes dentures to fit poorly or cause discomfort

Prevention

- Don't smoke tobacco in any form (cigarettes, cigars, or pipe). Avoid smokeless (chewing) tobacco as well.

- Drink alcohol only in moderation.

- Get regular dental checkups.

When to Call a Health Professional

- If one or more of the above symptoms develops and persists longer than two weeks without explanation. Minor irritations that clear up with home treatment are usually not a cause for concern.

TMJ Syndrome

The olive-sized joint that connects your jawbone to your skull is called the temporomandibular joint (TMJ). TMJ syndrome is a set of symptoms that relate to damage, wear and tear, or unusual stress to the joint. The symptoms can include:

- Pain in and around the joint

- Noises such as clicking, popping, or snapping in the joint

- Limited ability to "open wide"

- Muscle pain and spasms where the jaw muscles attach to the bone

- Headache, neck and shoulder pain, ear or eye pain, and difficulty swallowing

The cause of TMJ syndrome is difficult to determine. The most likely causes include:

- Injury, such as a direct blow to the jaw, whiplash, or forceful stretching of the jaw during dental work

- Chronic tooth grinding, clenching, or gum chewing

- Arthritis in the joint

- Chronic muscle tension due to stress, anxiety, depression, or poor posture (usually affects the jaw muscles more than the joint)

- Teeth that do not meet when you bite

TMJ often responds well to home care, and most cases don't require surgery. In addition to the home treatments listed here, your family doctor, dentist, or a physical therapist may be able to recommend exercises or other treatment, depending on the cause of the problem. Surgery is needed for only a few TMJ problems.

Prevention

- Regularly practice progressive muscle relaxation, particularly before going to sleep. See page 368.

- Stop chewing gum or tough foods at the first sign of pain or discomfort in your jaw muscles.

- Avoid biting your nails and chewing on pencils or other objects which force your jaw into an awkward position and may cause pain.

- Maintain good posture with your ear, shoulder, and hip in a straight line to prevent muscle tension. See page 30.

- Good dentistry will allow your teeth to meet evenly when you bite down.

Home Treatment

- Continue the prevention tips.

- Avoid chewing gum and foods that are hard to chew.

- Avoid opening your mouth too wide.

- Do not cradle the telephone receiver between your shoulder and jaw.

- Rest your jaw, keeping your teeth apart and your lips closed. (Keep your tongue on the roof of your mouth, not between your teeth.)

- Put an ice pack on the joint for 10 to 15 minutes, four times a day. Gently open and close your mouth while the ice pack is on.

- If there is no swelling, use moist heat on the jaw muscle three to four times a day. Gently open and close your mouth while the heat is on. Alternate with the cold pack treatments.

- Use aspirin or ibuprofen to reduce swelling and pain.

- If you are under a lot of stress or if you are anxious or depressed, see Chapter 19 on Mental Self-Care.

When to Call a Health Professional

- If pain is severe.

- If TMJ symptoms occur after an injury to the jaw.

- If clicking or cracking sounds in your jaw continue without pain for over two weeks, tell your doctor or dentist at your next regular visit.

- If any jaw problem or pain continues without improvement for over two weeks.

- If other mild TMJ symptoms do not improve after four weeks of home treatment.

They aren't making mirrors like they used to.
Tallulah Bankhead

14

Skin, Hair, and Nail Problems

Our skin, hair, and nails are often where the first telltale signs of age begin to appear. As you age, your skin:

- Grows thinner.

- Gets dryer.

- Becomes less stretchy, so wrinkles appear.

- Takes longer to heal when it is cut or bruised.

These changes are more pronounced and come earlier in people whose skin has been repeatedly exposed to sun over the years.

The good new is, while some of the skin problems that arise with age may be a nuisance, few are dangerous. Except for certain skin cancers that are not caught early, death from skin problems is rare. Even though you can't slow down or prevent every change that occurs with age, good self-care can help you keep your hair, skin, and nails looking and feeling as healthy as ever.

Age Spots

Age spots are areas of skin that have changed color due to long-term exposure to sunlight. People used to think that the yellow, red, tan, or brown spots were a sign of liver ailments, hence the name "liver spots." However, the spots have nothing to do with your liver or any other organ.

Age spots are usually harmless. If you notice a spot that has become irritated or is changing in color, size, or shape, show it to your doctor during your next visit.

Skin Problems

Skin Symptoms	Possible Causes
Raised, red, itchy welt (may occur after an insect bite or taking a drug)	See Hives, p. 219; Insect and Tick Bites, p. 286.
Red, painful, swollen bump under the skin	See Boils, p. 214.
Red, flaky, itchy skin	See Dry Skin, p. 215; Fungal Infections, p. 217; Rashes, p. 221.
Rash that develops after wearing new jewelry or clothing, being exposed to poisonous plants, eating a new food, or taking a new drug	See Rashes, p. 221.
Red, itchy, blistered rash	Possible poison ivy, oak, sumac. See Rashes, p. 221.
Painful blisters in a band around one side of the body	See Shingles, p. 224.
Change in shape, size, or color of a mole, or persistently irritated mole	See Skin Cancer, p. 225.
Cracked, blistered, itchy, peeling skin between the toes	See Fungal Infections (athlete's foot), p. 217.
Red, itchy, weeping rash on the groin or thighs	See Fungal Infections (jock itch), p. 217.
Flaky, silvery patches of skin, especially on knees, elbows, or scalp	See "Psoriasis," p. 222.
Sandpapery skin rash with sore throat	Possible scarlet fever. See p. 91.
Reddish-yellow, scaly patches on scalp, forehead, sides of nose, eyelids, behind ears, center of chest	See Rashes (seborrheic dermatitis), p. 222.
Chafing rash between folds of skin (armpit, groin, under breasts)	See Rashes (chafing), p. 223.
Fingernails or toenails are thickened, discolored, or soft and crumbly	See Fungal Infections, p. 217.

Blisters

Blisters are usually the result of persistent or repeated rubbing against the skin. Some illnesses, like shingles (page 224), cause blistering rashes. Burns (page 269) can also blister the skin.

Prevention

- Avoid shoes that are too tight or that rub on your toes or heels.

- Wear gloves to protect your hands when doing heavy chores.

Home Treatment

- If a blister is small and closed, leave it alone. Protect it from further rubbing with a loose bandage, and avoid the activity or shoes that caused it.

- If a small blister is in a weight-bearing area, protect it with a doughnut-shaped moleskin pad. Put the open area over the blister.

- Blisters should be left unbroken. However, if a blister is large and you feel that draining it would make you more comfortable, here is a safe method:

  ○ Clean a needle with rubbing alcohol.

  ○ Gently puncture the blister at the edge.

  ○ Press the fluid in the blister toward the hole to drain it.

- Once you have opened a blister, or if it has torn open on its own, wash the area with soap and water.

- Gently smooth the flap of skin covering the blister over the tender skin underneath. Do not remove the skin flap unless it is very dirty or torn, or if pus is forming under the blister.

- Apply an antibiotic ointment and a sterile bandage. Do not apply alcohol or iodine. They will delay healing.

- Change the bandage once a day to reduce the chance of infection. Remove the bandage at night to allow the area to dry.

When to Call a Health Professional

- If blisters recur often and you do not know the cause.

- If signs of infection develop:

  ○ Increased pain, swelling, redness, or tenderness

  ○ Heat or red streaks extending from the blister

○ Discharge of pus

○ Fever of 100° or higher with no other cause

• If you have diabetes or peripheral vascular disease.

Boils

A boil is a red, swollen, painful bump under the skin, similar to an over-grown pimple. Boils are often caused by an infected hair follicle. Bacteria from the infection form an abscess or pocket of pus. The boil can become as large as a ping-pong ball and may be extremely painful.

Boils occur most often in areas where there is hair and chafing. The face, neck, armpits, breasts, groin, and buttocks are common sites.

Prevention

• Wash boil-prone areas often with soapy water. An antibacterial soap may help. Dry thoroughly.

• Avoid clothing that is too tight.

Home Treatment

• Do not squeeze, scratch, drain, or lance a boil. Squeezing can push the infection deeper into the skin. Scratching can spread bacteria, which can cause new boils to form.

• Wash yourself gently with anti-bacterial soap (Dial, Safeguard) to prevent boils from spreading.

• Use moist heat often. Try applying hot, wet washcloths to the boil for 20 to 30 minutes, three to four times a day. Do this as soon as you notice a boil. The heat and moisture can help bring the boil to the sur-face, but it may take five to seven days. A hot water bottle applied over a damp towel also may help.

• Continue using warm compresses for three days after the boil opens. Apply a bandage to keep draining material from spreading, and change the bandage daily.

When to Call a Health Professional

If needed, your doctor can drain a boil and treat the infection. Call a doctor:

• If a boil is on your face, near your spine, or in the anal area.

• If signs of worsening infection develop:

○ Increased pain, swelling, redness, or tenderness

○ Red streaks extending from the boil

○ Continued discharge of pus

○ Fever of 100° or higher with no other cause

- If any other lumps, particularly painful ones, develop near the infected area.

- If pain limits your normal activities or interrupts your sleep.

- If you have diabetes.

- If the boil is as large as a ping-pong ball.

- If the boil has not improved after five to seven days of home treatment.

- If many boils develop and persist.

Dandruff

Dandruff occurs when skin cells flake off your scalp. This flaking is natural and occurs all over your body. On the scalp, however, larger flakes can mix with oil and dust to form dandruff. Dandruff cannot be cured, but it can be controlled.

Home Treatment

- Try frequent and energetic shampooing with any shampoo. Wash hair daily if it helps control dandruff.

- If dandruff is excessive and itchy, try a dandruff shampoo (Head & Shoulders, Sebulex, Tegrin, T-Gel) three times a week, alternating with your regular shampoo. Experiment to find the dandruff shampoo that works best for you.

When to Call a Health Professional

- If frequent shampooing or use of a dandruff shampoo does not control dandruff. Your doctor may prescribe a stronger dandruff shampoo.

Dry Skin and Itching

As you age, your skin produces less of the natural oils that help retain its moisture. Dry air can cause your skin to become dry, as can excessive bathing with strong soaps and hot water.

Dry skin is often worse in the winter due to lower indoor humidity created by forced air heat. The lower legs, forearms, hands, and scalp are especially prone to dry skin. Without good home care, the skin can become red, cracked, and prone to irritation and infections.

Prevention

- Avoid overexposure to the sun. See page 227.

- Humidify your home, particularly the bedrooms.

- Use warm, not hot, water when you bathe. Hot water strips the skin's natural oil, which helps hold in moisture. If possible, bathe less frequently.

- Avoid strong detergents and deodorant soaps. Limit use of perfumes and perfumed products.

- Apply a moisturizer (Eucerin, Keri Lotion, Lubriderm, Vaseline) while skin is still damp to seal in moisture. A light layer of petroleum jelly is also an effective and inexpensive moisturizer. Reapply lotion often.

Home Treatment

- Follow the prevention guidelines above.

- Bathe every other day instead of every day. Use warm or cool water and a gentle soap (Basis, Dove, Oil of Olay). Use little or no soap on dry skin areas. Pat dry with a towel; don't rub skin.

- For very dry hands, apply a thin layer of petroleum jelly and wear thin cotton gloves to bed. (This may also help dry feet.) Severely dry skin may require several treatments.

- Avoid scratching, which damages the skin. If itching is a problem, see "Relief From Itching" in the box at right.

Relief From Itching

- Keep the itchy area cool and wet. Try a compress soaked in ice water. Apply a moisturizer to skin while damp.

- An oatmeal bath may help relieve itching. Wrap one cup of oatmeal in a cotton cloth and boil as you would to cook it. Using the oatmeal-filled cloth as a sponge, bathe in tepid water without soap. Or try an Aveeno Colloidal Oatmeal bath.

- Calamine lotion can be helpful for poison ivy or poison oak rashes.

- Try an over-the-counter one percent hydrocortisone cream for small itchy areas. Use sparingly on the face or genitals. If itching is severe, your doctor may prescribe a stronger cream.

- Try an over-the-counter oral antihistamine (Benadryl, Chlor-Trimeton).

- Cut nails short or wear cotton gloves at night to prevent scratching.

- Wear cotton clothing. Avoid wool and acrylic fabrics next to the skin.

When to Call a Health Professional

- If you itch all over your body and you do not have a rash or any other obvious cause for itching.

- If itching is so bad that you cannot sleep and home treatment methods are not helping.

- If the skin is badly broken due to scratching.

- If signs of infection develop:

  o Increased pain, swelling, or tenderness

  o Red streaks extending from the area

  o Discharge of pus

  o Honey-colored crust forms on the rash

  o Fever of 100° or higher with no other cause

Fungal Infections

Fungal infections of the skin most commonly affect the feet, groin, scalp, or nails. Fungi grow best in warm, moist areas of the skin such as between toes, in the groin area, and under breasts. If infection occurs in an area where hair grows, such as the scalp, hair loss may occur.

Athlete's foot (tinea pedis) is the most common fungal skin infection. Symptoms include intense itching, cracks, blisters, redness, and scaling on the soles of the feet, and peeling, moist areas between the toes. It often recurs and must be treated again each time.

Jock itch (tinea cruris) causes redness, scaling, severe itching, and moistness on the skin of the groin and upper thighs. There are usually red, scaly, raised areas on the skin that weep or ooze pus or clear fluid.

Fungal nail infections cause discoloration, thickening, and often softening of the fingernails and toenails. Often a build-up of yellow debris develops under the free edge of the nail. These infections are difficult to treat and often cause permanent damage to the nails. If treatment with medication does not work, the nail may have to be removed.

Some other infections cause inflammation of the nail bed or the tissue adjacent to the nail. Without treatment, these can lead to serious complications, including more widespread infection.

Prevention

- Keep feet clean and dry. Dry between the toes after swimming or bathing, and apply absorbent powder (Micatin, Zeasorb).

- Wear leather shoes or sandals that allow your feet to "breathe," and wear cotton socks to absorb sweat. Use powder on your feet and in your shoes. Give shoes 24 hours to dry between wearings.

- Do not go barefoot in public pools and showers. Wear thongs or shower sandals.

- Wash and dry the groin area well, especially after exercise, and apply powder to absorb moisture. Wear cotton underclothes and avoid tight pants and pantyhose.

- Don't share hats, shoes, combs, or hairbrushes.

Home Treatment

- Follow the prevention guidelines above.

- For athlete's foot and jock itch, use an over-the-counter antifungal powder or lotion such as Lotrimin AF or Micatin. Use the medication for a week or two after the symptoms clear up to prevent recurrence. Do not use hydrocortisone on a fungal infection.

- Consider wearing cotton socks, and change them twice a day to keep your feet dry. If possible, wear open sandals. When indoors, go in stocking feet.

When to Call a Health Professional

- If signs of infection are present: increased swelling and redness, pus, or a honey-colored crust on the rash.

- If you have diabetes and develop athlete's foot. People with diabetes are at increased risk of infection and may need professional care.

- If home treatment fails to clear up athlete's foot or jock itch after two weeks.

- If there is sudden hair loss associated with flaking, broken hairs, and inflammation of the scalp; or if several household members suddenly start losing their hair.

Hair Changes

As your skin ages and your hormones change, your hair also may undergo changes. Men tend to lose hair (see Baldness on page 247). After menopause, women tend to grow more facial and body hair. Both men and women tend to lose hair color. All of these changes are normal and do not pose medical problems.

Bald spots should be distinguished from baldness. Bald spots may be caused by repeated stress to the hair such as tight braids or habitual hair pulling. Bald spots that occur on a normal scalp sometimes indicate a more serious problem.

Some medications, vitamins, and illnesses may cause hair to break near the roots, change texture, or come out easily. Call your doctor if this occurs.

When to Call a Health Professional

- Call your doctor if you do not know the cause of any bald spot.

Hives

Hives (urticaria) are an allergic reaction of the skin. Hives are raised, red, itchy patches of skin (wheals or welts) that may appear and disappear at random. They range in size from less than a quarter-inch to an inch or more, and they may last as little as a few minutes or as long as a few days.

Multiple hives may occur in response to a drug, food, or infection. A single hive commonly develops after an insect sting. Other possible causes include plants, inhaled allergens, stress, cosmetics, and exposure to heat, cold, or sunlight. Often a cause cannot be found.

Prevention

- Avoid foods, medications, cosmetics, plants, insects, and animals that cause you to break out in hives.

- Reduce stress in your life. See page 363.

Home Treatment

- Continue to avoid the substance that causes hives.

- Cool water compresses will help relieve itching. Also see page 216.

- An oral antihistamine (Benadryl, Chlor-Trimeton) may help treat the hives and relieve itching. Once the hives have disappeared, decrease the dose of the medication slowly over five to seven days.

When to Call a Health Professional

Call 911 or emergency services immediately if hives occur with the following signs of a severe allergic reaction, especially soon after taking a drug, eating a certain food, or being stung by an insect:

- **Lightheadedness or feeling like you may pass out.**

- **Swelling around the lips, tongue, or face that may interfere with breathing.**

- **Wheezing or difficulty breathing.**

Call a health professional immediately:

- If there is swelling of the lips, tongue, or face that is not interfering with breathing.

- If many hives develop rapidly. If you commonly get hives, apply home treatment as your doctor has recommended.

Call a health professional:

- If hives persist for several days despite home treatment and avoiding suspected irritants.

Ingrown Toenails

An ingrown toenail is often caused by an improperly trimmed nail that cuts into the skin or by wearing shoes that are too tight. Because the cut can easily become infected, prompt care is needed.

Prevention

- Cut toenails straight across so the edges cannot cut into the skin.

- Wear roomy shoes.

- Wash your feet and change your socks often.

Caregiver Tips on Nail Care

People with poor eyesight, joint stiffness, or tremor may have difficulty providing proper nail care for themselves. Present them with the gift of a foot bath, foot massage, and toenail and fingernail trim every few weeks.

Use care when trimming toenails and fingernails for a person who has diabetes or peripheral vascular disease. See page 146.

Home Treatment

- Soak your foot in warm water.

- Wedge a small piece of wet tissue under the corner of the nail to help it grow out straight.

- Trim the nail straight across once it has grown out enough to do so.

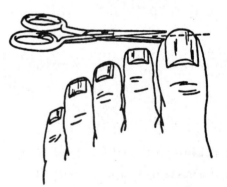

Cut toenails straight across to avoid ingrown toenails.

When to Call a Health Professional

- If signs of infection develop:

  - Increased pain, swelling, or tenderness

  - Red streaks extending from the area

  - Discharge of pus

  - Fever of 100° or higher with no other cause

- If yellow-brown discoloration, nail destruction, or other signs of fungal infection develop, tell your doctor at your next appointment.

- If you have diabetes or circulatory problems. The risk of infection is higher in people who have these conditions.

Rashes

A rash (dermatitis) is any irritation or inflammation of the skin. Rashes can be caused by illness, allergy, heat, and sometimes emotional stress.

Poison ivy and other plant rashes are often red, blistered, and itchy. Rashes appear in lines where the plant's leaves brushed against the skin.

When you first get a rash, ask yourself the following questions to help determine its cause (also see page 212):

Calluses and Corns

Calluses and corns are hard, thickened skin that builds up on parts of the foot that are exposed to friction and pressure. Calluses are common on the soles of the feet and heels. Corns usually form on the toes, where shoes press and rub skin against bone.

You can prevent corns and calluses by avoiding shoes that pinch or cramp your toes or by using insoles to cushion your feet. If you cannot avoid wearing shoes that rub your feet, use moleskin pads for protection.

If a callus or corn becomes painful, soak your feet in warm water and rub the callus or corn with a towel or pumice stone. You may need to do this for several days until the thickened skin is gone. If a corn or callus breaks open or becomes sore, see your doctor.

Do not try to cut or burn off corns or calluses. If you have diabetes or peripheral vascular disease, talk with your doctor about removing troublesome corns or calluses.

- Did a rash that is localized (in a small area of your skin) occur following contact with anything new that could have irritated your skin: poison ivy, oak, or sumac; soaps, detergents, shampoos, perfumes, cosmetics, or lotions; jewelry or fabrics; new tools, appliances, latex gloves, or other objects? The location of the rash is often a clue to its cause.

- Have you eaten anything new that you may be allergic to?

- Are you taking any new medications, either prescription or over-the-counter?

- Have you been unusually stressed or upset recently?

- Is there joint pain or fever along with the rash?

- Is the rash spreading? Does it itch?

Seborrheic Dermatitis

Older adults are particularly prone to a rash called seborrheic dermatitis. Small, reddish-yellow, scaly patches develop in areas that are particularly oily: the scalp, forehead, sides of the nose, eyelids, behind the ears, and in the center of the chest.

This common problem is caused by overactive oil glands in the skin. Emotional stress, physical exertion, and certain medications can trigger

Psoriasis

Psoriasis is a chronic skin condition that causes raised red patches topped with silvery, scaling skin on the knees, elbows, scalp, and back. The fingernails, palms, and soles of the feet also may be affected. It is not contagious.

The patches, called plaques, are made of dead skin cells that accumulate in thick layers. Normal skin cells are replaced every 30 days. In psoriasis, skin cells grow rapidly (they are replaced every three to four days) and are shed slowly.

Small patches of psoriasis can often be treated with regular use of hydrocortisone or tar-based cream.

Tar products (lotions, gels, shampoos) may also be useful, although they may increase sensitivity to the sun. Limited exposure to the sun also may help (protect unaffected skin with sunscreen). If psoriasis affects the scalp, try a dandruff shampoo.

Stress contributes to psoriasis. Stress reduction may help in some cases. See page 363.

Call your doctor if psoriasis covers much of your body or is very red. More extensive cases often need professional care.

flare-ups. It responds well to home treatment with dandruff shampoos and hydrocortisone creams.

Intertrigo (Chafing)

Intertrigo is a chafing rash that occurs between skin folds. Common sites are the armpit, groin, inner thighs, anal region, and under the breasts. Moisture, warmth, and friction combine to cause chafing.

Weight loss and home treatment can clear up the problem. If the rash is not treated, bacterial or fungal infections may develop.

Home Treatment

- If you come in contact with a substance that may cause a rash, such as poison ivy, wash all exposed areas thoroughly with detergent and water.

- Watch for early signs of rashes. Fast treatment can usually clear up the problem quickly, before it spreads.

- If a rash develops, wash affected areas with water only. Soap can be irritating. Pat dry thoroughly.

- Apply cold, wet compresses to the rash to reduce itching. Repeat frequently. Also see page 216.

- Leave the rash exposed to air. Baby powder can help keep it dry. Avoid lotions and ointments until the rash

heals. However, calamine lotion is helpful for plant rashes. Use it three to four times a day.

- Hydrocortisone cream can provide temporary relief of itching. Use sparingly on facial rashes and the genitals.

- Rashes on the feet or groin may be due to fungal infections. See page 217.

When to Call a Health Professional

- If signs of infection appear:

  - Pain, swelling, or tenderness

  - Heat and redness, or red streaks extending from the area

  - Discharge of pus

  - Honey-colored crust forms on the rash

  - Fever of 100° or higher with no other cause

- If you suspect a medication reaction caused the rash.

- If rash occurs with fever and joint pain.

- If rash occurs with sore throat. See page 91.

- If you aren't sure what is causing a rash.

- If rash continues after two to three weeks of home treatment.

Shingles

Some people who had chickenpox as children may develop shingles later in life. Shingles (herpes zoster) is caused by reactivation of the chickenpox virus in the body. The virus usually affects one of the large nerves that spreads outward from the spine, causing pain and a rash that appears in a band around one side of the chest, abdomen, or face.

The symptoms of shingles develop in a pattern. First, there will be a tingling, burning, throbbing, or stabbing pain in the affected nerve. Pain is usually worse when shingles affects the face or scalp.

A rash, which develops into blisters, will appear two to three days after the pain begins. The blisters will dry up in a few days and will drop off in two to three weeks.

About half of people over 60 who get shingles experience lingering pain (**post-herpetic neuralgia**) in the affected nerve for months or years.

No one is sure what causes the chickenpox virus to become active again. Shingles may be more likely to develop when illness or medications have weakened a person's immune system, and it can recur.

Prevention

• If you have never had chickenpox, avoid exposure to people with shingles or chickenpox.

• A vaccine to prevent chickenpox is available. It may prevent shingles if you have never had chickenpox. However, it *will not* prevent shingles if you already have had chickenpox.

Home Treatment

• Keep shingles blisters clean and dry to prevent infection.

• Reduce the pain caused by your clothing rubbing against the blisters by taping cotton gauze over the blistered area.

• Use aspirin or acetaminophen to control pain.

• See page 216 for relief from itching.

• Avoid contact with children, pregnant women, and adults who have never had chickenpox until the blisters have completely dried.

When to Call a Health Professional

• If you suspect shingles, call your doctor immediately. He or she can prescribe drugs that can limit the pain and rash.

- If shingles blisters appear in or near the eye or on the tip of the nose.

- If facial pain develops. Your doctor can determine if the eyes are involved.

Skin Cancer

Skin cancer is the most common type of cancer. Fortunately, many types of skin cancer are easy to cure.

Most skin cancer is caused by sun damage. Ninety percent of skin cancers occur on the face, neck, and arms, where sun exposure is greatest. Light-skinned, blue-eyed people are most likely to develop skin cancer. Dark-skinned people have less risk.

Most skin cancers are slow-growing, easy to recognize, and easy to treat. A small percentage of skin cancers are more serious.

Basal cell and **squamous cell skin cancers** (carcinomas) tend to develop in sun-exposed areas. They differ from non-cancerous growths in several important ways. Skin cancers:

- Tend to bleed more and are often open sores that do not heal.

- Tend to be slow-growing.

Most moles are harmless. However, **malignant melanomas** (one type of cancerous mole) can be fatal and should be treated promptly.

Prevention

Most skin cancers can be prevented by avoiding excessive exposure to the sun. See page 227. Unfortunately, sun damage from earlier years is often the cause of skin cancer later in life. However, some skin cancers occur without sun exposure or damage.

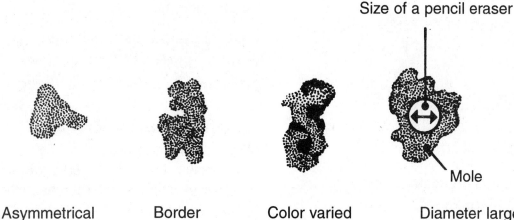

| Asymmetrical shape | Border irregular | Color varied or multi-colored | Diameter larger than a pencil eraser |

Watch for these mole changes.

Home Treatment

Examine your skin with a mirror or with another person's help. Look for unusual moles, spots, or bumps. Pay special attention to areas that get a lot of sun exposure: hands, arms, chest, neck (especially the back of the neck), face, ears, etc. Report any changes to your doctor.

When to Call a Health Professional

If your moles do not change over time, there is little cause for concern. If you have a family history of malignant melanoma, let your doctor know. You may be at higher risk. Call your doctor if you notice any of the following changes:

- A sore that bleeds or won't heal.

- Changes in moles:

  - Asymmetrical shape: one half does not match the other half.

  - Border irregularity: the edges are ragged, notched, or blurred.

  - Color: the color is not uniform. Watch for shades of red and black, or a red, white, and blue mottled appearance.

  - Diameter: larger than a pencil eraser (harmless moles are usually smaller than this).

- Scaliness, oozing, bleeding, or spreading of pigment into surrounding skin.

- Appearance of a bump or nodule on a mole, or any changes in a mole's appearance.

- Persistent itching, tenderness, or pain.

- Unusual skin changes or growths, especially if they bleed and keep growing.

Skin Growths

Most bumps and lumps that occur as we age are harmless growths, spots, or skin tags that remain stable once they have appeared.

Seborrheic keratoses are oval-shaped, brown or black, waxy, wart-like, flat-topped growths on the face, neck, and trunk.

Cherry angiomas (ruby spots) are small, reddish-purple spots most often found on the trunk and upper legs, but also on the face, neck, scalp, and arms. These harmless bumps are clusters of dilated tiny blood vessels (capillaries) and will bleed profusely if punctured. They are increasingly common after age 40.

Skin tags are fleshy, tag-like growths of skin on the face, neck, chest, underarms, and groin.

Sebaceous gland growths are small, yellowish bumps on the forehead and face.

Pre-Cancerous Growths or Patches Solar or **actinic keratoses** are small red patches caused by long-term exposure to sunlight. These patches have a crusted, scaly, yellow-brown surface. They are considered to be pre-cancerous. If protected from the sun, the patches may grow smaller and disappear. If sun exposure continues, they may eventually change into skin cancers.

Prevention

- Non-cancerous growths such as skin tags, sebaceous gland growths, and seborrheic keratoses usually cannot be prevented.

- To help prevent actinic keratoses, always use a sunscreen that has a sun protective factor (SPF) of 15 or greater.

When to Call a Health Professional

- If any skin growth appears to change in size, shape, texture, or color.

- If any sore persists for four to six weeks without healing.

- If signs of skin cancer develop. See page 225.

Sunburn

A sunburn is usually a first- or second-degree burn that involves just the outer surface of the skin. Sunburns are uncomfortable but usually are not dangerous unless they are extensive. Repeated sun exposure and sunburns increase the risk of skin cancer.

Prevention

Sunburn is completely preventable. If you are going to be in the sun for more than 15 minutes, take the following precautions:

- Use a sunscreen with a sun protection factor (SPF) of at least 15. Apply the sunscreen 15 minutes before exposure. Reapply every two hours or as directed.

- If you are allergic to PABA, the active ingredient in some sunscreens, ask your pharmacist about non-PABA alternatives.

- Wear light-colored, loose-fitting clothes (preferably long-sleeved shirts and slacks) and a broad-brimmed hat to shade your face.

- Avoid the sun between 10 a.m. and 2 p.m., when burning rays are strongest.

Please note: A minimal amount of sunshine on the skin is needed to produce vitamin D. Vitamin D and calcium are needed to strengthen bones and prevent osteoporosis. Sunscreens block vitamin D production, so if you use them all the time you may want to consider boosting the amount of vitamin D in your diet. You can do this by drinking lots of vitamin D-fortified milk or by taking a low-dosage vitamin D supplement (no more than 1000 IU per day).

Home Treatment

- Watch for signs of heat exhaustion (page 283). Drink lots of water.

- Cool baths or compresses can be very soothing. Take acetaminophen or aspirin for pain.

- A mild fever and headache may accompany a sunburn. Lie down in a cool, quiet room to relieve headache.

- There is nothing you can do to prevent peeling; it is part of the healing process. Lotion can help relieve itching.

When to Call a Health Professional

- If signs of heat stroke develop (dry, flushed skin, confusion). See page 283.

- If there is severe blistering (blisters cover more than half of the affected body part) with fever, or if you feel very ill.

- If there is fever of 102° or higher.

- If lightheadedness or vision problems persist after you have cooled off.

Warts

Warts are infectious growths that are caused by a virus. They can appear anywhere on the body. Warts usually are not dangerous, but they can be bothersome.

Little is known about warts. Most are contagious. They can spread to other places on the person who has them, and they can be spread from person to person. However, some people seem to be more susceptible to warts, while others appear to be immune to them.

Genital and anal warts are easily spread through sexual contact and may increase the risk of cervical cancer. See page 261.

Plantar warts appear on the soles of the feet. Most of the wart lies under the skin surface, so it may feel like you are walking on a pebble.

Warts seem to come and go for little reason, and they appear to be sensitive to slight changes in the immune system. Although there is no scientific explanation of why it works, in some cases you can "think" them away.

When necessary, your doctor can remove warts. Unfortunately, they often come back.

Home Treatment

- Warts appear and disappear spontaneously. They can last a week, a month, or even years. To get rid of your warts, it helps to believe in the treatment. If something works for you, stick with it.

- If the wart bleeds a little, cover it with a bandage and apply light pressure to stop the bleeding.

- If the wart is in the way, reduce its size with a pumice stone or an over-the-counter salicylic acid solution (Compound W). This drug can be irritating in high concentrations; you may need to use a milder form for a longer period of time. Apply salicylic acid solution to the wart at night, and rub off the whitened skin in the morning. Do not use salicylic acid if you have diabetes or peripheral vascular disease.

- If you use a pumice stone, both the scrapings from the wart and the area of the pumice stone that touched the wart can be infectious. Do not touch this material. Discard both the wart scrapings and pumice stone promptly.

- Apply a doughnut-shaped pad to cushion the wart and relieve pain.

- Don't cut or burn off a wart.

- Try the least expensive method of treating warts that you can think of. You may save a trip to your doctor.

When to Call a Health Professional

- If a wart looks infected (increasing pain, swelling, redness, warmth, or discharge of pus) after being irritated or knocked off.

- If a plantar wart is painful when you walk and foam pads do not help.

- If a wart causes continual discomfort, or if warts are numerous enough to be a problem.

- If a wart develops on the face and is a cosmetic concern.

- If you have warts in the anal or genital area, see page 261.

The most creative force in the world
is the menopausal woman with zest.
Margaret Mead

15
Women's Health

Women have special health needs when it comes to self-care. They often must cope with health care problems that are unique to them. This chapter covers health issues of special concern to older women and what can be done to manage them better.

Breast Health

After lung cancer, breast cancer is the second leading cause of cancer deaths in women. However, breast cancer is highly treatable if it is detected early. There are three methods to use for early detection: breast self-exams, clinical breast exams, and mammograms.

Breast Self-Exam

Most breast lumps are discovered by women themselves. The breast self-exam is a simple technique to help you learn what is normal for you and to become aware of any changes.

Set up a regular time each month to examine your breasts. The first day of each month is an easy time to remember.

Most women's breast tissue has some lumpiness or thickening. This is common. When in doubt about a particular lump, check the other breast. If you find a similar lump in the same area on the other breast, it may be less concerning. Be on the lookout for a lump that feels much harder than the rest of the breast.

Have any areas of concern or doubt checked by your doctor. The important thing is to learn what is normal for you and to report changes to your doctor.

The breast self-exam takes place in two stages.

Stage 1: In front of the mirror

Look at your breasts in a mirror. Few women have breasts that match exactly. It is normal for one breast to be slightly larger than the other. Learn what is normal for you.

Stand and look at your breasts in four positions:

- With your arms at your sides

- With your hands on your hips

- With your arms raised overhead

- While bending forward

In each position, look for changes in the contour and shape of your breasts, the color and texture of the skin and nipples, and any discharge from the nipples. Squeeze the nipple of each breast gently between thumb and index finger. A discharge is common, but in rare cases it may be significant.

Stage 2: Lying down

To examine your right breast, place a pillow or folded towel under your right shoulder. If your breasts are large, lie on your left side and turn your right shoulder back flat to spread the breast tissue more evenly over your chest wall. Use the pads of the three middle fingers of your left hand to examine your right breast. Move your fingers in small, dime-sized circles. Use light to medium pressure in each spot to feel the full

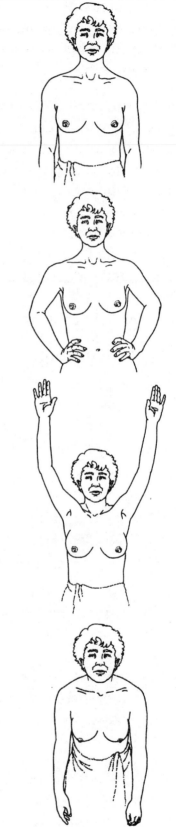

Breast self-exam, stage 1

thickness of the breast tissue. Don't lift your fingers away from the skin. You are feeling for lumps, thickening, or changes of any kind.

To make sure you cover the whole area, imagine that your breast is a clock. Start on the outside of the breast at 12:00, move slowly to 1:00 and then around the clock back to 12:00. Then move one inch in toward the nipple and go around the clock again. Be sure to include the nipple, the breastbone, and the armpit in your exam.

Move the pillow or towel to the other shoulder and repeat this procedure for the other breast.

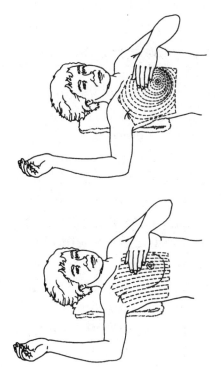

Breast self-exam, stage 2

If you discover a new lump, thickening, or change of any kind, or if there is a discharge from the nipple when you are not squeezing it, report it to your doctor. Most lumps are not cancerous (malignant), but be sure to tell your doctor about anything you find.

When you examine your breasts each month, you will learn what is normal for you and quickly recognize if something changes. The breast self-exam takes some practice. If you have questions, ask your doctor for help in learning the technique.

Clinical Breast Exam

The second method for early detection of breast problems is the clinical breast exam. This is when your doctor or nurse practitioner uses a technique like the breast self-exam to check your breasts. A clinical breast exam is recommended every one to two years after age 40.

Mammogram

A mammogram is a breast X-ray that can reveal breast tumors too small to be detected by a breast self-exam. Mammograms can detect breast cancer earlier when it may be more successfully treated. Studies have shown that mammograms save lives in women over 50, reducing breast cancer death rates by up to one-third. After age 50 (more specifically, after menopause), mammograms are recommended every one to two years.

After age 70, discuss with your doctor whether a different schedule is appropriate.

Less than a third of older women follow recommended guidelines for regular mammograms. Don't put it off. Your local hospital or American Cancer Society chapter can provide information on where to get a mammogram.

Preparing for a Mammogram

• Do not wear deodorant, perfume, powder, or lotion, because they can affect the quality of the X-ray.

• Wear clothing that allows you to remove only your shirt or blouse.

Breast Health Tips

• Do your breast self-exam every month. Most breast lumps are discovered by women themselves. When detected early, breast cancer usually can be successfully treated.

• Have a mammogram every one to two years after age 50.

• Have a clinical breast exam every one to two years.

• Limit alcohol to one drink per day. Heavy drinking increases the risk of breast cancer.

• Eat a low-fat diet. Cut down on fried foods and high-fat meats and dairy products.

• Eat foods containing vitamins A and C (dark green and orange vegetables and fruits). Eat more cruciferous vegetables (broccoli, cabbage, kale). There is some evidence that a diet that includes these foods may reduce the risk of breast cancer.

Gynecological Health

Pelvic exams and Pap smears are vital components of women's health. These exams can give you early signs of any abnormalities in your reproductive organs. It is better to catch any disease in its early stages, when it is much easier to treat.

Self-Exam

Examine your entire genital area periodically. Look for any sores, warts, red swollen areas, or unusual vaginal discharge. A healthy vaginal discharge will be white to yellowish-white and smell slightly like vinegar. It can be either thick or thin and present in large or small amounts; every woman is different. A normal vaginal discharge will change gradually with age and at menopause. If your discharge seems unusual in amount, smell, or consistency, see Vaginitis and Yeast Infections on page 240.

There should be no pain or straining on urination. If you experience pain or burning on urination, read about Urinary Tract Infections on page 139. If you have problems with bladder control, see Urinary Incontinence on page 137.

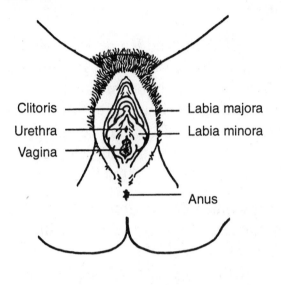

Clitoris

Urethra

Vagina

Labia majora

Labia minora

Anus

Female genitals

The Pelvic Exam and Pap Test

A pelvic exam given by a health professional will generally include an external genital exam, a Pap test, and a manual exam.

The Pap test is the screening exam for cancer of the cervix. Pap smears detect 90 to 95 percent of cervical cancers, making this a reliable and important test. (See Women's Cancers on page 242.)

The doctor will insert a tool called a speculum into your vagina to make it easier to see the cervix. There may be some discomfort. Tell the doctor if you feel any pain. The speculum can be adjusted to ease your discomfort. After doing a visual examination, she will use a special swab to gather some cells from your cervix and vagina.

For a manual exam, the doctor inserts two gloved and lubricated fingers into your vagina and presses on your lower abdomen with the other hand to feel the ovaries and uterus. The doctor may also insert one finger into the rectum and one into the vagina to examine other pelvic areas.

Pap smears are recommended every one to three years, depending on your risk factors. Women with a single sexual partner and several consecutive normal Pap smears need less frequent exams (every two to three years). Women with multiple sexual partners, other risk factors for cervical cancer (see page 244), or a history of abnormal tests need yearly exams.

After age 65 and two consecutive normal Pap smears, you can stop having Pap tests. It is important to continue to have regular pelvic exams.

Women who have had a hysterectomy may still need to have regular Pap smears and/or pelvic exams, even if the cervix has been removed. Even if your uterus and ovaries have been removed, you still need to be screened for cancer of the vagina and vulva. Ask your doctor about the best schedule for you.

Do not douche, have intercourse, or use feminine hygiene products for 24 hours before the exam because they can alter the results.

For more information on women's health, see Resources 59 and 60 on page 422.

Menopause

Menopause occurs when the production of the female hormones (estrogen and progesterone) is greatly reduced and menstrual periods stop. Most women go through menopause between the ages of 45 and 55 (the average age is 51). You are considered to have passed menopause after one year of no menstrual periods.

Hormonal changes may cause irregular menstrual periods before they stop altogether. You may also have hot flashes, vaginal dryness, and mood changes. The decreased estrogen level related to menopause is also directly linked to osteoporosis. See page 55.

Women can expect to live one-third of their lives after menopause, so it is important to manage any problems related to menopause.

Irregular periods may mean lighter or heavier than usual menstrual flows, shorter or longer intervals between flows, or spotting. Some women have regular periods until they stop suddenly, and others have irregular periods for a long time during menopause. Every woman is unique and will experience menopause differently.

Hot flashes are sudden periods of intense heat, sweating, and flushing. A hot flash usually begins in the chest and spreads out to the neck, face, and arms. They may occur as frequently as once an hour and last as long as three to four minutes.

Most women going through menopause (75 to 80 percent) will have hot flashes. Hot flashes usually cease within one or two years.

If hot flashes occur at night, they may disturb your sleep patterns. Disrupted sleep patterns can lead to insomnia, fatigue, irritability, or poor concentration.

Vaginal changes that occur with menopause include dryness and loss of elasticity, thinning of the vaginal walls, and shrinking of the labia, the outer lips of the vagina. Pain, irritation, and discharge resulting from these changes is known as atrophic vaginitis. These changes may also make vaginal infections more common. Vaginitis and yeast infections are discussed on page 240.

The loss of moisture and lubrication in the vagina may cause pain during and soreness after sexual intercourse.

However, vaginal changes do not have to lead to a decrease in sexual responsiveness or pleasure. There are things you can do to replace lost moisture.

Mood changes are caused by the hormonal and physical changes of menopause. Symptoms such as nervousness, lethargy, insomnia, moodiness, or depression are common.

With menopause, many women fear emotional upset and loss of sexuality. On the other hand, many women look forward to freedom from menstrual cycle discomfort and freedom from birth control. Understanding what is happening to you and using home care techniques to relieve any discomfort will help you through menopause.

Home Treatment

Irregular periods

• Keep a written record of your periods (the date, length, and amount of flow) in case you need to discuss them with a health professional.

Hot flashes

• Keep your home and work place cool.

• Wear layers of loose clothing that can be easily removed.

• Drink lots of water and juices. Avoid caffeine and alcohol if they worsen hot flashes.

• Exercise regularly to help stabilize hormone levels and ease insomnia.

Vaginal dryness

• Use a water-soluble vaginal lubricant such as K-Y Jelly or Surgilube to ease discomfort during sexual intercourse. Vegetable oil will also work. Do not use Vaseline or other petroleum-based products.

• Regular sexual activity improves circulation and suppleness in the vagina.

Birth Control During Menopause

Some women may continue to ovulate after menopause, which means there is a slight chance that they could become pregnant, even though they are no longer menstruating regularly.

Women who have their last period before age 50 and who do not want to become pregnant should continue using contraceptives (other than birth control pills) for two years. Some women may be able to take birth control pills with medical supervision. Women who have their last period after age 50 generally need to use birth control for only 12 months.

Mood changes

• Don't try to handle mood changes alone. Reach out to friends and discuss your symptoms. Give yourself, and ask from others, abundant amounts of love, caring, and understanding.

When to Call a Health Professional

• If you have any vaginal bleeding after you have gone six months without a period.

• If any vaginal bleeding is significantly heavier than normal for you (soaking a pad or tampon an hour for eight hours is often considered severe).

• If you have any vaginal bleeding while taking estrogen-only replacement therapy (ERT).

• If you have vaginal bleeding while taking estrogen and progestin (hormone replacement therapy, or HRT) that is unexpected or that you haven't discussed with your doctor.

• If vaginal bleeding persists longer than two to three weeks.

• If intermittent or irregular vaginal bleeding occurs for more than two to three months.

• If vaginal dryness is not relieved by using a vaginal lubricant. Your doctor may prescribe estrogen that you can apply directly to the vagina as a cream or suppository.

• If you are considering hormone replacement therapy.

Hormone Replacement Therapy

Hormone therapy helps relieve the short-term symptoms of menopause and reduces some long-term risks associated with lower estrogen levels. There are two types of hormone therapy.

Estrogen replacement therapy (ERT) is estrogen alone. ERT is usually prescribed only for women who have had a hysterectomy, since estrogen alone increases the risk of endometrial (uterine lining) cancer. Brand names include Estrace, Genesis, and Premarin. Women with a uterus who take ERT need regular checkups for uterine lining changes.

Hormone replacement therapy (HRT) combines estrogen with progestin, another hormone. HRT is usually prescribed only for women who have a uterus. The progestin protects the uterus from cancer. Brand names include Amen, Aygestin, Norlutin, and Provera.

Hormone therapy reduces some health risks and increases others. Consider the following factors in your decision.

Osteoporosis

Both ERT and HRT reduce the risk of osteoporosis and slow the rate of bone loss that occurs after menopause, which helps reduce the risk of fractures. It is estimated that ERT can reduce the risk of fractures caused by osteoporosis by up to 60 percent. See page 57 for information on preventing osteoporosis.

Heart Disease

ERT reduces a woman's risk of heart disease by increasing high-density lipoprotein (HDL or "good") cholesterol. Studies of HRT suggest it also has a significant "heart-protective" effect.

Because the risk of heart disease is much greater than other health risks for post-menopausal women, ERT or HRT may be a wise choice for many women.

Breast Cancer

Taking hormone therapy for up to five years *does not* appear to increase the risk of breast cancer. Longer-term use (10 to 15 years or longer) *does* appear to increase the risk.

Women who currently have breast cancer should not take ERT or HRT. Rarely, women who have had breast cancer in the past may be able to take ERT or HRT. Discuss this with your doctor.

If you choose to take hormones, it is important to get a yearly mammogram.

Endometrial (Uterine) Cancer

Estrogen alone (ERT) increases the risk of endometrial cancer (cancer of the lining of the uterus), although the risk is very low. Estrogen combined with progestin (HRT) protects against this increased risk.

Gallbladder Disease

Both ERT and HRT increase the risk of gallbladder disease.

Considerations

Hormone therapy reduces the discomfort caused by menopausal symptoms. However, ERT and HRT also have side effects that may be unacceptable to some women. They include periodic vaginal bleeding (HRT only), bloating, cramping, nausea, and breast tenderness. Your doctor may be able to ease these side effects by adjusting the dose.

To gain the long-term benefits of hormone therapy, the medications must be taken for many years. Women on long-term hormone therapy need regular visits to a health professional.

ERT and HRT must be taken daily, so you have to remember to take a pill every day (or on a specific cycle) for as long as you continue the therapy. Some forms may be available as skin patches.

Should *You* Take Hormones?

Discuss each of the above risks and benefits with your doctor. Few risks appear to be associated with short-term (up to one year) hormone therapy to relieve menopause symptoms. Long-term use reduces the risk of heart disease and osteoporosis. However, long-term use may increase the risk of breast cancer. If you are considering long-term therapy, keep the following in mind:

- If your risk for osteoporosis or heart disease is already very low, long-term hormone therapy may not give you enough additional benefits to justify the added risk and inconvenience.

- If you are at risk for osteoporosis or heart disease, the benefits of long-term therapy may outweigh the added risk and inconvenience. (If you scored over 19 on the osteoporosis risk factor scale on page 56, ERT may be particularly valuable.)

- For maximum benefit, hormone therapy should be started as soon as possible after menopause. To reduce the risk of osteoporosis, the most benefit occurs during the first five to seven years after menopause. Starting later may still provide some benefit. The risk of heart disease is reduced whenever you start taking hormones. In either case, the risk begins to increase again if hormone therapy is stopped.

Who Should *Not* Take Hormones?

Hormone therapy is not usually recommended for women who have had breast cancer, trouble with blood clots, liver disease, or undiagnosed vaginal bleeding.

Vaginitis and Yeast Infections

Vaginitis is a general term for any vaginal infection, inflammation, or irritation that causes a change in the normal vaginal discharge. It is a common problem, and some women are more susceptible than others. Postmenopausal women, who have lower estrogen levels, are more prone to vaginitis. An aggravating fact about vaginitis is that it can recur.

Symptoms include a marked change in the amount, color, odor, or consistency of the discharge, genital itching, painful urination, and pain during sexual intercourse. Common types of vaginitis include yeast infection, bacterial vaginosis, and atrophic vaginitis (see page 236). If you have burning and pain on urination and feel the need to urinate frequently, see Urinary Tract Infections on page 139.

Irritation caused by frequent douching, tight clothing, or use of strong soaps or perfumed feminine hygiene products may contribute to vaginal infections. Diabetes and the use of antibiotics or corticosteroids also increase the risk of vaginitis. Some types of sexually transmitted diseases can cause an unusual vaginal discharge (see page 261), but vaginitis is not usually a symptom of a sexually transmitted disease.

Yeast infections (candidiasis) are the most common kind of vaginitis among older women. A yeast infection is an excess growth of yeast organisms in the vagina due to an imbalance among the normal organisms in the vagina.

Yeast infections can cause severe discomfort but rarely cause serious problems. Common symptoms of yeast infections include itching (often severe) in the genital area; white, curdy, usually odorless vaginal discharge; painful urination; and pain during sexual intercourse.

Yeast infections are commonly associated with antibiotic or steroid use, diabetes, and illnesses that impair the immune system.

Prevention

- Wear cotton underpants. The organisms that cause vaginitis grow best in warm, moist places, and nylon underpants tend to trap heat and perspiration. Avoid clothing that is tight in the crotch and thighs.

- Wash your genital area once a day with a mild, non-perfumed soap. Rinse well and dry thoroughly. Avoid douching.

- Avoid feminine deodorant sprays and other perfumed products. They irritate tender skin.

- Wipe from front to back after using the toilet to avoid spreading bacteria from the anus to the vagina.

- Eat a cup of yogurt that contains live *Lactobacillus* organisms each day. They help restore the normal balance in the vagina and may help prevent a yeast infection. This is especially helpful if you are taking antibiotics.

- It is not clear whether a high-sugar diet may increase the risk of yeast infections, but limiting your sugar intake may help.

Home Treatment

- Bacterial vaginosis may go away by itself in three to four days. If symptoms persist, call your doctor.

- Avoid sexual intercourse for two weeks to give irritated vaginal tissues time to heal.

- Avoid scratching. Use cold water compresses to relieve itching.

- Use an over-the-counter medication for yeast infections (Gyne-Lotrimin, Monistat 7) as directed. Be sure your symptoms are due to a yeast infection before you begin self-treatment. If symptoms persist, call your doctor.

When to Call a Health Professional

- If you have pelvic or lower abdominal pain, fever, and unusual vaginal discharge.

- If you think you have a yeast infection for the first time, or if you aren't sure whether your symptoms are due to a yeast infection.

- If home treatment with an over-the-counter product fails to clear up a yeast infection within three to four days, or if you are using antifungal creams repeatedly.

- If you have pain with intercourse that is not eased by use of a vaginal lubricant.

- If any unusual discharge lasts more than two weeks.

If you plan to see a health professional, do not douche, use vaginal creams, or have intercourse for 48 hours or longer before your appointment, because they may make the diagnosis difficult.

Women's Cancers

Cancer of the breast and of the female reproductive organs can often be detected early by regular screening exams, such as mammograms, Pap tests, and pelvic exams. See pages 233 to 235 for information on these screening tests, including how often they are recommended. When detected early, women's cancers can often be treated successfully.

The main risk factors for each type of cancer are listed on page 244. If you have risk factors for a particular cancer, discuss with your doctor whether you should have more frequent screening tests.

Breast Cancer

Breast cancer is the second leading cause of cancer deaths in women. By age 85, one out of every nine women will have developed breast cancer. However, breast cancer is highly treatable if it is detected early. Regular mammograms (page 233) are very effective in detecting breast cancer early. Monthly breast self-exams are also important (page 231). Because most cases of breast cancer occur in women who don't have any known risk factors, regular screening is important.

Hysterectomy Guidelines

A hysterectomy is the surgical removal of the uterus. It is sometimes needed to save a woman's life. However, it is often performed unnecessarily. Hysterectomy is often the best solution for:

- Endometrial or cervical cancer
- Severe uterine bleeding of unknown cause
- Ovarian cancer
- Large fibroids with severe bleeding and pain
- Severe prolapse of the uterus
- Severe and recurrent pelvic inflammatory disease (PID)

Hysterectomy is generally *not* the best solution for:

- Non-invasive cervical cancer before menopause
- Fibroids with mild or no symptoms
- Endometriosis without severe symptoms
- Prolapsed uterus that responds to exercise and other treatments
- Pelvic inflammatory disease that responds to other treatments
- Abnormal uterine bleeding

The guidelines above may not apply to you. Work with your doctor to decide if a hysterectomy is the best solution for your problem.

Cervical Cancer

The cervix is the opening to the uterus, sometimes called the "neck of the womb." The Pap test (page 235) is very effective in detecting cervical cancer early. When it is detected early, cervical cancer is often curable.

Endometrial Cancer

Endometrial (uterine) cancer affects the lining of the uterus. It can be successfully treated if it is detected early. Irregular vaginal bleeding may be a warning sign. The Pap test can detect some cases. Pelvic exams are also important. Estrogen-only replacement therapy (ERT) increases the risk of endometrial cancer (see page 239). Women who take ERT and who have a uterus may have small tissue samples taken from their uterine lining (endometrial biopsy) to check for cancerous changes once a year.

Ovarian Cancer

Ovarian cancer is the second most common cancer of the female reproductive organs. It may be detected with regular pelvic exams. When detected early, it may be successfully treated. Unfortunately, it is difficult to detect until it has spread.

Home Treatment

Good home care can help you stay in a positive frame of mind, which will make your treatment as effective as possible.

Risk Factors for Women's Cancers				
Risk Factor	**Breast Cancer**	**Cervical Cancer**	**Endometrial Cancer**	**Ovarian Cancer**
Family history of cancer (mother, sister, or aunt)	✓			✓
Breast cancer				✓
Menstruation before age 11	✓		✓	
Intercourse before age 18		✓		
Never having children or having the first child after age 30	✓			✓
History of infertility			✓	
History of multiple sex partners		✓		
Genital warts (HPV infection)		✓		
Late menopause (after age 55)	✓		✓	
Estrogen replacement Long-term or high-dose therapy*	✓		✓	
Obesity*			✓	
Cigarette smoking*		✓		
*Risks that can be changed.				

Some risk factors are more significant than others. If you have any of the risk factors above, ask your doctor to assess your risk of cancer. Work together to develop a screening schedule that takes your individual situation into account.

- See "Winning Over Serious Illness" on page 376.

- Take good care of your mental health. Depression is a common response to a diagnosis of cancer.

- Learn as much as you can about different treatment options. Work with your doctor to develop a treatment plan that will best meet your needs and desires. If you are not comfortable with the treatment options offered, ask your doctor about other options or consider a second opinion.

- If surgery is suggested, see page 10 for questions you may want to ask your doctor.

When to Call a Health Professional

Talk with your doctor about the best schedule of screening tests for you. Screening tests for women's cancers include mammograms, Pap tests, and pelvic exams.

Screening tests do not prevent cancer. However, many cancers can be treated more successfully if they are detected early.

*My doctor says I'm on the verge of
becoming an old man. I place no stock in that.
I've been on the verge of becoming an angel all my life.*
Mark Twain

16
Men's Health

At first glance, men appear to be at a great disadvantage when it comes to life expectancy. On average, women outlive men by seven years. In fact, by age 75 only two men are alive for every three women. Health problems such as heart disease, emphysema, cirrhosis, lung cancer, and fatal accidents are much more common in men than in women.

However, there is some good news lurking behind these facts. Most of the health problems that rob men of their years can be prevented or successfully managed with simple lifestyle changes. There is no hormonal cause for cigarette smoking, heavy drinking, lack of exercise, or not using seat belts. These are habits that can be unlearned the same way they were learned. If you can identify any life-shortening habits and work

on developing healthy practices, you will likely add years to your life and surely add life to your years.

This chapter covers health problems that are of particular concern to men.

Baldness

Heredity is the biggest factor in determining when you will begin to lose your hair, but age comes in a strong second. By age 60, most men have some degree of baldness. Natural hair loss cannot be prevented.

Hair loss can also be caused or accelerated by a variety of medications. These include some drugs for high blood pressure, high cholesterol, arthritis, and ulcers, as well as cancer chemotherapy.

Baldness increases the risk of sunburn and skin cancer on the scalp. Wear a hat or use a sunscreen with an SPF of 15 or more. Bumps on the head can be more painful when you have less hair to cushion the blow.

When to Call a Health Professional

• If your hair loss is sudden, rather than gradual.

• If spots of baldness appear, rather than symmetrical, localized thinning.

• If a rash or scaliness on your scalp occurs with hair loss.

• If you are concerned that hair loss may be a side effect of medication. Ask your doctor or pharmacist if the medication could be the cause.

Erection Problems

Erection problems are common and can often be solved with self-care. As a man ages, the speed of his sexual response slows, his drive to reach orgasm is delayed, and the force of his orgasm gradually lessens. This is normal. These physical changes need not be seen as problems. In many cases, they can prolong sensual enjoyment prior to orgasm.

An erection problem, sometimes called impotence, is a *persistent* difficulty in achieving or maintaining an erection capable of intercourse. Note the word persistent; occasional episodes of impotence are perfectly normal and are nothing to worry about.

One out of every four men experiences a significant erection problem by age 65. However, it is not an inevitable part of getting older. Although occasional erection problems are common, there is no age limit to the ability of healthy men to have erections.

Many erection problems have at least some physical cause. Diabetes, heart and circulation problems, medication side effects, alcohol and drug abuse, and other physical problems contribute to impotence.

In other cases, erection problems can be traced to psychological factors, such as stress, anxiety, grief, depression, and negative feelings. Psychological and physical causes interact. Stress or anxiety will often combine with a minor physical problem to cause an erection problem. Worrying about the erection problem increases the likelihood that it will happen again.

If a physical cause for an erection problem can't be found, psychological counseling may help. After all other options have been tried for several months without success, you may wish to talk with your doctor about erection-producing injections or a vacuum device. A penile implant may be appropriate as a last resort.

Prevention

Erection problems can usually be prevented by taking a more relaxed approach to lovemaking and watching for possible side effects from medications or illnesses.

Home Treatment

- Rule out medications first. Many drugs have side effects that can cause erection problems, especially blood pressure medicines, diuretics, and mood-altering drugs. Look up the side effects of your medications (see Resource 2 on page 418). If an erection problem may be a drug side effect, discuss it with your doctor. An alternative medication may be an option. Do not stop taking any medication without talking to your doctor.

- Avoid alcohol. Even small amounts of alcohol can cause temporary impotence. Alcohol also interacts with many medications.

- Don't smoke. Smoking reduces blood flow, which can interfere with your ability to have an erection.

- Take time for more foreplay. Let your partner know that you would enjoy more stroking. Slow down; then slow down some more.

- Relax. If you experience occasional bouts of impotence, worrying about how you will perform next time may only aggravate the problem.

- Make sure you're ready. If you are grieving over a loss, you may not be ready for erections and intercourse. Give yourself some time.

- Find out if you can have erections at other times. If you can have an erection on awakening, or at other times, the problem may be stress-related or due to an emotional problem.

When to Call a Health Professional

- If you think that a medication may be causing the problem. Substitutes may be available.

- If there is a loss of pubic or armpit hair and your breasts enlarge.

- If a few months of home treatment has not brought relief, see your doctor to discuss treatment options.

Genital Health

Daily cleaning of the penis, particularly under the foreskin of an uncircumcised penis, can prevent bacterial infection and reduce the already low risk of penile cancer. Because the risk of testicular cancer is very low in older men, testicular self-exams are usually not recommended after age 50.

Experts do not agree on the most appropriate schedule of screening tests for prostate cancer. See page 254.

When to Call a Health Professional

- If you notice any new lumps, nodules, or unexplained enlargement in the testicles, or if a lump is getting larger or changing.

- If you have unexplained groin pain.

- If you notice any penile discharge. Also see page 261.

Hernias

A hernia occurs when part of the intestine bulges out through a weak spot in the abdominal wall. Hernias are more common in men but do occur in women. They commonly occur in the groin and may bulge into the scrotum. An inguinal hernia occurs when a part of the intestine protrudes down the inguinal canal, which leads from the abdomen to the scrotum.

Hernias are often caused by a weakness in the abdominal wall. They may be made worse by increased

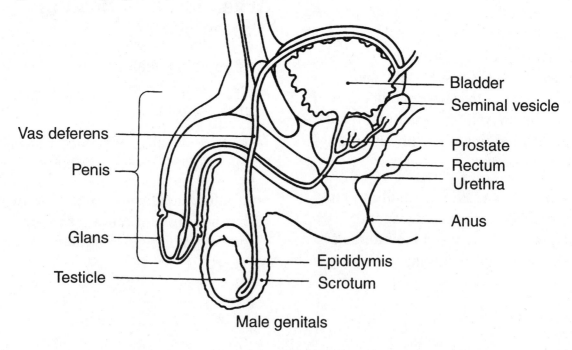

Male genitals

abdominal pressure resulting from lifting heavy weights, coughing, or straining during a bowel movement.

The symptoms of a hernia may come on suddenly or gradually. There may be a feeling that something has given way and varying amounts of pain. Symptoms may include:

- Feeling of weakness, pressure, burning, or pain in the groin or scrotum.

- A bulge or lump in the groin or scrotum. The bulge may be easier to see when the person coughs and may disappear when he lies down.

- Pain in the groin when straining, lifting, or coughing.

(Symptoms of a hernia in women are the same and may occur in the groin or lower abdomen just above the crease of the thigh.)

A hernia is called reducible if the bulge can be pushed back into place inside the abdomen. If a hernia becomes trapped outside the abdominal wall, it is said to be irreducible or incarcerated. If the blood supply to the tissue is cut off, it is said to be strangulated, and the tissue will swell and die. The dead tissue quickly becomes infected. Rapidly increasing pain in the groin or scrotum is a sign that a hernia has become strangulated. Immediate medical attention is needed.

Prevention

- Use proper lifting techniques (see page 31) and avoid lifting weights that are too heavy for you.

- Avoid constipation and do not strain during bowel movements and urination.

- Stop smoking, especially if you have a chronic cough.

When to Call a Health Professional

If you have been diagnosed with a hernia, call a health professional immediately:

- If you experience sudden, severe increasing pain in the area of the hernia, scrotum, or groin.

- If the hernia cannot be reduced with gentle pressure when lying down.

- If there are signs of a blockage in the intestine, such as vomiting or inability to pass stools or gas.

Call a health professional:

- If you suspect a hernia, to confirm the diagnosis and discuss treatment options. Not all hernias require surgery.

- If mild groin pain or an unexplained groin bump or swelling continues for more than one week.

Prostate Problems

The prostate is a doughnut-shaped gland that lies at the bottom of the bladder, about halfway between the rectum and the base of the penis. It encircles the urethra, the tube that carries urine from the bladder out through the penis. This walnut-sized gland produces some of the fluid that transports sperm during ejaculation.

The three most common prostate problems in older men are: prostate enlargement, prostate cancer, and prostate infection (prostatitis).

Prostate Enlargement (Benign Prostatic Hypertrophy)

As men age, the prostate may enlarge. This seems to be a natural process and is not really a disease. However, as the gland gets bigger, it tends to squeeze the urethra and cause urinary problems, such as:

- Difficulty in getting urine started and completely stopped (dribbling)

- The urge to urinate frequently, or being awakened by the urge to urinate

- Decreased force of urine stream

- Painful urination

- Incomplete emptying of the bladder

An enlarged prostate gland is not a serious problem unless urination becomes extremely difficult or backed-up urine causes bladder infections or kidney damage. Some dribbling after urination is very common and not necessarily a sign of prostate problems.

Surgery is usually not necessary for an enlarged prostate. Although surgery used to be a common treatment, research shows that most cases of prostate enlargement do not get worse over time. Many men find that their symptoms are stable and sometimes even clear up on their own. In these cases, the best treatment may often be no treatment at all.

Drugs are available that may help improve symptoms in some men. Your doctor can advise you on the various treatment options.

Prevention

- Since the prostate produces seminal fluid, a long-standing belief exists that regular ejaculations (two to three times per week) will help prevent an enlarged prostate. There is no scientific evidence of this, but it is without risk.

Home Treatment

- Avoid antihistamines and decongestants, which can make urinary
  problems worse.

- If you are bothered by a frequent
  need to urinate at night, cut down
  on beverages before bedtime,
  especially alcohol and caffeine.

- Don't postpone urinating, and take
  plenty of time. Try sitting on the
  toilet instead of standing.

- If dribbling after urination is a
  problem, wash your penis once a
  day to prevent skin infections.

- See Urinary Incontinence on
  page 137.

When to Call a Health Professional

- If fever, chills, or back or abdominal
  pain develops. Also see Prostate
  Infection on page 254.

- If the symptoms of an enlarged
  prostate come on quickly, are bothersome enough that you want help,
  or last longer than two months.
  Early examination allows you to be
  sure of the diagnosis.

- Diuretics, tranquilizers, antihistamines, and antidepressants can
  aggravate urinary problems. If you
  take these drugs, ask your doctor if
  there are alternative medications that
  do not worsen urinary problems.

Prostate Cancer

Prostate cancer is the most common
cancer and the second leading cause
of cancer deaths in men. However, it
is usually a small and slow-growing
cancer. Risk increases with age, and
most cases are in men over 65. Since
it usually develops late in life and
grows slowly, it usually does not
shorten a man's life. However, when
it is large, advanced, or develops at a
younger age, it can be very serious.
When detected early, before it has
spread to other organs, the cancer
may be curable.

There are no early symptoms of
prostate cancer. Most men have no
symptoms at all. In some cases, it can
cause urinary symptoms very similar
to those of prostate enlargement. In
advanced cases, other symptoms may
be caused by spread of the cancer to
other organs or to the bones.

Risk factors for prostate cancer
include family history and a high-fat
diet. Black men are at increased risk.

Prevention

Maintaining a low-fat diet is the
only known way to reduce the risk
of prostate cancer.

Home Treatment

Prostate cancer treatment is tailored to each individual. Work with your doctor to be sure that you will receive long-term benefit from treatment.

Learn all you can about the available treatment options, which may include watchful waiting, so that you and your doctor can select the one best suited for you. Your age, overall health, other medical conditions, and the characteristics of the cancer are all important factors to consider in making treatment decisions.

See "Winning Over Serious Illness" on page 376.

When to Call a Health Professional

• If any urinary symptoms come on quickly, are bothersome enough that you want help, or last longer than two months. Early evaluation allows you to be sure of the diagnosis and consider treatment options.

There are mixed opinions about the value of using digital rectal (prostate) exams and the prostate-specific antigen (PSA) blood test to screen for prostate cancer in men who do not have any urinary symptoms. Detecting and treating early prostate cancer has not been shown to improve the quality of life or to prolong life.

Therefore, many experts are uncertain whether routine rectal exams or PSA tests are appropriate for all men.

Talk with your doctor for more information about screening.

Prostate Infection (Prostatitis)

There are two types of prostate infections: chronic and acute. Chronic infections are more common, and symptoms may include:

• Pain and burning on urination and ejaculation

• A strong and frequent urge to urinate while passing only small amounts of urine

• Lower back or abdominal pain

• Blood in the urine (occasionally)

Acute prostatitis comes on suddenly and occurs with fever and chills in addition to some or all of the symptoms of a chronic infection. Either infection may occur with a urinary tract infection. See page 139.

Prostate infections will usually respond well to home care and antibiotics. If the infection recurs, long-term antibiotics may be necessary.

Prevention

- Drink plenty of fluids, both water and fruit juices. Extra fluids help flush bacteria from the urinary tract. Try to drink two quarts a day.

- Avoid alcohol and caffeine. Caffeine can cause a strong and frequent urge to urinate. Remember that colas, coffee, and tea contain caffeine.

- Keep stress under control. A high level of stress may be associated with prostate infections.

Home Treatment

- Drink as much water as you can tolerate.

- Eliminate all alcohol and caffeine from your diet.

- Hot baths help soothe pain and reduce stress.

- Aspirin or ibuprofen may help ease painful urinary symptoms.

When to Call a Health Professional

- If urinary symptoms occur with fever, chills, vomiting, or pain in the lower back or abdomen.

- If there is blood in the urine.

- If your symptoms get worse.

- If you have pain on urination or ejaculation and a discharge from your penis.

- If new urinary symptoms continue for more than two days despite home care.

- If any chronic urinary symptom has not been evaluated by a doctor.

Age may well offer the opportunity to understand sex
as intimate communication in its finest sense.
Norman M. Lobsenz

17

Sexual Health

Sex and sexuality communicate a great deal: affection, love, esteem, warmth, sharing, and bonding. These gifts are as much the birthright of those in their 80s and 90s as those who are much younger.

Three aspects of sexuality are covered in this chapter: the changes that come with aging, suggestions on how to adjust to these changes, and information about sexual health problems.

Sexuality and Physical Changes With Aging

In most healthy adults, pleasure and interest in sex do not diminish with age. Age alone is no reason to change the sexual practices that you have enjoyed throughout your life. However, sexual response does slow down as you age, and you may have to make a few minor adjustments.

Common Physical Changes in Men

• It may take longer to get an erection, and more time needs to pass between erections.

• Erections will be less firm. However, a man with good blood flow to his penis will be able to have erections that are firm enough for intercourse for his entire life. For information on erection problems, see page 248.

• Older men are able to delay ejaculation for a longer time.

Common Physical Changes in Women

Most physical changes take place after menopause and are due to lower estrogen levels. These changes can be altered if a woman is taking hormone replacement therapy.

- It may take longer to become sexually excited.

- Skin may feel more sensitive and irritable, making caressing and skin-to-skin contact less pleasurable.

- The walls of the vagina become thinner and drier and are more easily irritated during intercourse. (Use a water-based vaginal lubricant or K-Y Jelly to reduce the irritation. Do not use petroleum jelly. Your doctor can also prescribe a vaginal cream containing estrogen, which will help reverse the changes in the vaginal tissues.)

- Orgasms may be somewhat shorter than they used to be and the contractions experienced during orgasm can be uncomfortable.

Sexuality and Cultural and Psychological Changes

In addition to physical changes that affect sexuality in later years, there are cultural and psychological factors too. Take ageism, for example. In our culture, sexuality is equated with youthful looks and youthful vigor. Too many people seem to think that as a person ages, he or she becomes less desirable and less of a sexual being. Older adults may accept this stereotype and buy into the notion that they are not permitted or expected to be sexual.

Joy in sex and loving knows no age barriers. Almost everyone has the capacity to find lifelong pleasure in sex. To believe in the myth that "old people have no interest in sex" is to miss out on wonderful possibilities.

Being single through choice, divorce, or widowhood can present a problem as well. By the time you reach age 60, there are five single women for every single man, and that ratio goes up with increasing years. Women and men who are single may not know how to deal with their sexual feelings. Generally speaking, it is better to take some risks and express your desires than to suppress them until you are no longer aware that they exist.

Physical and emotional needs change with time and circumstance. Intimacy and sexuality may or may not be important to you. The issue here is one of choice. If you freely decide that sex is no longer right for you, then that is the correct decision. It is possible to live a fulfilling life without sex. However, if you choose to continue enjoying your sexuality, you deserve support and encouragement. You may still find uncharted sensual territories to explore.

Use It or Lose It: Keeping Sexual

Just as exercise is the key to maintaining fitness, sexual activity on a regular basis is the best way to maintain sexual capacity. On the other hand, it is never too late to get started. Many older people who have been celibate for years develop satisfying sexual practices within new loving relationships. For others, self-stimulation is common and poses no health risks or side effects.

Other considerations:

- To enhance sexual response, use more foreplay and direct contact with sexual organs.

- The mind is an erogenous zone. Fantasy and imagination help arouse some people. Try setting the mood with candlelight and soft music, or whatever else "turns you on."

- Many medications, especially high blood pressure medications, tranquilizers, and some heart medications, inhibit sexual response. Check with your doctor about lower doses or alternative medications.

- Colostomies, mastectomies, and other operations that involve changes in physical appearance need not put an end to sexual pleasure. Communicating openly about your fears and expectations can bring you and your partner closer together and help you overcome barriers. If necessary, a little counseling for both of you can help you adjust.

- People with heart conditions can enjoy full, satisfying sexual lives. Most doctors recommend that you abstain from sex for only a brief time following a heart attack. If you have angina, ask your doctor about taking nitroglycerine before sexual intercourse.

- If arthritis keeps you from enjoying sex, experiment with different positions. Try placing cushions under hips. Also work to relieve arthritis pain. See page 45.

- Drink alcohol only in moderation. Small amounts may heighten sexual responsiveness by squelching inhibitions. Larger amounts may increase sexual desire, but they decrease sexual performance.

Other Aspects of Sexuality

Sexuality goes far beyond the physical act itself. It is part of who we are. It involves our needs for touch, affection, and intimacy.

Touch

Touch is a wonderful and needed sense. Babies who are not touched do not thrive. Children who are not touched develop emotional problems. Touch is important to older adults as well. Touch helps us feel connected with others and enhances our sexuality.

- Get a massage. Professional massages are wonderful, but simple shoulder and neck rubs feel great too. Find a friend who will trade shoulder rubs with you. See page 367 for instructions.

- Look for hugs. Everybody needs them. Some people are a little shy about hugs, but it's okay to ask, "Would you like a hug?"

- Consider getting a pet. Caring for a pet can help meet your needs for touch. Some studies have shown that older people who have pets to care for live longer.

Affection

To give and receive affection is a wonderful feeling. If you like someone, be sure to let them know. If someone seems to like you, appreciate it. It is never too late to make new friends and strengthen bonds with longtime companions.

Intimacy

Intimacy is the capacity for a close physical or emotional connection with another person. Intimacy is a great protector against depression.

Talking with a confidant can help ease life's problems. When you lose

a loved one, intimacy may be what you miss most. You may not find someone to fully replace a loved one who died, but you can begin to rebuild intimacy in your life in the following ways:

- Turn to your children, siblings, or old and new friends.

- Look for another person in your same situation. One of the richest benefits of support groups is that members often find intimacy with one another.

- Be available to others. Just as you need people, there are people who need you too.

Sexually Transmitted Diseases

Sexually transmitted diseases (STDs) or venereal diseases (VD) are infections passed from person to person through sexual intercourse or genital contact. Chlamydia, gonorrhea, genital herpes, genital warts, and syphilis are among the most common STDs. AIDS (acquired immune deficiency syndrome), which can affect men and women of all ages, is discussed on page 263.

Chlamydia (kla-MID-ee-uh) is a disease that infects millions of men and women each year. It may be difficult to detect chlamydia since about 80 percent of women and 10 percent of men with the disease have no symptoms.

If symptoms do show up, they occur two to four weeks after exposure. In women, symptoms may include vaginal discharge, painful urination, genital itching, or lower abdominal or pelvic pain. If untreated, pelvic inflammatory disease (infection of the ovaries and fallopian tubes) may develop. In men, there may be a penile discharge and painful urination.

Chlamydia is easily treated with antibiotics.

Gonorrhea is caused by bacteria spread through sexual contact. Symptoms include painful urination, vaginal discharge, or a thick discharge from the penis. However, many people who are infected with gonorrhea have no symptoms. If untreated, gonorrhea can lead to pelvic inflammatory disease. It can sometimes spread to the joints and cause arthritis.

Genital herpes is caused by a virus that is easily spread through sexual contact and other direct skin contact. Symptoms occur two to thirty days after contact with an infected person.

The first symptoms include itching, burning, or tingling sensations in the genitals. Afterward, sores and blisters will appear on the genitals. Once

infected, you may suffer from recurrent outbreaks. Some people have the virus but do not have any symptoms.

Genital warts are caused by a virus. In women, the warts may appear on the vagina, the cervix, or around the anus. Warts on the cervix are usually detected by a Pap test (page 235). Genital warts in men are usually found on the penis or scrotum. All genital warts need to be evaluated by a health professional.

Women who have had genital herpes or genital warts are at higher risk for cervical cancer. See page 244, "Risk Factors for Women's Cancers."

Syphilis is a bacterial infection that is spread through sexual contact. Symptoms appear two weeks to one month after contact. The first symptom is a small red blister, ulcer, or sore (chancre) that appears on the genitals, anal area, or mouth. This sore is painless and may go unnoticed. The lymph nodes in the groin may also swell.

If syphilis is not treated early, it can proceed to a second phase in two to eight weeks. Symptoms of the second phase can include skin rash, patchy hair loss, fever, swollen lymph nodes, and flu-like symptoms, which are easily confused with other illnesses.

Syphilis can be treated with antibiotics. If untreated, it can cause serious problems and premature death.

Prevention

No matter what your age, when sexual intimacy becomes part of a new relationship, you need to exercise caution to protect yourself against sexually transmitted diseases.

Preventing a sexually transmitted disease is easier than treating an infection once it occurs. Only monogamy between uninfected partners or sexual abstinence completely *eliminates* the risk.

- Use condoms with any new partner until you are certain that person does not have any sexually transmitted diseases.

- Keep in mind that a person may not have any symptoms of an STD, but he or she can still transmit the disease to you. Condoms will help prevent transmission of an STD by a person who has no visible symptoms.

- If you or your partner has herpes, avoid sexual contact when a blister is present, and use condoms at all other times.

- The same behaviors that reduce your risk of HIV infection also reduce your risk of getting other STDs. See page 264 for additional prevention guidelines, including condom use.

When to Call a Health Professional

If you notice any unusual vaginal or penile discharge, sores, redness, or growths on the genitals, or if you suspect that you have been exposed to an STD, make an appointment as soon as possible. Avoid sexual contact while waiting for an appointment.

All STDs need to be diagnosed and treated by a health professional. Your sexual partner will probably need to be treated as well even if he or she has no symptoms. Otherwise, your partner may reinfect you or become ill from the untreated infection.

Symptoms such as vaginal or penile discharge and irritation may also simply be normal changes associated with aging. Consider whether you may have been exposed to an STD, and if you have any concerns, talk with your doctor.

HIV Infection and AIDS

About 10 percent of the AIDS (acquired immune deficiency syndrome) cases reported in the United States involve people over age 50. AIDS is caused by the human immunodeficiency virus (HIV). HIV destroys the immune system, making it impossible for the body to fight off disease. This leads to AIDS and its associated complications.

HIV spreads when blood, semen, or other body fluids from an infected person enter the body of someone else. HIV infection is not easy to catch. It is *not* spread by mosquito bites, dirty toilets, being coughed on or touched by an infected person, or by donating blood. In older adults, HIV infection is most commonly spread through:

- Blood transfusions, especially those that were received before donated blood was tested for the HIV virus. Because all blood and blood products are now tested for the HIV virus, the risk of getting HIV from blood transfusions is very low.

- Unprotected sexual intercourse or oral sexual contact with an infected person.

The HIV virus can also be spread by sharing injection needles and syringes with someone who is HIV-positive.

A simple, confidential blood test can determine if you are HIV-positive (meaning your body has developed antibodies to the virus). It can take up to six months after infection for HIV antibodies to develop. The virus can be transmitted to someone else before antibodies have developed.

Older adults who become infected with HIV become ill and tend to progress to AIDS faster than those who are younger.

Symptoms of HIV infection and AIDS

There are few early symptoms of HIV infection. Common symptoms of later HIV infection are:

- Rapid, unexplained weight loss

- Persistent, unexplained fever and night sweats

- Persistent, severe fatigue

- Persistent diarrhea

- Swelling of glands in the neck, armpits, and groin

As the immune system breaks down, a variety of other symptoms may appear, including:

- Unusual sores on the skin or in the mouth; white patches in the mouth

- Increased outbreaks of cold sores

- Unexplained shortness of breath and dry cough

- Severe numbness or pain in the hands and feet

- Personality changes or mental deterioration

- Unusual cancers and infections

These symptoms can be caused by many illnesses other than HIV infection or AIDS. However, if any symptom develops or persists without a good explanation, especially if your behavior puts you at risk of HIV infection, call your doctor.

Prevention

Only monogamous sexual relations between uninfected partners or sexual abstinence completely *eliminates* the risk of HIV and other sexually transmitted diseases. The following actions will *reduce* your risk:

- Use condoms with any new partner until you are certain that he or she does not have any STDs. Remember, it can take up to six months for antibodies to the HIV virus to develop and be detected in the blood. The virus can still be spread to another person during this time.

- Keep in mind that a person may not have any symptoms of an STD, including HIV infection, but he or she can still transmit the disease to you. Condoms will help prevent transmission of an STD by a person who has no visible symptoms.

- Use latex condoms from the beginning to the end of sexual contact. "Natural" or lambskin condoms do not prevent against HIV infection. For even greater protection, use a spermicide in addition to condoms. Apply the spermicide directly into the vagina, not into the condom.

- Do not rely on spermicides to protect against STDs. They add some protection when used with a condom but do not provide adequate protection when used alone. They do not protect against HIV.

- Never share toothbrushes, razors, needles, syringes, or other personal items that could be contaminated with blood.

- For more information, call the National AIDS Hotline at 1-800-342-AIDS.

It is by the presence of mind in untried emergencies that the native metal of a man (or woman) is tested.
James Russell Lowell

18

Injury Prevention and First Aid

What can you do to avoid injuries and be prepared for emergencies?

- Read this chapter before you need it. Review the symptoms of heart attack and stroke in Chapter 6 so that you will recognize them if they occur and be ready to take action. Consider taking a CPR and first aid class in your community.

- Keep a well-stocked first aid kit at home and in your car. See "Self-Care Supplies" on page 414.

- Know who to call in an emergency. Keep the numbers next to every phone.

- If you live alone, keep in touch with neighbors, relatives, or friends every day. Ask them to check up on you if they haven't heard from you.

- Wear a medical bracelet or necklace that gives information about any medical conditions or drug

allergies you have and any medications you are taking.

What to Do in an Emergency

If you are faced with an emergency, try to stay calm. Take a deep breath and count to 10. Tell yourself you can handle the situation.

- First, protect yourself and the injured person from any immediate dangers such as fire or an explosion.

- If you think the person might have a back or neck injury, do not try to move him unless the danger is great.

- Check the injured person for the ABCs: Airway, Breathing, and Circulation (see page 100). If the person is not breathing, call 911 or emergency services. If you have taken a CPR course, do rescue breathing.

- Treat life-threatening injuries like bleeding (page 274) or shock (page 291) first. Check for broken bones (page 292) and other injuries.

- If there are any serious injuries, call 911 or emergency services. Give them complete information about the situation: what happened, where it happened, and the injuries that occurred.

Injury Prevention

Accidents do happen, but they don't have to happen to you. Ninety-five percent of all injuries to older adults involve automobile accidents, fires, and falls. Follow these safety precautions to accident-proof yourself and your home.

Automobile Safety Checklist

❐ Always wear a seat belt, even if your auto has air bags.

❐ Never drink and drive.

❐ Check with your doctor or pharmacist about driving while on medications, especially if you take insulin or an oral hypoglycemic medication. Medications, including some over-the-counter drugs, can cause drowsiness, impaired judgment, and balance problems.

❐ Drive only in areas where you are comfortable driving. Keep trips short and try to avoid heavy traffic times.

❐ Be sure that your car is properly tuned and equipped with emergency supplies.

❐ Practice the flexibility exercises on pages 330 to 339 so you can get the widest range of vision possible.

❐ Consider updating your driving skills by taking a driver's safety course. (AARP offers a good one.)

❐ Check and correct your vision regularly.

❐ Wear good (quality) sunglasses to reduce glare.

❐ If your night vision is limited, avoid night driving.

❐ If your hearing is limited, keep a window open and the radio volume low.

Fire Safety Checklist

❐ Install smoke alarms outside bedrooms, at least one per floor.

❐ Keep multipurpose fire extinguishers in the kitchen and near fireplaces or woodstoves.

❐ Replace frayed or damaged electrical cords.

❐ Remove cords from under rugs and furniture.

❐ Do not nail or staple electrical cords. If a cord has a nail through it, throw the cord away.

❐ Remove electrical wires that are near tubs, showers, and sinks.

❐ Install special safety outlets in your bathroom. Ask for a ground fault circuit interrupter.

❐ Never smoke in bed or when you are sleepy.

❐ Have a plan for leaving your home in case of a fire. Practice it.

❐ Don't tuck electric blankets in or cover them with other blankets. Turn the temperature down before you go to bed.

❐ Avoid small electric, kerosene, and propane heaters. If you must use them, keep them away from curtains, rugs, and furniture.

❐ Follow building codes for installing wood stoves and fireplace inserts.

❐ Clean wood stove and fireplace chimneys at least annually.

❐ Keep towels away from the kitchen stovetop.

❐ Roll up loose, long sleeves when cooking.

❐ Select stovetop controls that clearly show when the burners are on.

❐ To avoid burns, set water heaters at 120° or lower.

Fall Prevention Checklist

❐ Have a lamp or light switch that you can easily reach without getting out of bed.

❐ Use night lights in the bedroom, bathroom, and hallways.

❐ Keep a flashlight handy.

❐ Have light switches at both ends of stairs and halls. Install handrails on both sides of stairs.

❐ Turn on the lights when you go into the house at night.

❐ Add grab bars in shower, tub, and toilet areas.

❐ Use bathmats with suction cups.

❐ Use non-slip adhesive strips or a mat in the shower or tub.

❐ Consider sitting on a bench or stool in the shower.

❐ Consider using an elevated toilet seat.

❐ Wear non-slip, low-heeled shoes or slippers that fit snugly. Don't walk around in stocking feet.

☐ Keep telephone and electrical cords out of pathways.

☐ Tack rugs and glue vinyl flooring so they lie flat. Remove or replace rugs or runners that tend to slip, or attach non-slip backing.

☐ Make certain carpet is firmly attached to the stairs.

☐ Purchase a step stool with high and sturdy handrails. Repair or discard wobbly step stools. Do not stand on a chair to reach things. Store frequently used objects where you can reach them easily.

☐ Paint the edges of outdoor steps and any steps that are especially narrow or are higher or lower than the rest.

☐ Paint outside stairs with a mixture of sand and paint for better traction. Keep outdoor walkways clear and well lit.

☐ Keep snow and ice cleared from entrances and sidewalks.

☐ Use helping devices, such as canes, when necessary.

☐ Learn how to get out of a chair safely (see "Sofa Safety" on page 279) and lift objects correctly (see page 31).

☐ Review medications with your doctor or pharmacist. Some drugs, including over-the-counter drugs, can make you drowsy, dizzy, and unsteady.

☐ Watch your alcohol intake. More than two drinks per day can cause unsteadiness.

☐ Have your hearing and eyesight tested. Inner ear problems can affect balance. Vision problems make it difficult to see potential hazards.

☐ Exercise regularly to improve muscle flexibility and strength.

☐ If you feel dizzy or lightheaded, sit down or stay seated until your head clears. Stand up slowly to avoid unsteadiness.

For more safety information, see Resource 50 on page 422.

Bruises

Bruises (contusions) are usually caused by a bump or fall, which can rupture small blood vessels under the skin. Blood seeps into the surrounding tissues, causing the black and blue color of a bruise.

Aging and sun damage over the years weaken the tiny veins in the skin. The weakened veins are easily broken. This causes you to bruise more easily as you age. The bruises also take longer to heal.

People who take aspirin or blood thinners (anticoagulants) may bruise easily. A bruise may also develop after blood is drawn.

Home Treatment

- Apply ice or cold packs for 15-minute intervals during the first 48 hours to help vessels constrict and to reduce swelling (see page 294). The sooner you apply ice, the less bleeding and bruising will result.

- If possible, elevate the bruised area. Blood will leave the area and there will be less swelling.

- Rest the bruised area so you don't injure it further.

- If the area is still painful after 48 hours, apply heat with warm towels, a hot water bottle, or a heating pad.

- If you bruise easily, ask your doctor or pharmacist to review your medications to see if bruising may be a side effect.

When to Call a Health Professional

- If you suspect a medication may be causing bruises.

- If the following signs of infection develop:

  o Increased pain, swelling, redness, or tenderness

  o Heat or red streaks extending from the area

  o Discharge of pus

  o Fever of 100° or higher with no other cause

- If you suddenly begin to bruise easily or if you have unexplained recurrent or multiple bruises.

Burns

Burns are classified as first-, second-, or third-degree depending on their depth. A first-degree burn, such as a mild sunburn (see page 227), involves only the outer layer of skin. The skin is dry, painful, and sensitive to touch.

A second-degree burn involves several layers of skin. The skin becomes swollen, puffy, weepy, or blistered, and is very painful.

A third-degree burn involves all layers of skin and underlying tissue or organs. The skin is dry, pale white or charred black, swollen, and sometimes breaks open. Nerves are destroyed or damaged, so there may be surprisingly little pain except on the edge of the burn, where there may be a second-degree burn.

Chemical burns to the eye occur when something caustic, such as a household cleaning product, is splashed into the eye. The vapors or fumes of strong chemicals can also burn the eyes. The eye becomes red and watery and may be sensitive to light. If the damage is severe, the eye appears whitish.

Prevention

- See the Fire Safety Checklist on page 266.

If your clothing catches fire:

- Do not run, as it will fan the flames. Stop, drop, and roll on the ground to smother the flames, or smother the flames with a blanket, rug, or coat.

- Use water to douse the fire and cool the skin.

To prevent chemical burns to the eyes:

- Wear goggles or safety glasses when working with substances that may burn the eyes.

Home Treatment

- Run cold tap water over the burn for 10 to 15 minutes. Cold water is the best immediate treatment for minor burns. The cold lowers the skin temperature and lessens the severity of the burn. Do not use ice, as it may further damage the injured skin.

- Remove rings, bracelets, watches, or shoes from the burned limb. Swelling may make them difficult to remove later.

For first-degree burns and second-degree burns with intact blisters:

- Leave the burn alone for 24 hours. Don't cover the burn unless clothing rubs on it. If it rubs, cover it with a gauze pad taped well away from the burn. Do not encircle a hand, an arm, or a leg with tape. Change the bandage after 24 hours and then every two days.

- Do not put salve, butter, grease, oil, or ointment on a burn. They increase the risk of infection and don't help heal the burn.

- After two to three days of healing, the juice from an aloe leaf can soothe minor burns.

- **For minor second-degree burns**: Do not break blisters. If the blisters break, clean the area by running tap water over it. Apply an antibiotic ointment, such as Polysporin or

Bacitracin, and cover the burn with a sterile dressing. Don't touch the wound with your hands or any unsterile objects. Remove the dressing every day, clean the wound, and cover it again.

- Aspirin or ibuprofen can help relieve pain from minor burns.

Large second-degree burns and third-degree burns require immediate medical treatment. Call a health professional and apply home treatment:

- Make sure the source of the burn has been extinguished.

- Have the person lie down to prevent shock.

- Cover the burned area with a clean sheet soaked in cool water.

- Do not apply any salve or medication to the burn.

For chemical burns to the eye:

- Immediately flush the eye under running water. Open and close the eyelids (with the fingers, if necessary) to force the water to all parts of the eye.

- Continue flushing for 15 to 20 minutes or until the eye stops hurting, whichever takes longer.

- After flushing the eye, cover it with a clean bandage or cloth.

When to Call a Health Professional

Call immediately:

- For all third-degree burns.

- If in doubt as to the extent of a burn, or in doubt if it is a second- or third-degree burn.

- If a second-degree burn involves more than 10 percent of the face, hands, feet, or genitals, especially in a person who has diabetes.

- If the burn encircles an arm, a leg, or a joint or covers more than one-quarter of the thigh, lower leg, upper arm, or forearm.

- If it is an electrical burn. Electrical burns are often deeper and more extensive than they appear.

- If a chemical burn to the eye was caused by an acid (battery acid) or an alkali (drain cleaner, ammonia).

- If the following symptoms persist after you have flushed a chemical from the eye for 10 to 30 minutes:

  ○ Pain, persistent redness, discharge, or watering

  ○ Any visual impairment, such as double vision, blurring, or sensitivity to light

  ○ Colored part of the eye (iris) appears white

Call a health professional:

- If the pain lasts longer than 48 hours.

- If signs of infection develop:

  - Increased pain, swelling, redness, or tenderness

  - Heat or red streaks extending from the area

  - Discharge of pus

  - Fever of 100° or higher with no other cause

Choking

Choking is usually caused by food or an object stuck in the windpipe. A person who is choking cannot cough, talk, or breathe and may turn blue or dusky. The **Heimlich Maneuver**, described at right, can help pop out the food or object.

Prevention

- Don't drink too much alcohol before eating. It may dull your senses and you might not chew food properly or might try to swallow too large a portion of food.

- Take small bites. Cut meat into small pieces. Chew your food thoroughly.

Choking Rescue Procedure (Heimlich Maneuver)

WARNING: Do *not* begin the choking rescue procedure unless the person *cannot breathe* or is turning blue and cannot speak, and you are *certain* the person is choking.

If an object is not easily dislodged by the Heimlich maneuver or if the victim is unconscious, have someone call 911 or emergency services while you continue trying.

Adults and Children Over One Year

If victim is standing or sitting:

- Stand behind the victim and wrap your arms around her waist.

- Make a fist with one hand. Place the thumb side of your fist against her abdomen, just above the navel but well below the breastbone. See Illustration A on page 273.

- Grasp your fist with the other hand. Give a quick upward thrust into the victim's abdomen. See Illustration B on page 273. This may cause the object to pop out. Use less force for young children.

- Repeat until the object pops out or the victim loses consciousness.

- If you choke while alone, do abdominal thrusts on yourself or lean hard over the back of a chair to pop out the food.

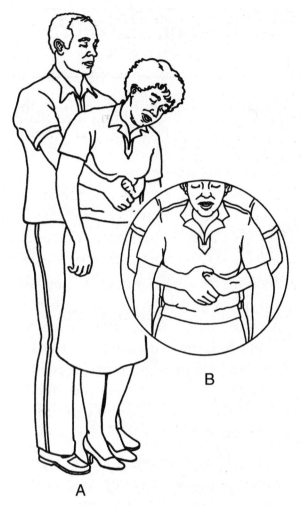

A

B

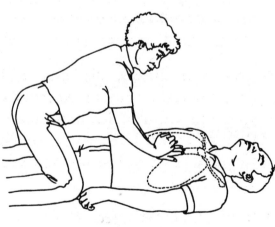

C

If victim is on the floor:

- Turn the victim face up and straddle him on your knees next to his hips.

- Place the heel of one hand against the victim's abdomen, just above the navel but well below the breastbone. Place your other hand directly over the first. See Illustration C.

- Give a quick upward thrust into the victim's abdomen. Use less force for children. Repeat until the object pops out.

If the victim loses consciousness, call 911. If you've been trained in how to do the mouth sweep, do it and continue the Heimlich maneuver.

When to Call a Health Professional

- **Call 911 or emergency services immediately if you are unable to dislodge the object or the person loses consciousness.** If you have been trained in CPR, attempt rescue breathing.

- Call a health professional if the object has been dislodged by the Heimlich maneuver or if the throat, chest, or abdomen is tender after an object has been dislodged. There could be injuries from the object or the maneuver.

Are Sutures Necessary?

To prevent infection, cuts that need stitches should be sutured within eight hours. Wash the cut well and stop the bleeding, then pinch the sides of the cut together. If it looks better, you may want to consider stitches. If stitches are needed, avoid using an antibiotic ointment until after a health professional has examined the cut.

Sutures may be needed for:

- Cuts more than ¼ inch deep that have jagged edges or gape open.

- Deep cuts on a joint: elbow, knuckle, knee.

- Deep cuts on the palm side of the hand or fingers.

- Cuts on the face, eyelids, or lips, or in an area where you are worried about scarring.

- Cuts that go down to the muscle or bone.

- Cuts that continue to bleed after 15 minutes of direct pressure.

Cuts like these that are sutured usually heal with less scarring.

Sutures may not be needed for:

- Cuts with smooth edges that tend to stay together when you move the affected body part.

- Shallow cuts less than ¼ inch deep that are less than one inch long.

Cuts and Puncture Wounds

When you have a **cut** (laceration), the first steps are to stop the bleeding and determine whether or not stitches (sutures) are needed.

If the cut is bleeding heavily or spurting blood, apply direct pressure to stop the bleeding.

Bleeding from minor cuts will usually stop on its own or with a little direct pressure. To decide whether stitches are needed, see "Are Sutures Necessary?" at left. If stitches are needed, apply home treatment and seek medical care as soon as possible, within eight hours.

If stitches are not needed, you can clean and bandage the cut at home.

Puncture wounds are caused by sharp, pointed objects that penetrate the skin. They are easily infected because they are difficult to clean.

Home Treatment

- Wash the cut well with soap and lots of water. Do not use rubbing alcohol, hydrogen peroxide, iodine, or mercurochrome, which can harm tissue and slow healing.

- Stop any bleeding from a cut by applying direct pressure with a clean cloth for 10 to 15 minutes. If blood soaks through the cloth, apply another one without lifting the first. If direct pressure does not slow or stop bleeding after 15 minutes, press firmly on a pressure point between the wound and the heart.

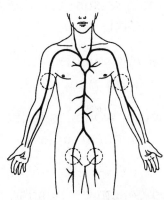

Pressure points. Press firmly to help stop bleeding.

- Leave small cuts unbandaged, unless they will become irritated. They heal best when exposed to the air.

- If a cut needs bandaging, apply antibiotic ointment (Polysporin or Bacitracin) to keep the cut from sticking to the bandage.

- Use an adhesive bandage (Band-Aid) to continue the pressure. Always put an adhesive strip across a cut rather than lengthwise. A butterfly bandage (made at home or purchased) can help hold cut skin edges together:

  - Cut a strip from a roll of one-inch adhesive tape and fold it sticky side out. Cut notches into the tape as shown in A.

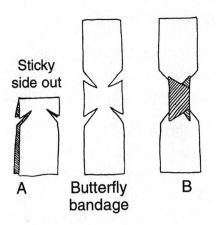

Sticky side out   A   Butterfly bandage   B

  - Unfold the tape, then fold the notched pieces together sticky side in as in B. The center of the tape will be non-sticky. Keep the part that will be over the cut clean.

  - Place one end of the tape on the skin; then pull the other end across the cut to close the wound tightly. If the cut is long, use more than one bandage.

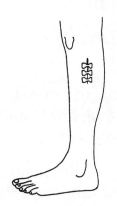

Use several butterfly bandages for a long cut.

- Apply a clean bandage at least once a day, or when it gets wet. Leave the bandage off whenever possible.

For puncture wounds:

- Make sure that nothing is left in the wound, such as the tip of a needle. Check to see if the object is intact.

- Allow the wound to bleed freely to clean itself out unless there has been a large loss of blood or the blood is squirting out. If bleeding is heavy, apply direct pressure over the wound.

- Clean the wound thoroughly with soap and water.

- For the next four to five days, soak the wound in warm water several times a day. This will clean the wound from the inside out. If the wound is closed, an infection under the skin may not be detected for several days.

When to Call a Health Professional

Call 911 or emergency services immediately:

- **If the person goes into shock, even if bleeding has stopped. See Shock on page 291.**

- **If blood flows continuously from a wound and cannot be significantly reduced or stopped with direct pressure.**

Call immediately:

- If there is blue, white, or cold skin, numbness, tingling, or loss of feeling, or if the person is unable to move a limb below the wound.

- If bleeding that can be controlled with direct pressure continues longer than one hour.

- If a cut needs stitches. They need to be done within eight hours.

- If a puncture wound is in the head, chest, or abdomen, unless it is minor.

- If a deep puncture wound to the foot occurred through a shoe.

- If you are unable to remove an object from a cut or puncture wound, or if the wound may contain a foreign object.

Call a health professional:

- If signs of infection develop:
  - Increased pain, swelling, or tenderness
  - Heat and redness or red streaks extending away from the wound
  - Discharge of pus
  - Fever of 100° or higher with no other cause

- If your tetanus shots are not up to date (see page 21), especially if an object that caused a puncture wound was dirty, such as a rusty nail or a farm implement. Call within 48 hours of the injury.

Fainting and Unconsciousness

Fainting is usually a short loss of consciousness lasting only a few seconds. It is most often due to a momentary drop in blood flow to the brain. When you fall or lie down, blood flow is improved and you regain consciousness. Fainting is usually not serious if it lasts only a few seconds and the person completely regains consciousness. If it happens more than once, there may be a more serious problem and it should be checked out by a doctor. Dizziness (page 197) and fainting can also be brought on by sudden emotional stress or injury.

An **unconscious** person is completely unaware of what is going on around him and is unable to move on his own. Fainting is a form of brief unconsciousness; a coma is a deep, prolonged state of unconsciousness.

Causes of unconsciousness include stroke, epilepsy, heat exhaustion, diabetic coma, insulin shock, head or spinal injury, suffocation, drunkenness, shock, bleeding, and heart attack.

Home Treatment

- Check the pulse. If there is none, call 911 or emergency services.

- Make sure the unconscious person can breathe. Check for breathing. If the person is not breathing and you have been trained in CPR, open the airway and begin rescue breathing.

- Keep the person lying down.

- Look for a medical identification bracelet, necklace, or card that identifies a medical problem such as epilepsy, diabetes, or drug allergy.

- Treat any injuries.

- Do not try to give the person anything to eat or drink.

When to Call a Health Professional

Call 911 or emergency services immediately:

- **If an unconscious person has no pulse.**

- **If someone has completely lost consciousness. If someone faints but immediately regains consciousness, call your doctor.**

- **If unconsciousness follows a head injury. A head injury victim needs to be carefully observed. See page 281.**

- **If a person with diabetes loses consciousness. He or she may have insulin shock (low blood sugar) or be in a diabetic coma (too much sugar in the blood).**

Call a health professional:

- If a person has fainted more than once.

Falls

Many older adults are concerned about falling. One-third of people over age 65 fall each year. Falling can cause serious injuries, especially in older adults who have weaker bones, and the injuries may take longer to heal.

Many falls are related to poor eyesight or household hazards such as loose rugs, slippery sidewalks, loose electrical cords, and dark stairways. Falls may also be caused by health problems or medications that make you dizzy, unsteady on your feet, or sleepy. Any fall that was caused by dizziness, a seizure, or loss of consciousness needs to be evaluated by a doctor.

Prevention

- Exercise regularly to keep your muscles and bones strong and flexible. This may help prevent falls and will also help you recover faster from a fall.

- Have your vision and hearing checked regularly. Also see a doctor about anything that makes it hard for you to walk, such as joint pain or foot problems.

- Talk to your doctor or pharmacist about any medications you are taking. Have a "brown bag" medication review (see page 396) to find out if any of your medications have side effects like drowsiness or dizziness.

- See "Sofa Safety" on page 279 and the Fall Prevention Checklist on page 267. Also see Vertigo and Dizziness on page 197.

Home Treatment

If you fall and you are not seriously injured, you may be able to treat yourself at home. To get up from the floor safely:

- Roll to your hands and knees and crawl to a piece of furniture that will support your weight, such as a sofa or an armchair.

- Use the furniture to pull yourself up gently. Sit for a minute before trying to stand up.

If you have any minor injuries, such as a bruise or sprain, see the home treatment in this chapter.

Sofa Safety

Many hip fractures happen when older adults with bone or joint problems get up from a sofa or low chair. To reduce your risk of falls and hip fractures, avoid sitting in sofas and chairs that put your hips lower than your knees. Get up from a sofa or chair in the following way:

1. If you are getting up from a sofa, sit next to the arm rest. If the chair has arms, use them for support.

2   Before standing up, put your feet parallel, with your toes pointing straight ahead.

3. Stand slowly, using the arm rest to help you. If the chair doesn't have arm rests, use the edge of the chair.

4. Hold on to the chair or sofa until you have your balance.

When to Call a Health Professional

Call 911 or emergency services immediately:

- **If a person remains unconscious after a fall.**

- **If a person is having a seizure that is not stopping.**

Call immediately:

- If a person lost consciousness and fell but has now regained consciousness.

- If a person fell due to a seizure but the seizure has now stopped. If the seizure is due to a chronic condition and your doctor has recommended treatment, begin the treatment.

- If someone is not able to get up after a fall.

- If you have severe bleeding or bruising.

- If you suspect a broken bone. See page 292.

- If pain develops in the hips, lower back, or wrists. These areas are especially likely to fracture in older adults.

- Call your doctor if you think a fall was caused by a medical problem or a medication.

Frostbite

Frostbite is freezing of the skin or underlying tissues that occurs as a result of prolonged exposure to cold.

Frostbitten skin is pale or blue, stiff or rubbery to touch, and feels cold and numb. There may be loss of function in the frozen area. Blisters may develop as the frostbitten area warms.

Prevention

Stay dry and out of the wind in extreme cold and cover areas of exposed skin. Keep the body's core temperature up:

- Wear layers of clothing. Wool and polypropylene are good insulators. Wear wind- and waterproof outer layers. Wear wool socks and well-fitting, waterproof boots.

- Wear a hat to prevent heat loss from your head. Wear mittens rather than gloves to protect fingers.

- Keep protective clothing and blankets in your car in cold weather in case of a breakdown in an isolated area.

- Don't drink alcohol or smoke when out in extreme cold.

Home Treatment

- Get inside or take shelter from the wind.

- Check for signs of hypothermia (page 284) and treat it before treating frostbite.

- Don't rewarm the area if refreezing is possible. Wait until you reach shelter.

- Warm small areas (ears, face, nose, fingers, toes) with warm breath or by tucking hands or feet inside warm clothing next to bare skin. Protect the frozen body part from further exposure. If possible, immerse it in warm water (104° to 108°) for 15 to 30 minutes.

- Don't rub or massage the frozen area, as it will further damage tissues. Avoid walking on frostbitten feet if possible.

- Keep the frostbitten part warm and elevated. Wrap with blankets or soft material to prevent bruising.

- Blisters may appear as the skin warms. Do not break them. The skin may turn red, burn, tingle, or be very painful. Aspirin or acetaminophen may help.

When to Call a Health Professional

- Call immediately if skin is white or blue, hard, and cold. Careful rewarming and antibiotic treatment are needed to prevent infection and permanent tissue damage.

- If blisters develop during rewarming. Do not break blisters. The risk of infection is very high.

- If signs of infection develop:

  - Increased pain, swelling, redness, or tenderness

  - Heat or red streaks extending from the area

  - Discharge of pus

  - Fever of 100° or higher with no other cause

Head Injuries

Most bumps to the head are minor and heal as easily as bumps anywhere else. Head injuries that cause cuts often bleed heavily because the blood vessels of the scalp are close to the surface. This bleeding is alarming but does not always mean that the injury is severe.

However, head injuries that do not cause visible external bleeding may cause life-threatening bleeding and swelling inside the skull. Anyone who has experienced a head injury should be watched carefully for 24 hours for signs of a severe head injury.

Occasionally there may be bleeding inside the skull that causes increasing pressure over days to weeks. Watch for slight changes in behavior after a head injury.

Prevention

- Wear your seat belt when in a motor vehicle.

- Wear a helmet while biking, motorcycling, and skating.

- Don't dive into shallow or unfamiliar water.

- See the Fall Prevention Checklist on page 267.

Home Treatment

- If the victim is unconscious, make sure there is no spinal injury before moving him. Check for other injuries.

- If there is bleeding, apply firm pressure directly over the wound with a clean cloth or bandage for 15 minutes. If the blood soaks through, apply additional cloths over the first one, without removing it.

- Apply ice or cold packs to reduce the swelling. A "goose egg" may appear anyway, but ice will help ease the pain.

- Watch for the following signs of a severe head injury immediately afterwards and then every two hours for the next 24 hours:

  - Confusion. Ask the person his name, address, age, the date, etc.

  - Inability to move arms and legs on one side of the body, or slower movement on one side than the other.

  - Lethargy, abnormally deep sleep, or difficulty waking up.

  - Vomiting that continues after the first two hours.

- Continue observing the person every two hours during the night. Wake him up and check for any unusual symptoms. **Call 911 or seek emergency care immediately if you cannot wake him or if he has any of the above signs of a severe head injury.**

- Check for injuries to other parts of the body, especially if the person has fallen. Often the excitement and alarm that accompanies a head injury will cause you to miss other injuries that also need attention.

When to Call a Health Professional

Call 911 or emergency services immediately:

- **If the person loses consciousness or is difficult to wake up (arouse) or is lethargic anytime after the injury.**

- **If double vision or speech difficulty occurs after the first minute.**

- **If there are seizures or convulsions or if there is weakness, or numbness, or inability to move arms and legs on one side of the body.**

Call immediately:

- If blood or clear fluid drains from the ears or nose following a blow to the head (not due to a cut or direct blow to the nose). If there is bleeding due to a cut on the scalp or face, see page 274.

- If the person is very confused or has any loss of memory after the first few minutes.

- If vomiting occurs after the first two hours or violent vomiting persists after the first 15 minutes. Mild nausea or vomiting at first is usually not serious.

- If a severe headache develops: "The worst headache I've ever had."

Call a health professional:

- If there are subtle changes in behavior or in ability to use part of the body, or if a new and different headache develops days to weeks after a head injury.

Heat Exhaustion and Heat Stroke

Heat exhaustion occurs when your body cannot sweat enough to cool you off. It generally happens when you are working or exercising in hot weather. Symptoms include:

- Fatigue, weakness, dizziness, or nausea

- Cool, clammy, pale, red, or flushed skin

Heat exhaustion can sometimes lead to **heat stroke**, which requires emergency treatment. Heat stroke happens when your body stops sweating but the body temperature continues to rise, often to 105° or higher. Symptoms include:

- Confusion, delirium, or unconsciousness

- Hot, dry, red, or flushed skin, even under the armpits

Prevention

- Avoid strenuous outdoor physical activity during the hottest part of the day.

- Avoid sudden changes of temperature. Air out a hot car before getting into it.

- If you take water pills (diuretics), ask your doctor about taking a lower dose during hot weather.

- Drink 8 to 10 glasses of water per day. Drink even more if you are working or exercising in hot weather.

- If you exercise or work strenuously in hot weather, drink more liquid than your thirst seems to require.

Home Treatment

- Get out of the sun to a cool spot and drink lots of cool water, a little at a time.

- If you are nauseated or dizzy, lie down.

- Sponge the body with cool water.

- If the body temperature reaches 105°, immediate cooling is essential. Use cold, wet cloths all over the body or a cool water bath.

- If the temperature is lowered to 102°, use care to avoid overcooling.

When to Call a Health Professional

Heat exhaustion can sometimes lead to heat stroke, particularly in older adults. Work fast to lower the temperature. **Call 911 or emergency services if signs of heat stroke develop**:

- **The skin is dry, even under the armpits, and bright red or flushed.**

- **The body temperature reaches 104° and keeps rising.**

- **The person is delirious, disoriented, or unconscious.**

Call immediately:

- If signs of heat exhaustion are not improving quickly with home treatment.

Hypothermia

Hypothermia occurs when the body loses heat faster than heat can be produced by muscle contractions and shivering and the body temperature drops below normal.

Early symptoms include:

- Shivering

- Cold, pale skin

- Sleepiness or lethargy

- Impaired judgment

Later symptoms include:

- Cold abdomen

- Slow pulse and breathing

- Weakness or drowsiness

- Confusion

Shivering may stop if body temperature drops below 96°.

People who have heart disease or diabetes, or who are inactive due to arthritis, stroke, or other conditions are at increased risk of hypothermia. Certain medications (including those used to treat high blood pressure, antidepressants, narcotics, barbiturates, sleeping pills, and anxiety drugs) increase the risk of hypothermia.

Some older adults, especially those who have chronic health problems, may be less likely to notice cool temperatures, and their bodies may not maintain a normal body temperature as well. Indoor temperatures below 65° also increase the risk.

Hypothermia is an emergency. It can quickly lead to unconsciousness and death if the heat loss continues.

Prevention

Whenever you plan to be outdoors for several hours in cold weather, take the following precautions:

- Dress warmly and wear wind- and waterproof clothing. Wear fabric that remains warm even when wet, such as wool or polypropylene.

- Keep protective clothing and blankets in your car in cold weather in case of a breakdown in an isolated area.

- Wear a warm hat. An unprotected head loses a great deal of the body's total heat production.

- Head for shelter and put on warm, dry clothing if you get wet or cold.

- Eat well before going out and carry extra food. Your body needs calories to produce heat.

- Don't drink alcohol while in the cold. It makes the body lose heat faster. It may also make you less likely to notice that you are becoming chilled.

To prevent hypothermia indoors:

- Keep your thermostat set at 65° or higher. If keeping the whole house heated is a problem, arrange to keep just a few rooms heated and close off others.

- If you must keep your home below 65°, wear several layers of warm clothing and a hat.

- Eat regularly. Your body needs food to produce heat.

- Get up and move around regularly if you must be indoors during cold weather. If moving around is a problem, do chair exercises or other activities that will get your blood moving.

- Wear warm clothes to bed and use warm bedding.

Home Treatment

The goal of home treatment is to stop additional heat loss and slowly rewarm the person. Warming one degree per hour is best.

- For mild cases, get the person out of the cold and wind, and give him dry or wool clothing and warm fluids to drink. If the person is indoors, increase the temperature in the room.

- For more serious cases, remove cold, wet clothes first; then warm the person with your own body heat by wrapping a blanket or sleeping bag around both of you.

- Give warm liquids to drink and high-energy foods, such as candy. Do not give food or drink if the person is disoriented or unconscious. Do not give alcoholic beverages.

- Rewarming the person in warm water can cause shock or heart attack. However, in emergency situations when help is not available and other home treatments are not working, you can use a warm water bath (100° to 105°) as a last resort.

When to Call a Health Professional

Call 911 or emergency services immediately:

- **If the person loses consciousness or is extremely confused.**

Call immediately:

- If late symptoms of hypothermia (page 284) are present.

Call a health professional:

- If the body temperature is 95° or lower or if early symptoms of hypothermia (page 284) are not improving after one hour of home treatment.

- If the victim is a frail or weak older person. It's a good idea to call regardless of the severity of the symptoms.

- If the body temperature does not return to normal after four hours of warming.

Insect and Tick Bites

Insect and spider bites and bee, yellow jacket, and wasp stings usually cause swelling, redness, and itching around the bite. In some people the redness and swelling may be worse, and the local reaction may last up to a day. In most cases, bites and stings are not serious.

Some people have severe skin reactions to insect or spider bites or stings, and a few have allergic (anaphylactic) reactions that affect the whole body. Symptoms may include hives all over the body, shortness of breath and tightness in the chest, dizziness, wheezing, or swelling of the tongue and face. If these symptoms develop, *immediate* medical attention is needed.

Few spider bites cause serious problems, although any bite may be serious if the person has an allergic reaction.

Black widow spider bites may cause chills, fever, nausea, and severe stomach pain. **Brown recluse** (fiddler) spider bites cause intense pain and may result in a blister that turns into a larger open sore.

Ticks are small arachnids (related to spiders) that fasten themselves to the body. A tick should be removed as soon as you discover it.

Lyme disease is a bacterial infection spread by deer ticks, which are tiny, about the size of the period at the end of this sentence. If you can see the tick easily, it is probably not a deer tick.

Early symptoms of Lyme disease include a red "bull's-eye" rash with a white center around the bite. The rash develops four days to three weeks after the bite. Fever, fatigue, headache, muscle aches, and joint pain may also occur. Lyme disease is treated with antibiotics.

Jellyfish are common on some ocean beaches. If touched, their tentacles release a stinging poison that causes a painful reaction.

Prevention

- To avoid bee stings, wear white or light-colored solid fabrics. Bees are attracted to dark colors and flowered prints.

- In tick-infested areas, wear light-colored clothing and tuck pant legs into socks.

- Avoid wearing perfumes and colognes when you are outside.

- Apply an insect repellent containing DEET to exposed areas of skin or to clothing every few hours when in insect-, spider-, or tick-infested areas. Apply carefully around eyes and mouth. Wash DEET off when you come inside. Alpha-Keri and Skin-So-Soft bath oils also seem to repel insects.

- Wear gloves and tuck pants into socks when working in woodpiles, sheds, and basements where spiders are found.

Home Treatment

For bee stings and insect and spider bites:

- Remove a bee stinger by scraping or flicking it out (if the stinger isn't visible, assume there isn't one). Don't squeeze the stinger; you may release more venom into the skin.

- If the bite is from a black widow or brown recluse spider, apply ice to the bite and call your doctor.

- Apply a cold pack or ice cube to the bite or sting. Some people also find that a paste of baking soda, meat tenderizer, or activated charcoal mixed with a little water helps relieve pain and decrease the reaction.

- An oral antihistamine (Benadryl, Chlor-Trimeton) may help relieve pain and swelling and relieve itching if there are many bites.

Calamine lotion, hydrocortisone cream, or a local anesthetic containing benzocaine (Solarcaine) may also help. If a rash develops, stop using the lotion or cream.

- If you have had a severe allergic reaction to insect venom, carry an emergency kit containing a syringe and adrenalin (epinephrine). Ask your doctor or pharmacist how to use the kit.

For tick bites:

- Check regularly for ticks when you are out in the woods and thoroughly examine your skin and scalp when you return home. Check your pets too. The sooner ticks are removed, the less likely they are to spread bacteria.

- Remove a tick by gently pulling with tweezers, as close to the skin as possible. Pull straight out and try not to crush the body. Save the tick in a jar for identification if symptoms of Lyme disease develop.

For jellyfish stings:

- Rinse the area immediately with saltwater. Do not use fresh water and do not rub; it will release more poison.

- Splash vinegar, alcohol, or meat tenderizer dissolved in saltwater on the area to neutralize the poison.

- Remove any attached tentacles carefully. Protect your hand with a towel and apply a paste of sand or baking soda and saltwater to the area. Scrape the tentacles off with the towel or the edge of a credit card.

- Apply calamine lotion to relieve pain and itching.

- If you are stung by a Portuguese man-of-war jellyfish, scrape the stinging tentacles off with sand and seek medical care immediately.

When to Call a Health Professional

Call 911 or emergency services immediately if signs of a severe allergic reaction (anaphylaxis) develop soon after an insect bite:

- **Lightheadedness or feeling like you may pass out.**

- **Swelling around the lips, tongue, or face that may interfere with breathing.**

- **Wheezing or difficulty breathing.**

Call a health professional immediately:

- If there is swelling of the lips, tongue, or face that is not interfering with breathing.

- If there is significant swelling around the site of the insect bite (e.g., the entire arm or leg is swollen).

- If there is a skin rash, itching, feeling of warmth, or hives.

- If you are stung by a Portuguese man-of-war jellyfish.

- If you are bitten by a black widow or brown recluse spider.

Call a health professional:

- If a blister appears at the site of a spider bite, or if the surrounding skin becomes discolored.

- To talk with your doctor about adrenalin kits or allergy shots (immunotherapy) if you have had a serious allergic reaction.

- If you are unable to remove a tick or part of a tick.

- In areas where Lyme disease is common, see a doctor if a deer tick has been attached for more than 24 hours.

- If a red "bull's-eye" rash, fever, fatigue, or flu-like symptoms develop up to three weeks after a tick bite.

| Nosebleeds |

Nosebleeds can usually be stopped with home treatment. Some common causes of nosebleeds are low humidity, colds and allergies, blows to the nose, medications (especially aspirin), high altitudes, and blowing or picking the nose.

Prevention

- Low humidity is a common cause of nosebleeds. Humidify your home, especially the bedrooms, and keep the heat low (60° to 64°) in sleeping areas.

- If your nose becomes very dry, breathe moist air for a while (e.g., from a shower) and then put a little petroleum jelly on the inside to help prevent bleeding. A saline nasal spray may also help.

- Limit your use of aspirin, which can contribute to nosebleeds.

Home Treatment

- Sit up straight and tip your head slightly forward. Tilting the head back may cause blood to run down the throat.

- Blow all the clots out of the nose (this may increase the bleeding). Pinch the nostrils shut between your thumb and forefinger or apply firm pressure against the bleeding nostril for *10 full minutes.* Watch the clock and resist the urge to peek after a few minutes to see if it has stopped bleeding.

- After 10 minutes, check to see if the nose is still bleeding. If it is, hold it for 10 more minutes. Most nosebleeds will stop after 10 to 30 minutes of direct pressure.

- Stay quiet for a few hours and do not blow the nose for at least 12 hours after the bleeding has stopped.

When to Call a Health Professional

Call immediately:

- If the bleeding hasn't stopped after 30 minutes of direct pressure.

- If blood runs down the back of your throat even when the nose is pinched.

Call a health professional:

- If the nose is deformed after an injury and may be broken.

- If nosebleeds recur often.

Objects in the Eye

A speck of dirt or small object in the eye will often wash out with your tears. If the object is not removed, it may scratch the covering of the eye (cornea). Most corneal scratches are minor and heal on their own in a day or two.

Home Treatment

Do not try to remove an object that is on the colored part of the eye or that is stuck in the white of the eye. Cover both eyes and call a health professional.

- Don't rub the eye.

- Wash your hands before touching the eye.

- If the object is at the side of the eye or on the lower lid, moisten a cotton swab or the tip of a twisted piece of tissue and touch the end to the speck. The object should cling to the swab or tissue. Some minor irritation is common after you have removed the object.

- Gently wash the eye with cool water. An eyedropper helps.

- Never use tweezers, toothpicks, or other hard items to remove any object.

When to Call a Health Professional

- If the object is on the colored part of the eye or is embedded in the white of the eye. Do not pull out an object that is stuck in the eye.

- If you cannot remove the object.

- If pain is severe or persists, if it feels like there is still something in the eye, or if vision is blurred after the object is removed. The cornea may be scratched. Keep the eye closed.

Shock

Shock may occur due to sudden illness or injury. When the circulatory system is unable to get enough blood to the vital organs, the body goes into shock. Sometimes, even a mild injury will lead to shock.

The signs of shock include:

- Cool, pale, clammy skin

- Dilated pupils

- Weak, rapid pulse

- Shallow, rapid breathing

- Thirst, nausea, or vomiting

- Confusion or anxiety

- Faintness, weakness, lightheadedness, or loss of consciousness

- Low blood pressure

Shock is a life-threatening condition. Call for help immediately if signs of shock develop.

Home Treatment

- After calling for emergency care, have the person lie down and elevate his legs 12 inches or more. If the injury is to the head, neck, or chest, keep the legs flat. If the person vomits, roll him to one side to let fluids drain from the mouth. Use care if there could be a spinal injury.

- Control any bleeding (see page 274) and splint any fractures (see page 292).

- Keep the person warm, but not hot. Place a blanket underneath him and cover him with a sheet or blanket, depending on the weather. If the person is in a hot place, try to keep him cool.

- Take and record the person's pulse every five minutes. Comfort and reassure him to relieve anxiety.

When to Call a Health Professional

- **Call 911 or emergency services if signs of shock develop.**

Strains, Sprains, and Fractures

A **strain** is a pulled muscle.

A **sprain** is an injury to the muscles, ligaments, tendons, and soft tissues around a joint. Generally, sprains hurt more and take longer to heal than strains.

A **fracture** is a broken bone. Most fractures also involve strains and sprains to the connecting muscles and ligaments. A **stress fracture** is a weak spot or small crack in a bone, often due to an increase in an activity that pounds the bone.

A **dislocation** occurs when one end of a bone is pushed or pulled out of place at a joint.

Unless a broken bone is obvious, it can be difficult to tell if an injury is a strain, sprain, or fracture. Injuries often involve all three. Rapid swelling often indicates a more serious injury.

Most minor strains and sprains can be treated at home, but severe sprains, fractures, and dislocated joints need professional care. Taking the time for good home treatment will often prevent further damage to an injured limb on the way to the doctor.

Splinting

Splinting immobilizes a limb that may be broken so that it isn't injured more. There are two ways to immobilize a fracture: tie the injured limb to a stiff object, or fasten it to some other part of the body. Do not tie too tight.

For the first method, tie rolled-up newspapers or magazines, a stick, a cane, or anything that is stiff to the injured limb with a rope, a belt, or anything else that will work.

Position the splint so the injured limb cannot bend. A general rule is to splint from a joint above the fracture to a joint below it. For example, splint a broken forearm from above the elbow to below the wrist.

For the second method, tape a broken toe to the next toe or immobilize an arm by tying it across the victim's chest.

Prevention

Many strains, sprains, and fractures in older adults are the result of falls. To reduce the chance of falls, see the Fall Prevention Checklist on page 267.

Home Treatment

Generally speaking, if the injury is to a muscle, ligament, tendon, or bone, the basic treatment is the same. It is a two-part process: **RICE** (rest, ice, compression, elevation) to treat the acute pain or injury; and **MSA** (movement, strength, alternate activity) to help the injury heal completely and to prevent further problems.

Check for other injuries, such as a bump on the head, especially if the person fell.

For sprains and strains of the back, see page 28. For sprains and strains of the neck, see page 40.

Begin the RICE process immediately for most injuries. If you suspect a fracture, splint the affected limb to prevent further injury. See page 292.

If the sprain is to a finger or part of the hand, remove all rings immediately. See box at right.

R. Rest. Do not put weight on the injured joint for at least 24 to 48 hours. Do not splint a joint or wear a sling for longer than 48 hours.

- Use crutches or a wheelchair to rest a badly sprained knee or ankle.

- Support a sprained wrist, elbow, or shoulder with a sling, which helps the injury heal faster.

- Rest a sprained finger or toe by taping it to a healthy one.

Removing a Ring

To remove a ring from a sprained or swollen finger:

- First, try soapy water. Ice water will also decrease the swelling.

- Stick the end of a slick piece of string, such as dental floss, under the ring toward the hand.

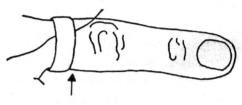

Start wrapping here

- Starting at the side of the ring closest to the end of the finger, wrap the string snugly around the finger toward the nail, wrapping past the knuckle. Each wrap should be right next to the one before.

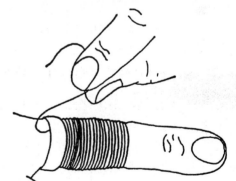

- Grasp the end of the string that is under the ring and start unwrapping it. Push the ring along ahead of the string as you unwrap it until the ring passes the knuckle.

I. Ice. Cold will reduce pain and swelling and promote healing. Heat feels nice, but until all of the swelling is gone, it does more harm than good. Apply ice or cold packs immediately to prevent or minimize swelling. See "Ice and Cold Packs" at right.

C. Compression. Wrap the injury with an elastic (Ace) bandage or compression sleeve to immobilize and compress the sprain. Don't wrap it too tightly, which can cause more swelling. Loosen the bandage if it gets too tight.

E. Elevation. Elevate the injured area on pillows while you apply ice and anytime you are sitting or lying down. Try to keep the injury at or above the level of your heart to help minimize swelling.

- Aspirin, ibuprofen, or naproxen may help ease inflammation and pain. Do not use drugs to mask the pain while you continue to use the injured joint.

- The use of heat (hot water bottle, warm towel, heating pad) after 48 hours of cold treatments is controversial. Some experts think it will increase swelling; others think it may speed healing. Do not apply anything that is uncomfortably warm.

Ice and Cold Packs

Ice can relieve pain, swelling, and inflammation from injuries and other conditions such as arthritis. Apply ice regularly as long as you have symptoms. Use either a cold pack or one of the following:

- Ice towel: Wet a towel with cold water and squeeze it until it is just damp. Fold the towel, place it in a plastic bag, and freeze it for 15 minutes. Remove the towel from the bag and place it on the affected area.

- Ice pack: Put about a pound of ice in a plastic bag. Add water to barely cover the ice. Squeeze the air out of the bag and seal it. Wrap the bag in a wet towel and apply to the affected area.

- Homemade cold pack: see page 411.

Ice the area at least three times a day. For the first 72 hours, ice for 10 minutes once an hour. After that, a good pattern is to ice for 15 to 20 minutes three times a day: in the morning, in the late afternoon, and about one-half hour before bedtime. Also ice after any prolonged activity or vigorous exercise.

To protect the skin, always keep a damp cloth between your skin and the cold pack. Press firmly against all the curves of the affected area. Do not apply ice for longer than 20 minutes at a time. Do not fall asleep with the ice on your skin.

Begin the **MSA** process as soon as the initial pain and swelling have subsided. This may be in two days or up to a week or longer, depending on the location and severity of the injury. Resume activities slowly. Any increased pain may be a sign you need to rest a while longer.

M. Movement. Resume a full range of motion as soon as possible after an injury. After one to two days of rest, begin moving the joint. If an activity causes pain, stop it and give the joint more rest. Gentle stretching will prevent scar tissue (formed as the injury heals) from limiting movement later.

S. Strength. Once the swelling is gone and range of motion is restored, begin gradual efforts to strengthen the injured area.

A. Alternate activities. After the first few days, but while the injury is still healing, phase in regular exercise using activities that do not place a strain on the injured part.

When to Call a Health Professional

Call immediately:

- If an injured limb is deformed, if a bone is poking through the skin, or if there is broken skin over the site of a suspected fracture.

- If there are signs that nerves or blood vessels have been damaged:

  - Numbness, tingling, or a "pins-and-needles" sensation in the limb below the injury.

  - The skin of the injured limb is pale, white, or blue, or feels colder than the uninjured limb.

Call a health professional:

- If you are not able to bear weight on or straighten the injured limb, or if the joint wobbles from side to side.

- If significant swelling develops within 30 minutes of the injury, or if swelling is not going down after two days of home treatment.

- If the pain is severe, or if it persists after two days of home treatment.

- If hip, low back, or wrist pain develops after a fall and you have or are at risk for osteoporosis. Even minor falls can break bones.

- If increased swelling, redness, and warmth develop in an injured area two days to two weeks after the injury.

To be seventy years young
is sometimes far more cheerful and hopeful
than to be forty years old.
Oliver Wendell Holmes on the
70th birthday of Julia Ward Howe

19
Mental Self-Care

Mental health problems are pretty much the same as other health problems: some can be prevented; others will go away on their own with a little care and home treatment; and some need professional attention.

Researchers have discovered that mental health problems often have underlying physical causes. Illnesses such as thyroid disease and chronic anemia can cause depression. Arthritis and other problems that cause chronic pain commonly lead to depression and, for some people, may increase the likelihood of drug or alcohol abuse.

We also know that mental health problems can begin when psychological or emotional stress (such as the loss of a loved one) triggers chemical imbalances in the brain. While some people can withstand more stress than others, nobody is immune to mental health problems.

Because mental health problems have both physical and psychological causes, both self-care and professional care are often needed. The goal of these treatment approaches is to reduce stress, identify and treat underlying physical problems, and restore the normal chemical balance in the brain.

Good mental self-care requires a keen awareness and understanding of symptoms. If you can recognize symptoms early and are willing to address their underlying causes, you can often prevent major mental health problems. Early recognition of symptoms can also allow you to seek help to resolve the problem before serious disruptions in your life occur.

Seeking Professional Help

This chapter does not cover all mental health problems. If you have mental or emotional symptoms that are not addressed here, contact your health professional. In general, if you have emotional symptoms such as anger, sadness or hopelessness, anxiety, or alcohol- or drug-related problems, it is a good idea to seek professional help when:

- You think your symptoms may have a physical cause.

- A symptom becomes severe or disruptive.

- A disruptive symptom starts to become a continuous or permanent pattern of behavior and does not respond to self-care.

- Symptoms become numerous, affecting all areas of your life, and they do not respond to self-care or communication efforts.

- You are thinking about suicide.

There is a wide range of professional and lay resources to choose from for mental health problems.

Family doctors: Mental health problems often have physical causes. Your doctor can review your medical history and medications for clues, provide some counseling, prescribe medications when necessary, or refer you to other resources.

Cost Management Tips

The old saying that "talk is cheap" does not apply to most professional psychotherapists and counselors. The following tips can help keep costs down.

- Don't just pick a name from the Yellow Pages. Ask someone you trust for a good referral.

- Use mental health professionals to help you identify the real problem and develop a self-management plan to resolve it.

- Emphasize the importance of self-care in the treatment plan.

- Ask about group therapy options.

- Check out 12-step programs such as Alcoholics Anonymous, Al-Anon, Overeaters Anonymous, and other groups that can help you deal with the problem. Such programs are usually free, effective, and available in most communities.

- Remember, if counseling is helping you feel better, it is well worth the time and money spent.

Psychiatrists: Psychiatrists are medical doctors who specialize in mental disorders. They counsel patients, prescribe medications, and order medical treatments.

Psychologists, social workers, and counselors: These professionals receive special training in helping people deal with mental health problems. They help patients identify, understand, and work through disturbing thoughts and emotions.

Pastors: People often turn to their clergy for counseling and advice in times of emotional distress. Some pastors have formal training in counseling.

Alcohol Problems

A person whose use of alcohol interferes with health or activities of daily living has an alcohol problem. A person who becomes physically and psychologically dependent on alcohol has developed alcoholism.

Long-term, heavy drinking can lead to liver, nerve, heart, and brain damage, as well as high blood pressure, stomach problems, sexual problems, and cancer. Alcohol abuse can also lead to violence, falls and accidents, social isolation, and difficulties at work, at home, and with the law.

For older adults, it is important to remember that:

- Alcohol slows brain activity.

- Alcohol impairs mental alertness, memory, judgment, physical coordination, and reaction time.

- Heavy alcohol use can lead to loss of employment, friends, and loved ones.

- As you get older, it takes your body longer to break down alcohol, and tolerance for it decreases. Drinking the same amount that you drank 20 years ago can cause a lot more damage.

- Alcohol complicates many medical problems.

- Tranquilizers, barbiturates, certain painkillers, and antihistamines all increase the intoxicating effect of alcohol.

- Alcohol interferes with the medical benefits of many drugs, including anticonvulsants, anticoagulants, and diabetic medications.

Symptoms of an alcohol problem or alcoholism include personality changes, blackouts, drinking more and more for the same "high," and denial of the problem. A person may gulp or sneak drinks, drink alone or early in the morning, and suffer from the shakes. He or she also may have family or work problems or get in trouble with the law as a result of drinking.

Alcohol abuse patterns vary. Some people drink excessively every day. Some drink large amounts of alcohol at specific times, such as weekends. Others may be sober for long periods, then go on drinking binges that last for weeks or months.

A person with alcoholism may suffer serious withdrawal symptoms (trembling, delusions, hallucinations, and sweating) if he or she stops drinking suddenly ("cold turkey"). Once alcohol dependency develops, it becomes very difficult, and possibly a health hazard, to abstain without outside help. Medical detoxification may be needed.

Screening Test

Many people will deny that they have problems with alcohol. The amount of alcohol a person drinks may be less important than the way he or she behaves when drinking and the effect that alcohol has on the person's life. The questions in the "Are You a Problem User?" chart on page 301 may help you or others recognize a problem.

Answering "yes" to two or more questions raises the possibility of an alcohol or drug problem and the need to seek help.

Prevention

- Recognize the importance of cutting back on alcohol as you age.

- If you drink, do so in moderation: fewer than two drinks a day for a man and one drink a day for a woman. One drink is 12 ounces of beer, 5 ounces of wine, or 1½ ounces of hard liquor.

- Provide nonalcoholic beverages at parties and meals.

- Seek friendships with people who do not rely on alcohol to enjoy themselves.

- Stay active and maintain daily responsibilities.

- Spend more time with friends or family after you have suffered any major loss or life change.

Home Treatment

- Recognize early signs that alcohol use is becoming a problem. See page 301.

- Look for other signs of mental stress. Try to understand and resolve sources of depression, anxiety, or loneliness.

- Attend an Alcoholics Anonymous meeting (a self-help group devoted to helping members get and stay sober).

- If you are concerned about another person's alcohol use:

  ○ Never ignore the problem. Discuss it as you would any other medical problem.

  ○ Do not attack the person's morals. Be nonjudgmental.

  ○ Talk about the problem, but don't nag about it.

  ○ Build up the person's self-esteem and reaffirm his value as a person. Help him see that his life can be successful without alcohol. Let him know that you will support his efforts to change.

Are You a Problem User?

Answer the questions honestly. Answer "yes" if the statement is true for alcohol or drugs (including prescribed or illegal substances that can be described as mood-altering or addictive).

1. Have you ever tried to stop using alcohol or drugs for a week or so but could stop for only a couple of days?

2. Do you resent the advice of others who try to get you to stop or cut down your use of alcohol or drugs?

3. Have you tried to control your use of alcohol or drugs by changing from one type of drink or drug to another?

4. Do you envy people who can use alcohol or drugs without getting into trouble?

5. Has your use of alcohol or drugs impaired your family relationships, your work, your driving safety, or any other aspect of your life?

6. During the past year, have you missed days of work because of your use of alcohol or drugs?

7. Do you tell yourself you can stop using alcohol or drugs any time you want?

8. Do you sometimes go on binges with alcohol or drugs?

9. Do you ever have blackouts related to your alcohol or drug use?

10. Have you ever felt that your life would be better if you did not use alcohol or drugs?

If you answer "yes" to two or more questions, you may have a problem with alcohol or drugs. If so, talk with a health professional.

○ Ask the person if he will accept help. Don't give up if the person's first response is "no." Keep asking. When he agrees, arrange for help that very day. Call a health professional or Alcoholics Anonymous for an immediate appointment.

○ Attend a few meetings of Al-Anon, a support group for family members and friends of alcoholics. Read some information about 12-step programs. See Resource 7 on page 419.

○ Remember, you cannot control another person's alcohol problem, but you can control how you are going to relate to that person.

When to Call a Health Professional

• If you answer "yes" to two or more questions on the "Are You a Problem User?" chart on page 301.

• If you recognize that you have an alcohol problem and are ready to accept help. Both outpatient and inpatient treatment programs are available.

Anger and Hostility

Anger signals your body to prepare for a fight. When you get angry, adrenalin and other hormones are released into the bloodstream. Blood pressure goes up.

Hostility is being ready for a fight all the time. Continual hostility keeps your blood pressure high and may increase your risk for heart attacks and other illnesses. Being hostile also isolates you from other people.

Home Treatment

• Notice when you start getting angry, and do something about it before it gets out of hand.

• Identify the cause of your anger. This may require the help of a professional.

• Express your anger in healthy ways:

○ Count to 10. Give yourself a little time for your adrenalin level to go down.

○ Try screaming or yelling in a private place, not at others.

○ Go for a short walk.

○ Talk about it with a friend.

○ Draw or paint to release the anger.

○ Write in a daily journal.

• Use "I" statements, not "you" statements, to discuss your anger. Say, "I feel angry when my needs are not being met," instead of, "You make me mad when you are so inconsiderate."

• Forgive and forget. Letting go helps lower blood pressure and eases muscle tension so you can feel more relaxed. Forgiveness is a gift you give to yourself as well as the person with whom you are angry.

When to Call a Health Professional

• If hostility has led or could lead to violence or harm to you or someone else.

• If anger or hostility interferes with your work, family, or friends.

• Also see Seeking Professional Help on page 298.

Anxiety

Feeling worried, anxious, and nervous is a part of everyday life. Everyone frets or feels anxious from time to time. However, when anxiety becomes overwhelming and interferes with daily life, it is not normal.

Anxiety can cause both physical and emotional symptoms:

Physical Symptoms

• Trembling, twitching, or shaking

• Muscle tension, aches, or soreness

• Restlessness

• Fatigue

• Insomnia

• Breathlessness or rapid heartbeat

• Sweating or cold, clammy hands

• Tingling in the hands or around the mouth

Emotional Symptoms

• Feeling keyed up and on edge

• Excessive worrying

• Fearing that something bad is going to happen

• Poor concentration and memory loss

- Excessive startle response

- Irritability or agitation

- Constant sadness

Anxiety about a specific situation or fear can cause some or all of these symptoms for a short time. This is normal as long as anxiety symptoms subside once the situation passes. Some people develop generalized anxiety disorders in which many of these symptoms occur without an identifiable cause.

Phobias and panic disorder are two common anxiety-related disorders. **Phobias** are irrational, involuntary fears of common places, objects, or situations.

Panic disorder is characterized by distinct periods of intense anxiety that occur when there is no clear cause or danger. Physical symptoms that may occur during a panic attack include hyperventilation, shaking, pounding heart, and feeling faint. Professional treatment is usually necessary in this situation and can often be effective in managing these disorders.

Hyperthyroidism (page 152) may also cause anxiety and other symptoms.

Home Treatment

The following home treatment tips can relieve simple anxiety. They also work well in combination with medical care.

- Recognize and accept your anxiety about specific fears or situations. Then say to yourself, "Okay, I see the problem. Now I'll start to deal with it."

- Be kind to your body:

  o Relieve tension with exercise. Getting a massage also may help.

  o Practice relaxation techniques. See page 365.

  o Get enough rest. If you have trouble sleeping, see Sleep Problems on page 315.

  o Avoid alcohol, caffeine, and nicotine. They increase your anxiety level.

- Engage your mind:

  o Get out and do something you enjoy, such as going to a funny movie or taking a walk or hike.

  o Plan your day. Having too much or too little to do can make you more anxious.

- Keep a record of your symptoms. Discuss your fears with a good friend. Confiding with others sometimes relieves stress.

- Get involved in social groups or volunteer to help others. Being alone makes things seem worse than they are.

- Develop positive expectations for the future.

- Consider whether medications might be making you anxious. See Resource 2 on page 418.

When to Call a Health Professional

- If anxiety interferes with your daily activities.

- If symptoms are severe and one week of home treatment has not helped.

- If you frequently have sudden, severe attacks of fear or anxiety with intense physical symptoms (shaking, sweating) when there is no apparent reason to be afraid.

- If intense, irrational fears of common places, objects, or situations interfere with your daily life.

- If you suffer from nightmares or flashbacks to traumatic events.

- If you are unable to feel certain about things (e.g., whether you unplugged the iron) no matter how many times you check, or if repetitive, compulsive behaviors interfere with your daily activities.

- If you are concerned that hyperthyroidism (page 152) may be causing the anxiety symptoms.

Depression

Most people experience depression at some point in their lives. Depression can range from a minor problem to a major, life-threatening illness. Depression is often treatable. For many people, treatment can mean a whole new life.

Medical science is getting closer to understanding depression. Most major depressions involve an imbalance of chemical messengers (neurotransmitters) in the brain. Many things can trigger these imbalances:

- Chronic stress or a stressful event

- Major illness

- Reaction to medications

- Alcoholism, drug abuse, dementia, and other mental health problems

- Reduced daylight during the winter seems to cause a form of depression called seasonal affective disorder in some people (see page 307).

- Loss of a loved one or something that is highly valued

Some people are genetically susceptible to chemical imbalances in the brain. Fortunately, effective treatments are available for them and others at high risk for depression.

Sadness or Depression?

If you have experienced four or more of the following symptoms nearly every day for more than two weeks, you may be suffering from depression:

- Feelings of sadness, anxiety, or hopelessness

- Lack of interest or pleasure in usual activities and pastimes

- Increase or decrease in appetite, or unexplained gain or loss of weight

- Frequent backaches, headaches, stomach problems, or other aches that don't respond to treatment

- Insomnia or excessive sleepiness

- Low energy, fatigue, tiredness

- Feeling restless or irritable

- Feeling worthless or guilty

- Inability to concentrate, remember, or make decisions

- Frequent thoughts of suicide or death

Home treatment may be enough for mild depression. However, if you are feeling suicidal, or if home treatment doesn't help within two weeks, call a doctor. With counseling, medication, and home treatment, most episodes of depression can be overcome.

Everyone gets sad. Gauging how deep and pervasive your sad feelings are can help you decide what you should do. See "Sadness or Depression?" at left to help determine if you are suffering from depression.

Feeling sad does not always mean that you are heading for a major depression. Bad news or disappointment can cause you to feel sad, perhaps for several days or weeks. This is normal and healthy as long as the sad feelings eventually go away. Grief (page 310) can also cause a normal sadness.

Home Treatment

Self-care may be all that is needed to pull you out of a mild depression. For more serious depression, self-care can add to the benefits of professional treatment.

- At the first sign of depression, ask a friend for some extra attention. You can lose objectivity about yourself when you feel blue.

- Consider what might be causing or adding to your depression:

  - Are medications causing it? Review your prescription and over-the-counter medications with a pharmacist or doctor.

  - If it's wintertime or you haven't been out in the sun for a while, read the information about seasonal affective disorder on page 307.

- Stay active. It's easier to **do** yourself into **feeling** better than to **feel** yourself into **doing** better.

- Get regular exercise. If nothing else, go for long walks. They help to clear the mind.

- Look for a laugh. Laughter, like exercise, can help restore balance to your system.

- Boost your self-esteem. Read the Mind-Body Wellness chapter beginning on page 371.

- Believe that this mood will pass. Then look for signs that it is ending.

- Surround yourself with happy, upbeat people.

- Books can help. See Resources 37 and 40 on page 421.

When to Call a Health Professional

Because many things can contribute to depression, combining self-care and professional treatment is often most effective. The most common form of treatment combines counseling (psychotherapy) with medication. Inpatient treatment is sometimes needed in severe cases. Call for help:

- If thoughts of suicide recur and persist. See Suicide on page 316.

Seasonal Affective Disorder (Winter Depression)

There is increasing evidence (not yet conclusive) that a lack of sunlight during winter months can cause depression in some people. Symptoms include melancholy moods, changes in sleeping habits, cravings for sweets and starchy foods, and chronic fatigue. If you notice such a pattern developing during the winter, consider the following:

- When the winter sun does shine, go outside and soak it up. Protect your skin—it's the eye's exposure to sunlight that makes the difference.

- Go south for a sunny vacation if you can.

- Some people may benefit from light therapy (phototherapy). This may consist of sitting in front of bright, full-spectrum fluorescent lights for one to five hours a day or other approaches. Depression often improves by the end of the first week of treatment.

Because it is a new approach to winter depression, the National Institutes of Health recommends that light therapy be supervised by a health professional.

- If you suspect you are very depressed. See "Sadness or Depression?" on page 306.

- If you suspect you are depressed, and two weeks of home treatment has not helped.

Caregiver Tips for Depression

- Help the person rebuild his self-esteem. Help him remember the positive things he has done and good times he has had.

- Help the person identify the situations in his life over which he has control.

- Encourage activity with others.

- Depressed people can lose objectivity about themselves. If signs of major depression are strong, insist that the person talk with a health professional.

- Caregivers get depressed too. If symptoms of depression develop, see Home Treatment for tips to help you get back on track.

- Remember that depression can often mimic dementia. Try to rule out depression if the person seems confused, withdrawn, or has other symptoms of dementia.

Drug Problems

Most people think of drug abuse as the illegal use of marijuana, cocaine, heroin, or other "street" drugs. Drug problems among older adults are more likely to be drug "misuse," the unintentional overuse of legal prescription drugs. Tranquilizers, sedatives, painkillers, and amphetamines are often misused unintentionally or accidentally.

The symptoms of drug misuse vary widely, depending upon the kind of drug. Often, they occur slowly over a long period of time, and they can be confused with symptoms of other health problems.

See page 410 for a list of symptoms that may be caused by adverse drug reactions.

Drug dependence or addiction occurs when you develop a physical or psychological "need" for a drug. You may not be aware that you have become dependent on a drug until you try to stop taking it. Sudden withdrawal from the drug can produce uncomfortable symptoms. The usual treatment for drug dependence is to gradually reduce the dose of the drug until it can be stopped completely.

Prevention

- Do not regularly use medications to help you sleep, lose weight, or relax. Look for non-drug solutions.

- Carefully follow the instructions for taking tranquilizers, sedatives, and painkillers. If your doctor prescribes these drugs, ask to start at the lowest dose possible. If you are already taking them, see if it is possible to slowly reduce the dose.

- Do not suddenly stop taking any medication unless your doctor tells you to do so. Serious symptoms can result if some medications are abruptly withdrawn.

- Do not take any medications with alcohol. It can react with many medications and cause serious complications.

Home Treatment

The best home treatment for drug misuse is to be on the lookout for early signs of adverse drug reactions or dependency.

- Ask your pharmacist if any of your current medications could potentially lead to overuse problems.

- Be especially cautious of the following types of medications:

  o Painkillers (codeine, Darvon, Demerol, Percodan, and others)

  o Tranquilizers (Ativan, Librium, Valium, and other benzodiazepines)

  o Sedatives or sleeping pills (Seconal, phenobarbital, Nembutal, and other barbiturates; Dalmane, Doriden, Halcion, and other nonbarbiturates; over-the-counter sleep aids)

- Discuss all medications you are taking, including over-the-counter products, with your doctor. Gradually reduce the dosages of any that you agree are not needed.

- See Chapter 26, Medication Management, for tips on how to take your medications correctly and avoid adverse reactions.

When to Call a Health Professional

- If you suspect that you or someone you know is becoming dependent on or misusing a medication. You may need a doctor's help to reduce the dosage or to stop taking the drug.

Grief

Grief is a natural healing process that enables you to adjust to significant change or loss. Although painful, grief is also of great benefit. It provides a period of adjustment and an opportunity to build a foundation for a meaningful future.

Grief can be expressed physically as well as emotionally. Physical symptoms include sighing, exhaustion, insomnia, restlessness, constipation, diarrhea, and nausea. Emotional responses to loss can consist of denial, anger, guilt, depression, and many other strong feelings.

It is not uncommon to be preoccupied with the image of a loved one who has died. Survivors often report seeing, having conversations with, or even being touched by the deceased person. This is normal.

No person or book can tell you what your grief "should" be like. How long and in what ways you grieve will be unique to you. However, there are stages of grief that are more or less common to many who suffer a loss.

The Stages of Grief

Grief is different for everyone. Your grief may not progress directly from one stage to the next. However, understanding what others have experienced can help you deal with your own emotions.

Shock and Denial: The "Not Me" Stage

If your loss is sudden, your first reaction may be shock. Shock is a natural anesthesia that protects you from overwhelming pain. You may even act as if nothing happened. You may feel numb. Later, you may not remember how you felt or acted during this period.

Denial is normal. You understand what has happened, but on a deeper level you don't really believe it.

Denial may pass quickly, or it may last for months or even years. Denial is all right for a while. It provides a brief respite before you have to gear up to deal with the loss. However, if denial lasts too long, it may separate you from reality.

Guilt and Anger: The "Why Me?" Stage

Few people experience the loss of someone or something important to them without some feeling of guilt. You tell yourself that you should have done things differently. "If only..." is a common thought. You may feel there was more you could have done. Eventually, feelings of guilt will be put in proper perspective.

Anger is also a normal response. Many people feel rage or at least mild anger. This anger needs to be expressed. However, lashing out at others can cause misunderstandings.

Some therapists recommend screaming or yelling in a private place to vent angry feelings without hurting those around you. See page 302 for other ideas.

Adjustment and Acceptance: The "Let's Get On With It" Stage

Life goes on. At some point in the grieving process, you will be better able to come to terms with your loss. Grief will loosen its hold on you, and in struggling to get on with life, you may discover new opportunities.

Loss teaches us new lessons. You may gain wisdom from your experience and be better able to help others.

Home Treatment

These home treatment guidelines are meant to help when you have lost a loved one. The same basic principles apply for other losses as well.

- Take as much time as you need to grieve. Review mementos, play nostalgic music, or read old letters.

- Let yourself cry.

- Talk about your grief with a friend. If your friend tells you to "snap out of it," find a more sympathetic listener. A minister, priest, rabbi, or other clergy member also may help you understand and deal with your loss.

Tips for Caregivers

At every stage of the grieving process, caregivers and friends can provide valuable support.

Shock and Denial Stage

- Give hugs; hold hands. Send cards, notes, flowers.

- Provide food, transportation.

- Do chores, but expect the person to help too.

- Help the person see the evidence of the loss.

Guilt and Anger Stage

- Listen, listen, listen. Show no judgment unless asked.

- Call or visit often. Be together in silence.

- Accept abrupt mood shifts.

- Provide assurance that the person was not to blame.

- Recommend and help arrange for support groups.

Adjustment and Acceptance Stage

- Invite the person to go places with you.

- Encourage exercise.

- Offer to listen.

- Reinforce your friendship.

- Encourage rebuilding friendships.

- Offer opportunities for recreation.

- Friends may feel awkward about mentioning your loss. Let them know it's all right to talk about it.

- Get regular exercise. Long walks are particularly healing.

- Write your thoughts down in a journal or paint or draw your grief. Find any way possible to express your feelings.

- Join a support group. Contact your local hospital to learn what's available.

- Postpone major decisions. Don't be rushed into decisions about moving or selling your possessions.

- See Resources 26 and 27 on page 420.

When to Call a Health Professional

If you have any of the following problems after a reasonable amount of time has passed since the loss occurred (This will vary from person to person. In some cases, normal mourning can last for years):

- You have not been able to grieve.

  ○ If you feel excessive anger towards specific people whom you blame for the loss.

  ○ If there is evidence of self-destructive behavior (either physical or financial).

  ○ If you have undiminished and overwhelming feelings of guilt.

- Social isolation increases.

- The grieving process seems to be taking longer than you expect.

Memory Loss

Contrary to what many people believe, normal aging does not contribute to memory loss. When you think about all the information your brain collects and stores over a lifetime, doesn't it seem logical that it should take more time to retrieve some memories? With a little training ("use it or lose it" definitely applies here), you can improve you ability to concentrate and keep your memory sharp.

Sometimes memory lapses indicate a medical problem. The following symptoms could be cause for concern:

- Increasing forgetfulness accompanied by personality changes

- Ignorance about familiar things like the alphabet, numbers, or the names of common objects

- Inability to remember a short name or phone number long enough to write it down. (This could also be due to a hearing problem or failure to pay attention.)

The Memory of Meanings

Most of us experience a memory trade-off as we age. What we lose is speed. It takes a little longer to retrieve names, dates, places, and other specific facts. What we gain has been called the "memory of meanings."

As we age we are better able to understand lessons learned from experience. We continually create new linkages between memories. These memory links may slow us down in retrieving facts. However, they are essential in connecting facts so that we understand the meanings behind them. For example, one study has described how younger school teachers remembered more facts about recently reported events, while older teachers better understood what the facts meant.

Another name for the memory of meanings is wisdom. The insight that comes with age and experience is well worth the trade-off in memory speed. Wisdom is a key to understanding people. It is essential too, if we are to help others to improve their lives.

Prevention

The best way to prevent memory loss is to stay healthy and actively use your memory. The following guidelines can be helpful:

- Eat well and drink plenty of fluids. A balanced, low-fat diet with ample sources of vitamins B_{12} and folate will help protect memory. Drinking plenty of water prevents dehydration, which can cause confusion and memory problems.

- Exercise regularly.

- Get plenty of rest. Many memory problems are the result of being over-tired. If you have difficulty sleeping, see page 315.

- Minimize your use of medications. Overuse of medications may be the single biggest cause of memory loss among older adults.

- Get help if you are depressed. Long-term depression has a powerful impact on memory and can cause other symptoms that mimic dementia.

- Limit your alcohol intake. Alcohol can affect memory long after you sober up.

- Develop a positive attitude about your memory. Reject the notion that memory declines with age. If you expect to keep a strong memory, it will be there when you need it. See Resource 36 on page 421.

Home Treatment

- Follow the prevention guidelines above. If you are concerned that memory loss may be due to dementia or Alzheimer's disease, see page 163.

- Deal with reversible causes of memory loss:

  - Acute illnesses will affect your memory. If you have a fever or any other signs of infection, see page 81.

  - Chronic problems with any major organ system, such as heart or kidney disease, can cause memory loss. If these problems are corrected through medical treatment, memory problems may improve.

  - Consider having your hearing or vision tested. If you do not hear or see well, your brain will have a more difficult time recording information that is heard or seen.

- Get help dealing with depression if you suspect it is a cause. See page 305.

- Learn new techniques to improve your memory:

  - Take a memory improvement course.

  - Strive to increase your attention span and ability to concentrate. Older people have more difficulty than younger people in dividing their attention between two or more activities. Concentrate on learning new things.

  - Keep written notes. Write all your plans on a calendar that you can refer to often.

  - To keep track of your eyeglasses, keep them on a cord around your neck.

  - To avoid misplacing your keys, keep them in a special place by the door.

  - Use a timer with a loud bell whenever you have something on the stove or in the oven.

  - To remember medications, use a medications box with compartments for each day.

When to Call a Health Professional

- If you are concerned that memory loss is caused by prescription drugs or specific medical problems.

- If there are obvious personality changes or memory problems related to immediate recall, or if a person has difficulty remembering familiar things like the alphabet. Also see "A Checkup From the Neck Up" on page 169.

- If memory loss starts to interfere with your work, hobbies, or friendships, or if it is becoming a safety hazard (such as forgetting to turn off the stove).

- If you are concerned about memory loss, or if memory loss has not responded to home treatment, discuss it with your doctor during your next appointment.

Sleep Problems

The term insomnia can mean:

- Trouble getting to sleep (taking more than 45 minutes to fall asleep).

- Frequent wakening with inability to fall back to sleep.

- Early morning awakening.

None of these are problems unless they make you feel chronically tired. If you are less sleepy at night, or if you wake up early, but you still feel rested and alert, there is little need to worry.

Short-term insomnia, lasting from a few nights to a few weeks, is usually caused by worry over a stressful situation. Long-term insomnia, which can last months or even years, is often caused by general anxiety, medications, chronic pain, depression, or other physical disorders.

Prevention

- Get regular exercise, but avoid strenuous exercise within two hours before bedtime.

- Avoid alcohol and smoking before bedtime. Drink caffeine in moderation, and not after noon.

- Drink a glass of warm milk at bedtime.

- Don't drink more than one glass of liquid at bedtime.

Home Treatment

- Don't take sleeping pills. They can cause daytime confusion, memory loss, and dizziness. Continued use of sleeping pills actually increases sleeplessness in many people.

- Try the following six-step formula for one month:

1. Use your bed only for sleeping. Don't eat, watch TV, or read in bed.

2. Sleep only at bedtime. Don't take naps. (However, naps are fine if you don't have sleep problems.)

3. Go to bed only when you feel sleepy.

4. If you lie awake for more than 15 minutes, get up and leave the bedroom.

5. Repeat steps 3 and 4 until it is time to get up.

6. Get up at the same time each day, no matter how sleepy you are.

- Review all of your prescription and over-the-counter medications with a pharmacist to rule out drug-related sleep problems.

- Read about anxiety and depression on pages 303 and 305.

When to Call a Health Professional

- If you suspect medications are causing sleep problems.

- If a month of self-care doesn't solve the problem.

Suicide

People who are very depressed or feel overwhelmed sometimes think of taking their own lives. This is particularly true of older adults who are facing retirement or major illness. Occasional thoughts of suicide do not put a person at high risk. However, if they recur often and persist, they should be treated seriously.

People who are considering suicide are often undecided about choosing life or death. With appropriate help, they can be protected while they are feeling suicidal, and they may choose to live.

Sleep Apnea

Apnea is a common problem that causes people to stop breathing for at least 10 seconds at a time during sleep. It is particularly common in older, overweight men. If apnea occurs frequently (more than 20 times in an hour) a person will complain of extreme daytime sleepiness in spite of seeming to sleep at night.

Apnea usually occurs when the pharynx muscles in the throat become too relaxed during sleep, allowing the pharynx to collapse and obstruct the airway. After a moment, the low level of oxygen causes an automatic response that triggers breathing to start again.

- Find out if you frequently stop breathing for 10 seconds or more while you sleep (having occasional episodes of apnea usually is not serious). Have your spouse monitor your sleep. Your doctor may also arrange for your sleep to be monitored at home or in a special sleep lab.

- Eat sensibly, exercise, and maintain a healthy body weight (obesity contributes to apnea).

- Avoid sleeping pills, alcohol, and antihistamines, which may worsen sleep apnea.

- If surgery is proposed, ask for a second opinion.

Prevention

When you are depressed, or when someone you know is depressed, be alert to the warning signs of suicide:

- Verbal warning. Up to 80 percent of people who commit suicide mention their intentions to someone.

- Preoccupation with death. A suicidal person may talk, read, draw, or write about death.

- Previous suicide attempt. Failed attempts are often followed by a successful attempt.

- Depression and social isolation. See page 305.

- Giving away prized possessions.

Home Treatment

- Use your common sense and a direct approach to determine if the suicide risk is high. Ask yourself or the person who you feel is at risk:

  ○ Do you feel there is no other way out of the crisis?

  ○ Do you have a suicide plan? How do you plan to do it? When do you plan to do it?

- Ask someone you trust to stay with you or the suicidal person until the crisis has passed.

- Encourage the person to seek professional help.

- Don't argue with or challenge someone who is thinking of suicide.

- Don't ignore warning signs thinking that you or another person will "snap out of it."

- Talk about the situation as openly as possible. Show understanding and compassion.

When to Call a Health Professional

- **Call 911 or other emergency services if a suicide attempt has been made.**

- Call your doctor or your local Suicide Prevention hotline (look in the Yellow Pages) immediately:

  ○ If you are considering suicide.

  ○ If you suspect someone has made suicide plans.

  ○ If someone you know has been talking about committing suicide and you are not sure what to do.

Even if you are on the right track,
you will get run over if you just sit there.
Will Rogers

20
Fitness

What would you say if someone told you there is a simple thing you can do that is guaranteed to:

• Make you stronger and more flexible?

• Reduce your risk of heart disease?

• Help you lose weight and look better?

• Give you more energy and enjoyment of life?

Would you do it? You bet you would! A famous doctor who studies older adults once said that if this thing could be put into a pill, it would be the most widely prescribed drug in the world. What is it? It's exercise!

But what if it's been years since you've exercised? Can you still benefit? You bet! Even if you have health problems that limit your mobility or your endurance, you can still find enjoyable activities to help you get results that will make a difference. It's absolutely guaranteed!

Your Personal Fitness Plan

No one can prescribe the perfect fitness plan for you. You have to figure out what you enjoy doing and what you will continue to do. If you enroll in an aerobic dance class, but you feel clumsy and uncomfortable with the music and movements, you're probably not going to stick with the program. On the other hand, if you enjoy walking, you might think about canceling your newspaper subscription so you can walk to the store each morning to pick up a paper. If you are unable to walk, try sitting in a chair and doing stretching and strengthening exercises while listening to your favorite music.

Benefits of Exercise

While regular exercise won't necessarily make you live longer, it will help you live *healthier*. In addition to making you feel good, exercise is one of your best weapons against problems that are commonly associated with aging.

Problem	Effects of Exercise
Arthritis	Improves flexibility and range of motion; improves muscle strength; helps protect joints
Constipation	Regular activity stimulates movement of waste through the intestines.
Chronic obstructive pulmonary disease (COPD)	Improves endurance and feeling of well-being
Depression	Improves self-image; increases energy level; often improves depressed mood
Diabetes (adult onset)	Helps the body use blood sugar more efficiently by making better use of the insulin it produces; helps control weight
Insomnia	Reduces stress, which promotes relaxation. Exercising early in the day often improves sleep.
High blood pressure	Lowers blood pressure; improves heart and lung function
Heart disease	Helps lower cholesterol; improves the heart's ability to pump blood
Obesity	Reduces weight by burning calories
Osteoporosis	Weight-bearing exercise (walking, lifting weights) helps maintain bone strength.

Fitness Assessment

Step 1: Where are you now?

On the scales below, a "10" is the highest fitness level that you could possibly expect to obtain. A "1" on the scale is no activity at all.

For each component, circle your current level of fitness.

Fitness Component

Endurance: 1 2 3 4 5 6 7 8 9 10

No activity   Very active

Muscle Strength: 1 2 3 4 5 6 7 8 9 10

Very weak   Very strong

Flexibility: 1 2 3 4 5 6 7 8 9 10

Very stiff   Very flexible

Step 2: How fit would you like to be?

For each component, circle the level of fitness that you would like to reach.

Step 3: Pick one area for improvement.

Put a "*" next to the fitness component that you want to improve first. Describe your long-term goal here:

_____

_____

Step 4: Set your one-month goal.

For the fitness area that you picked, what can you do to move your fitness up one point on the scale? Pick a one-month goal that you think you can accomplish with easy but consistent effort. Write your short-term goal here:

_____

_____

Step 5: Keep up the good work.

When you have reached your one-month goal, pick a new one. Each new goal can be an extension of the old one or a small step toward improving another fitness component. Good luck and happy fitness!

Personal Fitness Plan - cont.

What matters most is that you choose activities you enjoy and will do again and again.

Consistency is the most important, most basic, and the most often neglected part of fitness. It is the key to receiving all the benefits of fitness.

In general, a good fitness plan for a healthy adult includes exercises to improve endurance, strengthen muscles, and maintain flexibility. Depending upon your overall health and physical abilities, you may benefit from concentrating more on some of these areas, such as strength and flexibility, than others. Read about each of these aspects of fitness on the following pages. Then use the fitness assessment on page 321 to help you set your goals.

Getting Started: Tips for Beginners

If you are just starting a new exercise program, congratulations! You've already accomplished the most difficult task—deciding to do something to improve your fitness. Here are a few things to keep in mind as you begin your adventure.

- Start your new routine gradually. See "How Often and How Long Should I Exercise?" on page 323.

- Spend the first five minutes or so of your exercise routine warming up your muscles by doing some of the stretches on pages 330 to 339. Slowing your pace and adding some gentle stretches at the end of your routine will lower your heart rate gradually, improve flexibility, and reduce the chance of stiffness and injury.

- Expect some minor muscle and joint soreness and stiffness at first. Muscles that are not used to strenuous exercise will become sore shortly after you exercise. Adding new exercises and increasing the duration of your exercise routine also can cause soreness. This is normal and is not a cause for concern as long as the discomfort is not severe and does not persist. Stretching before and after you exercise will help prevent soreness and stiffness. See the box on page 328 for information about when to stop exercising.

- Drink water before, during, and after exercise to avoid dehydration.

- Let your doctor know that you plan to start a new fitness routine. He or she may have special recommendations for you if you have health problems. See the box on page 323.

- If you join an organized exercise class, let your instructor know about any health conditions you have. He or she may ask you to modify or avoid certain exercises that could cause you problems.

How Often and How Long Should I Exercise?

Be enthusiastic about your new fitness routine, but don't overdo it. Start an endurance-building activity by exercising for five to ten minutes twice a week. Add a few more minutes each week as you begin to feel more fit. You'll eventually want to work up to 30 minutes a day, three to four times a week. If this is an unrealistic goal for you, shorten the duration of your activity to 15 to 20 minutes, and do it six times a week.

If you are doing a repetitive activity, such as the strength-building exercises described at the end of this chapter, start by doing three to five repetitions. Increase the number of repetitions or begin adding resistance (weight), when you can do five repetitions with ease. Always take time to rest between exercises.

It's all right to exercise every day (after you've built up your endurance) as long as you don't start feeling extremely fatigued or have persistent muscle or joint pain. These problems are your body's way of telling you that it needs more rest.

Beginning a Fitness Program

For most people, moderate exercise is not a health hazard. However, if you can answer yes to any of the following questions, talk with your doctor before beginning an exercise program.

- Have you been told that you have heart trouble?

- Do you experience chest pains?

- Do you often feel faint or dizzy?

- Do you have arthritis or other bone or joint problems that might be aggravated by improper exercise?

- Do you have high blood pressure?

- Do you have diabetes? (You may wish to see your doctor to review the effects of increased exercise on your diabetic medications.)

- Are you unaccustomed to vigorous exercise and planning to do more than moderate activity (walking or bicycling)?

- Are there other reasons not mentioned here that raise doubts about the safety of exercise for you?

Fit Fitness Into Your Life

Whether you're just starting a new fitness routine or you've been physically active for years, there will be days when exercising just doesn't feel good. Oncoming illness, a poor night's sleep, worry, or a busy schedule can all keep you from getting the most out of your exercise routine. Listen to what your body and mind are trying to tell you. Try to keep going, but if you feel like you are struggling, stop and forget about it for that day. Don't feel guilty about taking a day off.

Unless you are ill, start your routine again the very next day. Chances are, you'll enjoy the activity even more because you've given your body the rest it was asking for. If you do end up taking a short break from your fitness routine, begin again at a lower level of exertion. Even a short layoff can result in a loss of conditioning, but you'll soon regain what was lost. Coming back gradually will reduce your risk of injury.

Endurance Training: Aerobic Fitness

Endurance is a measure of how well you can handle physical stress and strain. In fitness terms, it is how long you can dance, play with grandchildren, or garden without feeling tired or exhausted. Training to improve endurance is called aerobic conditioning. Aerobic means "with oxygen." The purpose of aerobic conditioning is to increase the amount of oxygen that is delivered to your muscles, which allows them to work longer. Any activity that raises your heart rate and keeps it up for an extended period of time is aerobic exercise. Examples include jogging, walking, swimming, dancing, bicycling, cross-country skiing, and rowing.

You may wish to choose an aerobic activity that is kind to your joints, such as walking, biking, or swimming. Aerobic exercise can be even more enjoyable if you have a partner. Ask a friend to join you for walks three times a week. If you love to dance, find out if your local community center or college offers ballroom dance or square dancing classes. You'll be having so much fun you won't even realize that you're exercising!

When it comes to aerobic conditioning, a longer workout is more beneficial than a more strenuous one (see "Pace Yourself" on page 326). Although you can benefit from as little as 10 minutes of aerobic exercise per session, extending your exercise time will increase your rewards. You benefit most from aerobic exercise when you can keep your heart rate up for 20 to 30 minutes.

Walking

Walking is a terrific form of aerobic exercise. It improves endurance and strength. It causes few injuries. It is inexpensive, and enjoyable whether you are alone or in a group.

If you want to start walking for health right now, great! Put this book down and go! It's as easy as that.

The following tips may increase the benefits and your enjoyment of walking:

- Walk at a steady pace, brisk enough to make your pulse and breathing increase, but not so fast that you can't talk comfortably. See the "talk-sing test" on page 326.

- Don't worry about your duration at the beginning. Consistency is what's important. As time goes by and your fitness improves, you'll likely find yourself walking longer (and picking up your pace).

- If there is a shopping mall in your area, find out if there is a morning walking program there. Mall walking is a popular way to exercise (and meet new friends) when the weather is bad.

- Find out about other organized walking groups in your community if you're looking for companionship. Ask at the local senior center, YMCA, or YWCA.

Aerobic Dance

If you like music and dancing, why not give aerobic dance a try? Many fitness centers offer aerobic dance classes for older adults.

How well you like aerobic dance may depend on the instructor. If the intensity of the workout is too high or the music is not to your taste, look for another group. The best way to judge both the instructor and the class is to observe the class and the participants before you sign up.

Swimming

Swimming, water aerobics, and water jogging are forms of aerobic exercise that are easy on your joints and muscles.

Check into what's available in your community. Organized classes are often available, as are open pool times when you can exercise by yourself.

Bicycling

Bicycling is another aerobic activity that is kind to joints and muscles. If you are not inclined to head out onto the open road (helmet firmly on your head), try a stationary bike. The health benefits are the same even if the scenery doesn't change.

Pace Yourself

Aerobic exercise does not have to be strenuous to be valuable. In fact, if you exercise too hard, you get less benefit than if you go at a moderate pace.

There are several ways to monitor your level of exertion. The simplest way is to **listen to your body**. Five to ten minutes into your activity, your body should begin to feel warm. You may begin to perspire. Your breathing should increase. If your pace seems too easy, increase it slightly until you feel as if you are pushing yourself. On the other hand, if you feel as if you are exercising too hard, ease up. You will reduce your risk of injury and enjoy the activity much more.

Another easy way to determine your ideal pace is the **"talk-sing test."**

- If you can't talk and exercise at the same time, you are working too hard.

- If you can talk while you exercise, you are doing fine.

- If you can sing while you exercise, it would be safe (and more beneficial) to exercise a little harder.

Your exercise is most effective when you can talk, but not sing, while doing it.

A more scientific way to monitor your pace it to check your **heart rate**. You can figure out your target heart

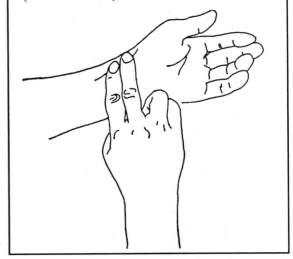

Taking Your Pulse

Your pulse can be felt most easily on the part of your wrist nearest your thumb. Place two fingers over the area with only slight pressure. You should feel a rhythmic beating. Count the number of beats you feel for 10 seconds. Multiply this by 6 to get the number of beats for 1 minute.

Example: 13 beats in 10 seconds gives a one minute pulse of 78 (13 x 6 = 78).

rate with the help of the box on page 327. If you are just starting an exercise program, gradually work up to a level of exertion that gets your heart rate into the low end of your target range. When exercising at a moderate pace, your target heart rate should be 65 to 80 percent of your maximum heart rate, depending on how fit you are.

If you are having a hard time catching your breath, check your heart rate. If you are exercising above your target rate, slow down. If you are in your target range, slow down, but try to reach your target heart rate the next time you exercise. If you continue to have difficulty exercising at your target heart rate, talk to your doctor. As your level of fitness increases (or if you have been exercising consistently for some time), you can try to reach a higher target heart rate.

Important note: The target heart rate method does not work for people who have pacemakers or are using pulse-altering medications. If you are not sure, ask your doctor or pharmacist.

Muscle Strengthening

As people grow older, they tend to lose muscle. Many think this muscle loss is strictly due to aging. Although age-related changes play a role in muscle loss, that's only part of the story.

When it comes to your muscles, the most important advice you can follow is: "Use it or lose it." Muscles become soft, flabby, and weak if they are not being used. Muscles that get regular use stay strong.

Suggested Heart Rate Range

Beginners should try to maintain a heart rate that is in the low end of the target range. Experienced exercisers will get more benefit from trying to reach the higher end of their target range.

Age	10-second heart rate*
50	18-23
55	18-22
60	17-21
65	17-21
70	16-20
75	16-19
80	15-19
85	15-18
90	14-17
95	13-17

*65% to 80% of maximum heart rate.

When to Slow Down or Stop Exercising

Exercising to stay fit may cause minor muscle and joint soreness. That's not a problem. However, it's a good idea to stop exercising if any of the following symptoms develop:

• Chest or upper abdominal pain that may spread to the neck, face, or arms

• Panting or extreme shortness of breath

• Nausea

• Persistent pain, joint discomfort, or muscle cramps

The effects of exercise last long after your workout is over. If you find you are having difficulty sleeping, you may be exercising too late in the day. Morning exercise boosts energy throughout the day and prepares you for a restful night's sleep.

Mild muscle aches and minor strains are to be expected when you first start an exercise program. However, if persistent muscle soreness does not go away after one to two weeks, you may need to modify your exercise routine.

Muscle strength is important to overall health:

• Strong muscles around joints may reduce arthritis pain.

• Strong ankle muscles reduce the chance of sprains.

• Strong abdominal and lower back muscles reduce the chance of back pain.

• Strong leg muscles protect against falls.

Keeping your muscles strong will keep you looking and feeling good and allow you to do all the things you enjoy. If you're not likely to join a gym or an organized fitness class, try exercising at home with inexpensive rubber tubing (see page 334), books, or soup cans while you are watching your favorite TV program. Walking up and down stairs is a great way to strengthen your legs (builds endurance too). Other simple, safe, and effective strengthening exercises can be found on pages 334 to 335. Most of the aerobic exercises discussed earlier will also help strengthen large muscle groups.

Flexibility

Many people notice a significant loss of flexibility as they grow older. The legs, back, neck, and shoulders all seem so much stiffer than before. Is this part of growing older? Maybe not.

Arthritis pain reduces joint mobility. However, if you want to be more flexible to avoid injuries, garden more comfortably, walk more smoothly, or get out of bed more easily, you can. Only minutes per day of slow, pleasant, relaxing stretching will give you results you can feel immediately. Stretching after exercise, when your muscles are warmed up, is particularly helpful.

There are many classes that teach stretching. Yoga and tai chi classes are particularly good. Swimming will help improve flexibility, and so will the exercises on pages 330 to 339.

- Stretch slowly and gradually. Stretch just to the point of muscle tension. If stretching hurts, you have gone too far or you are doing something incorrectly.

- Don't bounce. Maintain a continuous tension on the muscle you are stretching. Relax and hold each stretch for a count of 10.

- Exhale as you stretch to further relax your muscles.

- Try to stretch a little every day, even if you don't have a regular exercise session planned.

Exercises for Muscle Strength and Flexibility

The exercises on the following pages will help improve your muscle strength and overall flexibility. Try to do some of these exercises every day (try them first thing in the morning for an invigorating wake-up!).

- Do these exercises slowly.

- Breathe deeply and don't hold your breath.

- For exercises that are helpful for strengthening back and abdominal muscles, see pages 32 to 36.

Chair Exercises

For neck flexibility:

1. Slow Neck Stretches

- Gently lower your right ear toward your right shoulder. Hold for 5 counts.

- Bring head back to center.

- Gently lower your chin to your chest. Hold for 5 counts.

- Gently lower your left ear toward your left shoulder. Hold for 5 counts.

- Return to center.

- 5 repetitions.

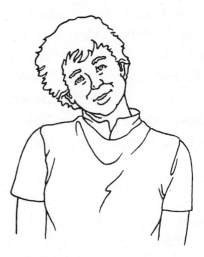

1. Slow neck stretches

2. Half-Circles

- Keep your chin level.

- Gently turn your head to the right. (Try to look over your shoulder.) Hold for 2 counts.

- Gently turn your head to the left. Hold for 2 counts.

- 5 repetitions.

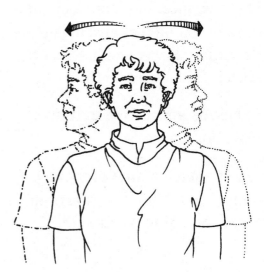

2. Half-circles

For shoulder flexibility:

3. Shoulder Rolls

- Keep your arms relaxed and at your sides.

- Trace large circles in the air with your shoulders.

- Roll forward 5 times, backward 5 times.

For hand and wrist flexibility:

4. Finger Squeezes

- Extend your arms in front at shoulder level, palms down.

- Slowly squeeze your fingers to form a fist, then release. 5 repetitions.

- Turn palms up. Squeeze and release. 5 repetitions.

5. Hand Circles

- Extend your arms in front at shoulder level. Keep your elbows straight, but not locked.

- Rotate your wrists in small circles.

- Do 10 circles forward, 10 backward.

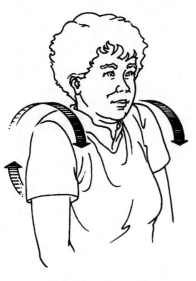

3. Shoulder rolls

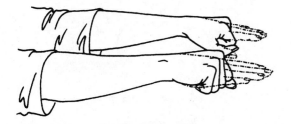

4. Finger squeezes

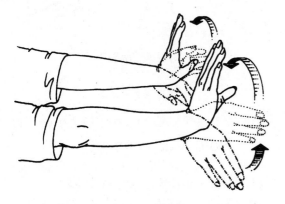

5. Hand circles

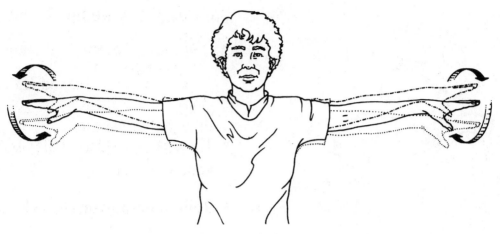

6. Arm circles

To strengthen shoulders and upper back:

6. Arm Circles

- Raise your arms at sides to shoulder level. Keep your elbows straight.

- Rotate your arms from shoulders in small circles.

- Do 10 circles forward, 10 backward.

For trunk flexibility:

7. Spine Twists

- Sit or stand with your back straight, head high.

- Raise your arms out to your sides at shoulder level. Bend your elbows upright, palms facing forward.

- Keep hips and knees facing forward.

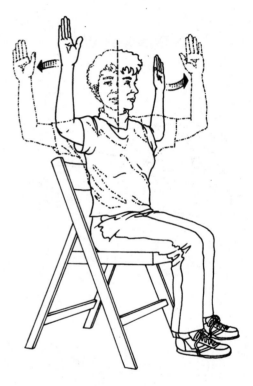

7. Spine twists

- Slowly twist your upper body to the right. Hold for 5 counts.

- Return to center, then twist to the left. Hold for 5 counts. Do 5 repetitions.

To strengthen knee flexors and lower abdomen:

8. Knee Lift

- Raise your right knee to your chest or as far upward as possible. Do not pull up or push down with hands.

- Return to starting position.

- Bring your left knee to your chest.

- Do 5 repetitions for each leg.

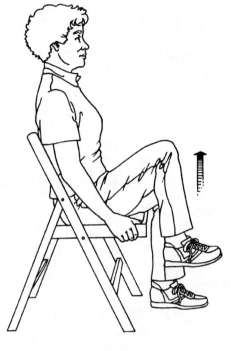

8. Knee lift

For ankle flexibility:

9. Ankle and Foot Circling

- Sit in a chair and cross your right leg over your left knee.

- Slowly rotate your right foot, making large circles.

- For each ankle, do 10 rotations to the right, 10 to the left.

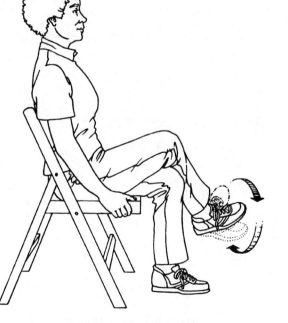

9. Ankle and foot circling

Rubber Tubing Exercises

For these exercises, you will need a 24-inch length of surgical latex tubing with knots tied at each end. Some exercise "stretchies" are sold at fitness stores.

When you use a "stretchie," go slowly and be careful not to overstretch.

At the start, hold each stretch for a count of 5. You may increase the time as you get stronger. Keep a firm grip too. You don't want the tubing snapping back at you!

These exercises will improve strength and flexibility in the arms and shoulders. They will also build strength in the chest and back.

10. Stretch and Reach

* Shorten the stretchie by holding one end with one hand and gripping the middle with the other hand.

* Raise both arms overhead, hands facing forward.

* Reach for the ceiling with alternate hands.

* Do 5 repetitions each hand.

11. Overhead Stretch

* Raise both arms overhead, hands facing forward.

* Tighten tubing by slowly pulling both arms away from center. Do not overstretch.

* Do 5 repetitions.

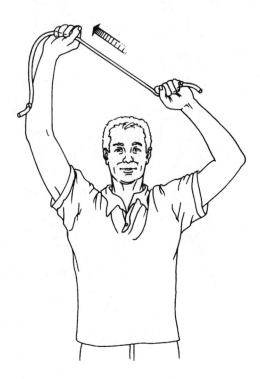

10. Stretch and reach

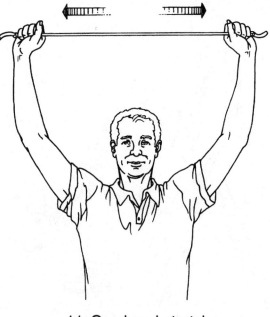

11. Overhead stretch

12. Up-down Stretch

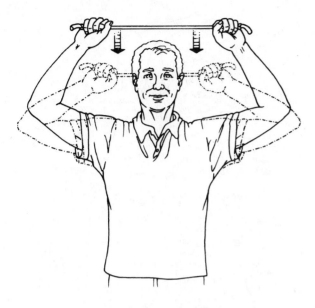

* Raise both arms overhead.

* Stretch the tubing slightly.

* Bend your elbows and lower arms; bring tubing to rest on shoulders behind your head.

* Do 5 repetitions.

12. Up-down stretch

13. Chest-level/Lap-level Stretch

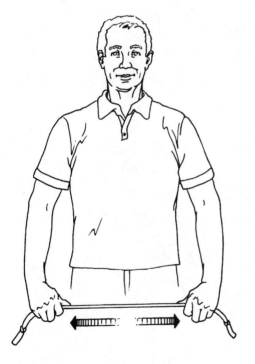

* Raise your arms out in front to shoulder level.

* Pull your hands apart, stretching tubing.

* Do 5 repetitions.

* Drop your arms to the level of your lap.

* Pull your hands and arms away from your body to the sides.

* Do 5 repetitions.

13. Lap-level stretch

Exercises Done While Standing

Hold onto a sturdy object, like the back of a chair, for these exercises.

For upper torso flexibility:

14. Side Stretch

- Hold onto the chair back with your right hand.

- Stand with your feet shoulder-width apart.

- Bring your left arm up and over your head. Slowly bend over to the right. Feel the stretch in your left side. Hold for a count of 10.

- Slowly return to an upright position. Do 5 repetitions for each side.

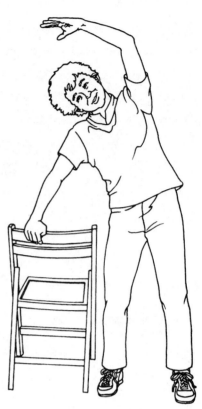

14. Side stretch

For stretching calf muscles:

15. Calf Stretch

- Face the back of the chair and point your toes straight ahead.

- Stretch your right leg behind you. Keep your left leg slightly bent.

- Press your right heel to the floor. (You should feel the stretch in your right calf muscle.)

- If you cannot get your heel down, move your legs closer together. Hold for a count of 5.

- Repeat 5 times for each leg.

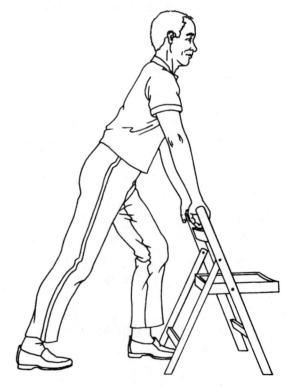

15. Calf stretch

To tone and strengthen legs and ankles:

16. Heel Raises

- Hold onto the chair back for support.

- Rise up on your toes. Hold for 5 counts.

- Repeat 10 times.

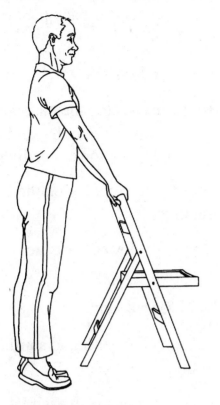

16. Heel raises

For balance and hip flexibility:

17. Leg Swings

- Stand up straight with your left side to the chair back. Hold on with your left hand.

- Gently swing your right leg to and fro. Repeat 10 times.

- Use controlled movements. Don't let your body move to the back or front when you swing your leg.

- Repeat 10 times with your left leg.

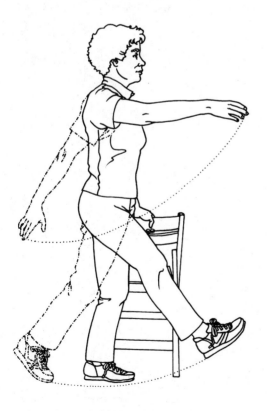

17. Leg swings

Floor Exercises

You may need to hold on to a piece of furniture that will support your weight (sofa, armchair) as you lower yourself and rise from the floor to do these exercises.

Some people become mildly dizzy when rising from the floor after exercising. To prevent a fall, sit up for a moment and let any dizziness pass before you try to stand up.

To stretch lower back and hamstrings:

18. Hamstring Stretch

- Lie on your back with your knees bent and feet close to buttocks.

- Bring your right knee to your chest, keeping your left foot flat on the floor (or your left leg straight, whichever feels better on your lower back).

- Keep your lower back pressed to the floor.

- Hold for 5 counts.

- To further stretch the hamstring, straighten your right leg and flex your right foot toward ceiling.

- Grasp your right leg on the back of the thigh.

- Keep your lower back pressed to the floor.

- Hold for 5 counts.

- Relax and lower leg to starting position.

- Repeat 5 times with each leg.

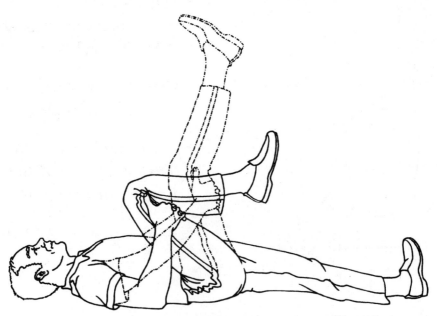

18. Hamstring stretch

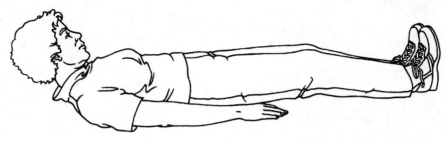

19. Head and shoulder curl

To strengthen stomach and neck muscles:

19. Head and Shoulder Curl

• Lie on your back with your knees slightly bent.

• Keep arms at sides.

• Curl your head and shoulders off floor. Hold for 5 counts.

• Return to starting position.

• Repeat 10 times.

To strengthen and tone hip and thigh muscles:

20. Side-lying Leg Lifts

• Lie on your right side, legs extended.

• Raise your left leg as high as is comfortable.

• Lower to starting position.

• Repeat 10 times for each leg.

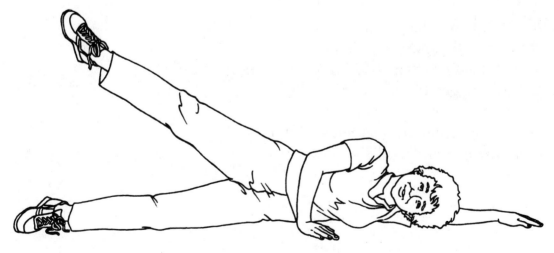

20. Side-lying leg lifts

You're On Your Way!

The exercises and advice outlined in this chapter are meant to give you a basic introduction to the world of physical fitness. There are literally hundreds of different activities that, when done regularly, will help you improve your endurance, muscle strength, and flexibility. One of them is right for you. If you would like to explore some more options, read Resources 24 and 25 on page 420.

One of the simplest ways to reward yourself for your work is to record your progress in a notebook or on a calendar. Each day write down:

- What you did.

- How long you did it.

- How hard you felt your effort was.

- Your attitude or motivation for that day.

A record like this will help you measure and improve the most important part of your fitness program—its consistency. As the pages fill up, your record will become an important reminder of how successful you have been in improving your health.

Eat less sugar
Eat less fat
Beans and grains
Are where it's at.
Unknown

21
Nutrition

As you age, certain things can happen that may change both what you need and what you choose to eat.

- Your metabolism slows down, so you need less energy from food.

- Physical changes may make different foods more attractive to you. For example, soft foods may be more appealing if you have dental problems. Sweet or salty foods may appeal to you if your senses of taste and smell have changed.

- Slowed digestion can cause constipation. You may find it helpful to increase the amount of fiber in your diet.

- Your lifestyle may change. You may eat alone more often, which may make you less inclined to prepare complete meals. Arthritis and other health problems may make shopping and meal preparation difficult.

Although your body needs fewer calories from food, it still needs plenty of vitamins, minerals, and fiber to maintain good health. That is why eating healthy foods becomes even more important as you get older. Use the checklist on page 344 to determine your nutritional health status.

Seven Simple Guidelines for Eating Well

(Dietary Guidelines for Americans, USDA, 1995)

1. Eat a variety of foods. Include a daily selection of:

- Whole-grain and enriched breads, cereals, and grain products

- Vegetables

- Fruits

- Milk, cheese, and yogurt

- Meats, poultry, fish, eggs, dried beans and peas, tofu

2. Balance the food you eat with physical activity. Maintain or improve your weight. See page 360.

3. Eat plenty of complex carbohydrates (grains, vegetables, starches, and fruits). These foods pack the most nutrients per calorie. See pages 345 to 346.

4. Choose a diet that is low in fat, saturated fat, and cholesterol. Fat has twice as many calories per gram as any other nutrient. A high-fat diet increases your risk for heart disease and some cancers. See pages 350 to 352.

5. Use sugars in moderation. Sugars have little, if any, vitamins, minerals, or fiber. See page 349.

6. Use salt and sodium in moderation. For some people, sodium increases blood pressure. See page 359.

7. If you drink alcoholic beverages, do so in moderation. Alcohol is high in calories and has no nutrients. As you age, your body breaks down alcohol more slowly, so it stays in your body longer. Drinking the same amount that you drank 20 years ago can cause a lot more damage.

Eating Alone?

Many older adults live and eat alone. This can affect your nutritional status, since you may not eat as well as when you are with others. You may not take the time to make balanced meals, or you may skip meals. If you often eat alone, consider the following:

- Plan your meals for the week and shop from a list. You are more likely to eat meals for which you have planned and have all the ingredients.

- Take turns with friends preparing meals for one another and eating together.

- Contact your local or state health department to find out about congregate meal sites in your area. They provide low-cost, nutritious meals and opportunities for socializing.

- Find out if your community has a Meals on Wheels program. If you are temporarily or permanently homebound, this service will deliver a hot, nutritious meal once a day.

- If you sometimes don't have enough money to buy the food you need, you may be eligible for Food Stamps or Supplemental Security Income (SSI).

Guide to Eating Well

Grains (breads, cereals, rice, pasta) form the foundation of a healthy diet. Serving sizes: 1 slice of bread, 1 oz. of cereal, ½ bagel, ½ cup of pasta or rice.

Eat plenty of fruits and vegetables. Serving sizes: ¾ cup fruit or vegetable juice; ½ cup raw, canned, or cooked fruits or vegetables; medium apple or banana; 1 cup raw leafy vegetables.

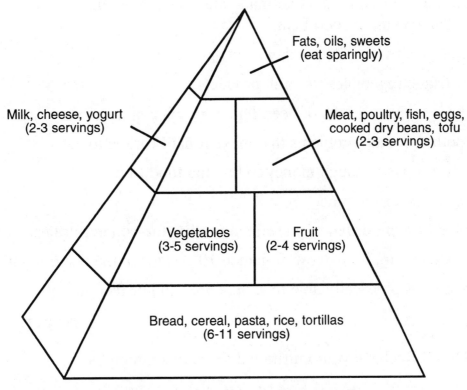

The Food Guide Pyramid (USDA)

Eat more fish, poultry, and cooked dry beans to reduce fat. Serving sizes: 2 – 3 oz. cooked lean meat, poultry, or fish; ½ cup cooked dry beans; 1 egg; 2 tbsp. peanut butter.

Choose nonfat or low-fat dairy products. Serving sizes: 1 cup milk or yogurt; 1½ – 2 oz. low-fat cheese; ½ cup cottage cheese.

Eat foods from the top of the pyramid only in moderation. Examples: cooking oil, butter or margarine, high-fat salty snacks, alcohol, candy.

Determine Your Nutritional Health

The warning signs of poor nutritional health are often overlooked. Use this checklist to find out if you or someone you know is at nutritional risk. Read the statements below. Circle the number in the yes column for those that apply to you or someone you know. Add up the numbers you circled for your total nutritional score.

	YES
I have an illness or condition that made me change the kind and/or the amount of food I eat.	2
I eat fewer than two meals per day.	3
I eat few fruits, vegetables, or milk products.	2
I have three or more drinks of beer, liquor, or wine almost every day.	2
I have tooth or mouth problems that make it hard for me to eat.	2
I don't always have enough money to buy the food I need.	4
I eat alone most of the time.	1
I take three or more different prescribed or over-the-counter drugs a day.	1
Without wanting to, I have lost or gained 10 pounds in the last 6 months.	2
I am not always physically able to shop, cook, and/or feed myself.	2

TOTAL _____

0-2   **Good!** Recheck your nutritional score in six months.

3-5   **You are at moderate nutritional risk.** See what you can do to improve your eating habits and lifestyle. Your office on aging, senior nutrition program, senior citizens center, or health department can help. Recheck your nutritional score in three months.

6 +   **You are at high nutritional risk.** Bring this checklist with you the next time you see your doctor, dietitian, or other qualified health or social service professional. Talk with them about any problems you have. Ask for help in improving your nutritional health.

Developed and distributed by the Nutrition Screening Initiative, a project of The American Academy of Family Physicians, The American Dietetic Association, and The National Council on the Aging, Inc., 1994.

Eating Well: A Basic Plan

Each day, eat a variety of foods from the Guide to Eating Well on page 343. Eat more from the bread and cereal and fruit and vegetable groups than from the other groups. Most people who follow this plan will get all the vitamins, minerals, and other nutrients that their bodies need.

Breads, Cereals, and Starches

Contrary to popular belief, bread, potatoes, rice, and pasta are not fattening. Starches are carbohydrates, which have less than half as many calories per gram as fat. Unprocessed starches (whole grains, vegetables) also contain large amounts of vitamins, minerals, fiber, and water.

These foods become fattening only when you add fat to them (or if you eat too much of them). Try substituting nonfat yogurt or salsa for butter and sour cream on baked potatoes. Use fresh vegetable and tomato sauces instead of rich cream sauces on pasta.

Fruits and Vegetables

Fresh fruits and vegetables provide vitamins, minerals, and fiber and are low in fat. Many fruits and vegetables contain a lot of vitamins A (beta carotene) and C, especially oranges and other citrus fruits, broccoli, sweet potatoes, winter squash, carrots, spinach, and other leafy greens.

Better Nutrition Can Be Easy

You don't have to change your whole diet at once. Just pick one improvement and stick with it:

- Buy only whole-grain bread.
- Buy only skim or low-fat milk.
- Use less oil for cooking and buy vegetable oil that is liquid at room temperature.
- Eat fish at least twice a week.
- Drink an extra glass of water when you wake each morning.

If you are generally healthy, you don't need to worry about maintaining a perfect diet. If you make healthy eating choices 80 percent of the time, occasionally enjoying high-fat or high-calorie foods the other 20 percent of the time won't be a problem.

A diet that includes lots of fruits and vegetables may help protect against heart disease and cancer.

Fruits and vegetables are most nutritious when they are eaten fresh and raw or lightly cooked. Steam or microwave vegetables to retain more vitamins.

Fruits and Vegetables Against Cancer

Fruits and vegetables are key elements of good basic nutrition. They contain lots of fiber, especially when eaten raw. A high-fiber diet may protect you against colon cancer.

Many vegetables and fruits contain the two antioxidant vitamins, A (beta carotene) and C, as well as other compounds that may protect against some cancers. Beta carotene is found in deep orange and dark green vegetables and fruits such as carrots, apricots, winter squash, sweet potatoes, cantaloupe, and broccoli. Vitamin C is found in citrus fruits and citrus fruit juices, such as oranges and orange juice, and in cantaloupe, strawberries, peppers, broccoli, and tomatoes.

Vegetables in the cabbage family, including broccoli, cauliflower, and brussels sprouts, appear to protect against several types of cancer.

The National Cancer Institute recommends that you eat at least five servings per day of fruits and vegetables to lower your risk of cancer.

While cooked or canned fruits and vegetables lose some nutrients during processing, they are better than not eating fruits and vegetables at all. Frozen raw or canned vegetables may have more nutrients than fresh vegetables that have been left in the refrigerator for several days.

Fiber

Fiber is the undigestible part of plants. It is not absorbed into the bloodstream like other nutrients. However, it plays an important role in keeping the digestive tract healthy by providing "bulk." There are two types of fiber:

Insoluble fiber, which can be found in whole-grain products like wheat flour, provides bulk for your diet. Together with fluids, insoluble fiber stimulates the colon to keep waste moving out of the bowels. Without fiber, waste moves too slowly, increasing your risk for constipation, colon cancer, and diverticulosis.

Soluble fiber, which is found in fruit, legumes (dry beans and peas), and oats, helps lower blood cholesterol, reducing your risk of heart disease. The fiber in legumes also can help regulate blood glucose levels.

Do you need more fiber in your diet? If your stools are soft and easy to pass, you probably get enough fiber. If they are hard and difficult to pass, more fiber and water may help. See page 118 for more information about constipation.

To increase fiber in your diet:

- Eat at least five servings of fruits and vegetables a day. Eat fruits with edible skins and seeds: figs, blueberries, apples, and raspberries. Eat more of the stems of broccoli and asparagus.

- Switch to whole-grain and whole-wheat breads, pasta, tortillas, and cereals. The first ingredient listed on the label should be *whole*-wheat flour. If it just says wheat flour, it means white flour from which most of the fiber has been removed.

- Eat more cooked dry beans, peas, and lentils. These high-fiber, high-protein foods can replace some of the high-fat, no-fiber meats in your diet.

- Popcorn is a good high-fiber snack. However, avoid adding oil, butter, and salt. Use an air or microwave popper to eliminate oil, and flavor with salt substitute or herb mixtures.

Water

As you age, your ability to sense thirst decreases, so you need to drink plenty of water to avoid dehydration. Along with fiber, water is important in preventing constipation.

One easy way to make sure you're getting enough water is to drink a big glassful when you first get up in the morning and continue to drink until you get six to eight 8-ounce glasses (two quarts) of water a day. If you drink other liquids, you can get by with less, but plain water is best. (Milk is a good choice, with the added bonus of a boost of calcium.)

If you are concerned about overloading your bladder, follow these tips:

- Gradually increase your water intake by a glass per week to give your body a chance to adjust.

- Drink most of your water in the morning and early afternoon.

Caffeine

There is no convincing evidence that a moderate amount of caffeine (two to three cups of coffee or cola per day) will do you any harm if you are healthy.

Caffeine is mildly addictive, and cutting back too quickly may cause a headache. Gradual reductions in caffeine work well.

Magic Elixir Promises Health Benefits!

Ladies and gentlemen, the miraculous magic elixir pictured here is essential to your continued good health. Not only does it taste great, but this magic tonic is guaranteed to protect your health in seven important ways.

1.   Aids Digestion! Helps to unlock the nutrients in your food.

2.   Prevents Constipation! At last, regularity is within your grasp.

3.   Keeps Vital Body Fluids in Balance!

4.   Helps Protect Against Colds, Coughs, Flu, and Sore Throats! You will stay healthier than ever before.

5.   Prevents Urinary Tract Infections! You will be "in the clear" and avoid troublesome irritations.

6.   Protects You From the Heat of the Sun! Helps cool your body to guard against heat stroke.

7.   Helps Weight Loss! Controls your appetite with no adverse side effects.

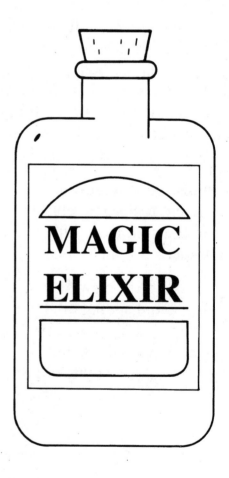

Yes, ladies and gentlemen, this miracle tonic is available today. It is one hundred percent natural and totally calorie-free. There are no artificial flavorings or preservatives whatsoever. Best of all, it can be delivered fresh to your home for less than a penny a day!

Drink one glass more today than you did yesterday, and two more than that tomorrow...until you are hooked on eight or more glasses a day. Order yours today by contacting your kitchen faucet, your Perrier dealer, or a mountain spring.

Yes, you guessed it right...the magic elixir is WATER!

Sugar

What's wrong with sugar? It comes from a vegetable (sugar beets or sugar cane), is relatively cheap, tastes good, is fat-free, and is even a carbohydrate. Can sugar be all that bad?

From a health point of view, the biggest problem with sugar is that it is stripped of all vitamins, minerals, and fiber. What is left are crystals of pure carbohydrate calories.

In moderation, sugar does little harm. However, if too many of your calories come from sugar, you will either gain too much weight or not get enough of the other nutrients you need. Sugar also contributes to cavities.

To reduce sugar in your diet:

- Be aware that all sugars are basically alike. Honey and brown or raw sugar have no advantage over other sugars.

- Processed foods can be full of hidden sugars. Flavored yogurt, breakfast cereals, and canned goods often have sugar added. Check the label for words that end with "-ose," like dextrose, fructose, sucrose, lactose, and maltose, which are forms of sugar. Corn syrup is another common form of sugar.

Artificial Sweeteners

Although artificial sweeteners do help you avoid sugar, losing weight depends more on reducing calories from fat. Avoid using artificially sweetened foods to justify eating more high-fat food.

Aspartame (NutraSweet) and saccharin are considered safe, but the effects of long-term use are not known. Use them in moderation. People who have PKU (phenyl-ketonuria—an inborn error of metabolism) should not use aspartame.

- Be aware that you lose taste buds as you age. Foods may need more sugar or other seasonings to taste like they used to. Try using more sweet spices, like cinnamon and nutmeg, in your favorite recipes.

- Limit foods that list sugar among the first few ingredients on the label.

- Look for breakfast cereals that have six grams or less of added sugar per serving.

- You can reduce the sugar in home-baked goods by up to one-half without affecting their texture.

- Make it a habit to eat a sweet piece of fruit instead of a sugary dessert most of the time.

Fats in Foods

Fat (the butter, cream, lard, oil, and grease in food) accounts for 37 percent of the calories in the average American diet. Fat has more than twice as many calories per gram as carbohydrates or protein.

How much fat is too much? The U.S. Dietary Guidelines recommend that less than 30 percent of total calories come from fat. Reducing dietary fat from 37 percent to 30 percent will slow the development of heart disease, reduce cancer risk, and improve your overall diet.

However, many scientists think a diet with 30 percent fat is still too high for a healthy heart. A diet that consists of 20 percent fat will further reduce the risk of heart disease and can also help inactive older adults maintain their weight.

There is some evidence that a 10-percent fat diet, along with other lifestyle changes can even reverse narrowing of the arteries (atherosclerosis). However, a 10-percent fat diet is hard to maintain. Based on your heart disease risks, you may wish to set a goal for how much fat to include in your diet. A registered dietitian (see page 356) can create a menu plan that will help you meet your goal.

Calculating Percent Fat

Each gram of fat contains 9 calories. To calculate the percent of a food's total calories that come from fat, multiply the grams of fat times 9 and then divide by the total number of calories. Multiply your result by 100 to get the percent.

For example, an 8-ounce serving of 2% milk has 5 grams of fat and 130 total calories.

$$\frac{5 \text{ grams fat x } 9 \text{ calories/gram x } 100}{130 \text{ calories}}$$

$$= \textbf{35\% calories from fat}$$

The new food labels contain information about the percentage of your daily fat allotment in a serving of food.

In a 2,000 calorie-per-day diet, the total daily fat allotment is 65 grams. Foods that get more than 30 percent of their calories from fat are not necessarily bad for you. A healthful diet combines higher-fat foods with lower-fat foods such as fruits, vegetables, and grains. It is recommended that no more than 30 percent of your total calories come from fat.

16 Simple Ways to Reduce Fat in Your Diet

When eating meat:

1. Reduce serving sizes to two or three ounces (about the size of a deck of cards), and don't eat seconds. If you like red meat, choose the leanest cuts, such as tenderloin, flank steak, chuck, top and bottom round, or lean veal.

2. Eat more poultry and fish. They contain less saturated fat than red meat.

3. Remove all visible fat before cooking. Poultry skin may be removed either before or after cooking.

4. Broil or bake instead of frying.

5. Replace some meat proteins with a combination of legumes (dried beans, peas, lentils) and grains.

When using dairy products:

6. Use skim, ½, or 1 percent milk.

7. Choose cheeses made with skim or part skim milk, or look for cheeses that have no more than five grams of fat per ounce (read the label).

8. Try low-fat or nonfat cottage cheese or yogurt in place of cream and sour cream, or use fat-free sour cream and cream cheese.

Types of Fat

Fats found in food are a mixture of three types: saturated, mono-unsaturated, and polyunsaturated. Saturated fats are found in meats (especially red meat), eggs, and dairy fats (butter, cheese, cream, etc.). Many processed foods contain saturated fats such as coconut oil, palm oil, or cocoa butter. A diet that includes a lot of saturated fat will cause increased levels of LDL ("bad") cholesterol in the blood (see page 352).

Monounsaturated fats (found in olive and peanut oil, avocados, most nuts, chicken, and fish) helps lower your LDL cholesterol level. Polyunsaturated fats (found in corn, sunflower, safflower, walnut, canola, and cottonseed oil) help lower your total cholesterol (both LDL and HDL).

Food labels indicate how many fat calories come from saturated fat and how many come from unsaturated fat. Try to limit your intake of saturated fats so that they are no more than one-third of your total daily fat intake (about 21 grams in a 2,000 calorie-per-day diet).

In cooking:

9. Steam vegetables. If you choose to saute them, use one table-spoon of oil (or less), or try using other liquids such as wine, defatted broth, or cooking sherry.

10. Use non-stick pans, or add oil to a preheated pan (less oil goes further this way).

11. Season vegetables with herbs and spices instead of butter and sauces, or try butter substitutes such as Butter Buds or Molly McButter.

12. Experiment with using less oil than is called for in recipes. You may need to increase other liquids. Use applesauce, prune puree, or mashed bananas to replace some or all of the fat in baked goods.

In general:

13. Avoid high-fat crackers, chips, non-dairy creamers, and mar-garines made with hydrogenated oil, palm oil, coconut oil, or cocoa butter.

14. Eat plenty of carbohydrates to fill you up (fruits, vegetables, grains, bread, pasta, etc.).

15. Let salads go naked, or eat them modestly dressed in lemon juice or fat-free mayonnaise or dressing.

16. Use fresh vegetable and tomato sauces instead of rich cream sauces on pasta.

Cholesterol

Cholesterol is a waxy fat that is produced by the human body and is also found in animal products. Your body's cells need cholesterol to function. Unfortunately, excess cholesterol builds up inside the arter-ies (atherosclerosis), increasing your risk for heart disease and stroke.

Good and Bad Cholesterol

Fat is carried in your blood attached to protein. The fat-protein combina-tion is called a lipoprotein. Two lipoproteins are the main carriers of cholesterol: low-density lipoprotein (LDL) and high-density lipoprotein (HDL).

LDL ("bad" cholesterol) acts like a fat delivery truck. It picks up choles-terol from the liver and delivers it to the cells. When more cholesterol is ready for delivery than the cells can take, LDL deposits the extra cholesterol on artery walls. A high concentration of LDL cholesterol in your blood *increases* your risk of heart disease and stroke.

HDL ("good" cholesterol) works like a garbage truck. It removes excess cholesterol from the bloodstream and takes it back to the liver. A high concentration of HDL cholesterol *decreases* your risk of heart disease and stroke.

Cholesterol Screening

Basic cholesterol screening tests are easy, quick, and inexpensive. They do not require fasting for accurate results. A test every five years is appropriate for most people. Call your local health department to learn if free or low-cost cholesterol tests are available.

If your total cholesterol is greater than 200 mg/dl (milligrams per deciliter), or if you have any of the following risk factors, have your cholesterol checked more often:

- Family history of early heart attack (before age 55 in father or brother; before age 65 in mother or sister)

- Current cigarette smoking

- High blood pressure (greater than 140/90)

- Diabetes

Experts don't agree on the best schedule for cholesterol testing. You and your doctor can determine the schedule that is best for you based on your risk factors.

If your total cholesterol is greater than 200, tests that measure your HDL and LDL levels can help further clarify your risk. See the chart on page 354 for an explanation of how HDL, LDL, triglycerides, and total cholesterol levels are related to risks.

For many people, a low-fat diet (see page 351) and exercise are all that is needed to lower blood cholesterol. People who have heart disease (or who are at very high risk) may need medication, as well as exercise and a low-fat diet, to lower their cholesterol.

Cholesterol in Foods

Only animal products (meat, poultry, fish, eggs, and dairy products) contain cholesterol. Of those, only egg yolks and organ meats are high in cholesterol. In fact, your cholesterol intake has less to do with raising blood cholesterol than does your fat intake (especially saturated fat), along with too many calories. To reduce blood cholesterol, eat a low-fat diet, specifically limiting saturated fat.

How to Reduce Your Cholesterol

- Eat less total fat, especially saturated fat. Follow the guidelines for eating less fat on page 351.

- Use cooking oil that is liquid at room temperature, and use it sparingly (one teaspoon at a time).

What Do the Numbers Mean?

Doctors don't agree on which cholesterol numbers are most useful in determining your risk of heart disease. The most commonly used values are listed here.

Desirable: All of the following:

- Total cholesterol below 200

- HDL cholesterol 45 or above

- LDL cholesterol below 130 (If you already have coronary artery disease, this should be below 100.)

- Total to HDL ratio below 4.5 (Below 3.5 is ideal)

Borderline high-risk: One or more of the following:

- Total cholesterol 200-239

- HDL cholesterol below 45

- LDL cholesterol 130-159

High-risk: One or more of the following:

- Total cholesterol 240 or higher

- HDL cholesterol below 35

- LDL cholesterol 160 or above

- Total to HDL ratio 4.5 or higher

For **triglycerides** (a type of fat):
Desirable: below 165

Borderline high-risk: 166-249

High-risk: 250 or above

- Eat two to three servings (two to three ounces per serving) of baked or broiled fish per week. Most fish contains omega-3 fatty acids, which may help lower blood cholesterol and triglycerides. In general, fish with darker flesh, such as mackerel, lake trout, herring, salmon, and halibut, have more omega-3 oils. The safety and value of fish oil supplements is not yet fully known.

- Get more exercise. Exercise increases your protective HDL cholesterol level.

- Quit smoking to increase your HDL levels and reduce your risk of heart disease.

- Lose weight if your doctor recommends it. Losing even 5 to 10 pounds can increase HDL levels and lower your total cholesterol.

Reversing Heart Disease

A low-fat diet and lifestyle changes may actually reverse the process of heart disease and help reopen arteries that are clogged by atherosclerosis.

Participants in the Lifestyle Heart Trial followed a vegetarian diet containing less than 10 percent of calories from fat and no caffeine. They also stopped smoking, got 30 minutes of exercise at least six days a week, and practiced a relaxation technique (deep breathing, stretching, muscle relaxation, etc.) for one hour each day. After a year, over 80 percent of the participants had lost weight, reduced their cholesterol, and most importantly, reduced the amount of blockage in their coronary arteries.

For more information, see Resource 28 on page 420.

- Eat more soluble fiber to help lower total cholesterol. See page 346.

- Attend a low-fat diet workshop or consult with a registered dietitian. A registered dietitian can help you lower your fat consumption to 30 percent, 20 percent, or less of total calories, based on your goal.

Medication for High Cholesterol

Several medications are effective in lowering cholesterol. However, they may have side effects, they are expensive, and they require lifelong use. Unless a person's LDL levels are very high, most doctors will recommend diet changes to try to lower cholesterol before prescribing medications.

Medications may be prescribed sooner for people with diabetes, high blood pressure, or other conditions that increase the risk of heart attack or stroke. Even if you are taking medication, you must still follow a low-fat diet.

Protein

Protein is important for maintaining healthy muscles, tendons, bones, skin, blood, hair, and internal organs. The need for protein does not decrease with age. Fortunately, most older adults get all the protein they need. In fact, most Americans get twice as much protein as they require.

If you eat animal products (milk, cheese, eggs, fish, meat), your diet will contain plenty of protein. If you eat little meat, poultry, or fish and use no dairy products, your diet will require careful planning to get all the protein and other nutrients you need.

Vitamins

Vitamins are tiny, unseen elements of food that have no calories; yet they are essential to good health. For most people, a diet that contains a variety of foods from the Guide to Eating Well (page 343) provides all the necessary vitamins.

Vitamins A, D, E, and K are fat-soluble and can be stored in the liver or in fat tissue for a relatively long time. The other nine vitamins are water-soluble and can be retained by the body only for short periods. They include:

- Thiamine (B_1)
- Riboflavin (B_2)
- Niacin (B_3)
- Pantothenic acid
- Biotin
- Folate
- Vitamin B_6 (pyridoxine)
- Vitamin B_{12} (cobalamin)
- Vitamin C

If you are eating less than 1,500 calories per day, you may wish to consider taking a vitamin-mineral supplement. Make sure the supplement you choose does not exceed 100 percent of the Recommended Dietary Allowance. Check the label to find this information. See page 357.

How to Contact a Registered Dietitian

If you have a health problem that requires you to maintain a strict diet, consider consulting a registered dietitian.

To locate a registered dietitian (RD) in your area, call the American Dietetic Association's Consumer Nutrition Hotline at 1-800-366-1655. You can listen to recorded messages about specific foods or nutritional guidelines, or you can speak with an RD or receive a referral to one in your area. The recorded messages are available weekdays from 9 a.m. to 9 p.m. (Eastern time). Dietitians are available between 10 a.m. and 5 p.m. This is a free service.

Personal consultations with a registered dietitian may not be covered by insurance. Check with your insurance carrier.

Minerals

Minerals in food help regulate the body's water balance, hormones, enzymes, vitamins, and fluids. Eating a variety of foods is the best way to get all of the minerals you need.

A total of 60 minerals have been discovered in the body, and 22 of these are essential to health. We know the most about calcium, sodium, and iron. All three are particularly important to older adults.

Calcium

Calcium is the primary mineral needed for strong bones. Women lose calcium from their bones most rapidly after menopause. A diet rich in calcium and vitamin D, combined with exercise, can help slow the loss of bone mass. This prevents or postpones osteoporosis (page 55) and the brittle bone fractures that it causes.

A total of 1500 milligrams of calcium per day is recommended for women after menopause. You can get this much from your diet if you consume three to four servings of items from the milk group each day (see the Guide to Eating Well on page 343 for serving sizes). Each serving contains about 300 milligrams of calcium (except cottage cheese). Try to choose low-fat and nonfat dairy

Vitamin-Mineral Supplement Buyer's Guide

Research shows that the vitamins found in certain foods may prevent some diseases, but it remains unproven whether supplements do the same. If you choose to take vitamin and mineral supplements, the following guidelines may be helpful:

- Choose a balanced, multiple-vitamin-mineral supplement rather than a specific vitamin or mineral, unless it has been prescribed by a doctor.

- Choose a supplement that provides about 100 percent of the RDA (Recommended Dietary Allowance) for vitamins and minerals.

- Avoid taking much more than 100 percent of the RDA for any vitamin or mineral unless prescribed by a doctor. This is particularly important for the fat-soluble vitamins A, D, E, and K, and for minerals. Because they are stored in the body, large doses can be toxic.

- High-priced brand-name vitamins are no better than store or generic brands.

products to avoid excess fat and calories. See the box at right if you have difficulty digesting milk (lactose intolerance).

Other foods such as tofu, soy milk, broccoli, greens, and calcium-fortified orange juice will also add calcium in smaller amounts.

While dietary calcium is preferred, low-dose calcium supplements may help slow bone loss. Any of the purified calcium compounds (calcium carbonate, calcium citrate, calcium gluconate, etc.) are well absorbed, as is calcium with amino acids (called chelates).

One 500-milligram TUMS (calcium carbonate) tablet provides about 200 milligrams of calcium. Taking a few TUMS tablets each day can help you meet your calcium needs.

Avoid bone meal, dolomite, and oyster shell calcium, as they are less well absorbed and are often contaminated with toxic minerals. Calcium absorption is improved by taking several small doses throughout the day, rather than one large dose once a day, and by taking calcium supplements with dairy products.

Men need 800 milligrams of calcium a day, which can be obtained from two servings from the milk group each day, plus the additional calcium found in other foods in the diet.

Milk or Lactose Intolerance

People whose bodies produce too little of the enzyme lactase have trouble digesting the lactose sugar in milk. In some people, lactose intolerance increases with age. Symptoms include gas, bloating, cramps, and diarrhea.

Tips for dealing with lactose intolerance include:

- Eat small amounts of dairy products at any one time.

- Drink milk only with snacks or meals.

- Try cheese, which usually does not cause symptoms. Yogurt made with active cultures causes fewer tolerance problems.

- Pretreated milk, enzyme treatments, and enzyme tablets (LactAid, Dairy-Ease) are available in most stores. Ask your pharmacist.

- If you cannot tolerate milk in any form, include other calcium-rich foods in your diet, including greens (mustard greens, kale, parsley, watercress), broccoli, tofu, corn tortillas, almonds, sesame seeds, and calcium-fortified orange juice. Consider a calcium supplement.

Sodium

Salt is the most familiar source of sodium. Other major sources of sodium are monosodium glutamate (MSG), baking soda, baking powder, soy sauce, and seasoning salts. Many canned and processed foods contain large amounts of sodium.

Most people get far more sodium than they need. Our bodies need only 500 milligrams per day. Anything over 2500 milligrams is probably too much. For some people, excess sodium causes high blood pressure. This "sodium sensitivity" increases with age.

If you want to cut back on the sodium in your diet:

• Read labels for sodium content.

Creative Salt Substitute

Mix together and put in a shaker:

½ teaspoon cayenne pepper

½ teaspoon garlic powder

1 teaspoon each:

Basil	Onion powder
Black pepper	Parsley
Mace	Sage
Marjoram	Savory
Thyme	

• Limit ready-mixed sauces and seasonings, frozen dinners, canned or dehydrated soups, and salad dressing. These foods are usually packed with sodium. Products labeled "low sodium" contain less than 140 milligrams of sodium per serving.

• Eat lots of fresh or frozen fruits and vegetables. These foods contain very little sodium.

• Don't put the salt shaker on the table, or get a shaker that allows very little salt to come out. Use salt substitute or Lite Salt sparingly.

• Always measure the salt in recipes and use half of what is called for.

• Avoid fast foods, which are usually very high in sodium. In a restaurant, ask the chef not to salt food during cooking.

Iron

The body needs small amounts of iron to make hemoglobin, which carries oxygen in the blood. Most older adults need about 10 milligrams of iron per day. An inexpensive blood test, done in your doctor's office, can determine if you need additional iron.

To get more iron in your blood:

• Get plenty of vitamin C, which helps you absorb more iron from food. Drink a glass of orange or other citrus juice while you eat a bowl of iron-enriched cereal. A high-iron cereal has at least 25 percent of the Daily Value (DV) for iron.

- The iron in animal tissues (heme iron) improves absorption of the iron in vegetables. Eat meat and veggies together to get an added boost of iron.

- Avoid caffeinated tea with meals. It interferes with iron absorption.

Iron-Deficiency Anemia

Iron-deficiency anemia in older adults is usually caused by chronic blood loss from the digestive tract.

Symptoms of iron-deficiency anemia include paleness and fatigue. If you have been diagnosed with iron-deficiency anemia, you will need to increase your iron intake. Your health professional will want to determine the cause of blood loss.

Iron Supplements

Older adults who eat fewer than 1,500 calories per day may wish to consider a vitamin-mineral supplement that contains iron. A low-dose ferrous-form iron supplement of no more than 20 milligrams per day is safe for most people. However, too much iron can cause a number of serious medical problems. Don't take more without consulting your doctor first. Take the supplement with orange or other citrus juice. Keep iron supplements away from children.

A Healthy Weight

People come in all shapes and sizes. Genetics, exercise, and the food you eat all play a role in determining your body's shape and size.

Eating well, enjoying physical activity, and accepting your body size are the keys to maintaining a sensible, nutritionally sound diet. Although excess body fat does increase your risk for heart disease, diabetes, and stroke, it is more important to focus on healthy habits rather than trying to achieve a certain body size or weight.

Exercise Makes It Easier

Regular exercise helps you maintain lean muscle mass while you are losing weight. This will help you feel stronger, more energetic, and in better overall health. As a bonus, regular exercise makes maintaining a healthy weight a little easier. See Chapter 20 for exercise guidelines.

Never Go Hungry

Skipping meals is not a good way to lose weight. Going hungry, even for a few hours, can cause your metabolic rate to drop and will make you more likely to overeat later. Eat a variety of nutritious low-fat foods. Take time to savor your food and relax during meals.

Get Help From Your Friends

The food customs and habits of friends and family affect what you eat. Those you spend time with can help you succeed with your weight-control plan. Ask friends and family to:

- Encourage you to respect yourself regardless of what you weigh.

- Celebrate events with a variety of nutritious foods and activities that everyone can enjoy.

- Serve meals that include low-fat or lower-calorie foods.

- Make water and low-fat snacks available.

- Offer small servings, and don't insist on second helpings.

- Join you in a walk, swim, or other enjoyable activity.

Help Yourself to Good Thoughts

Develop a positive attitude about yourself. Think of yourself as healthy, and take pride in making good nutrition and exercise choices. Focus on living a healthy life regardless of your weight.

Tips for People Who Are Underweight

If you have trouble gaining or maintaining your weight, try the following:

- Eat three meals plus three snacks a day. Don't skip meals.

- Use liquid supplements (such as Ensure) between meals to add calories.

- Choose the higher-calorie items from each food group (e.g., whole milk instead of skim milk).

- Eat the highest-calorie items first in a meal.

- Add extra fat to the foods you prepare.

We don't stop playing because we grow old.
We grow old because we stop playing.
Anonymous

22
Stress and Relaxation

Stress is the physical, mental, and emotional reactions you experience as the result of changes and demands in your life.

Stress is part and parcel of common life events, both large and small. It comes with all of life's daily hassles, traffic jams, long lines, petty arguments, and other relatively small irritations. Stress also comes with crises and life-changing events, such as illness or disability, marriage problems or divorce, loss of a spouse or other family member, retirement, children leaving home, and caregiving responsibilities.

All of these events may force you to adjust, whether you are ready to or not. Unless you can regularly release the tension that comes with stress, it can increase your risks for physical and mental illness.

Because many major life events are beyond your control, take charge of those aspects of your life that you can manage. One major change doesn't mean that all areas of your life must change. Continue to participate in the same activities you did before the event happened.

Not all stress is bad. Positive stress (eustress) is a motivator, challenging you to act in creative and resourceful ways. When changes and demands overwhelm you, negative stress (distress) sets in. This chapter has specific techniques that you can use to cope with stress in your life.

What Stress Does to the Body

At the first sign of alarm, chemicals released by the body automatically trigger the physical reactions. The physical reactions to stress are universal:

- Heart rate increases to move blood to the muscles and brain.

- Blood pressure goes up.

- Breathing rate increases.

- Perspiration increases.

- Digestion slows down.

- Pupils dilate.

- You feel a rush of strength.

Your body is tense, alert, and ready for action. For primitive people, these reactions were an advantage in the face of sudden danger, preparing them for survival by "fight-or-flight." Today, our bodies still react the same way, but it is not as acceptable to fight or run away from our stressors (although we often wish we could).

After the natural "alarm" reaction to a real or perceived threat, our bodies stay on alert until we feel that the danger has passed. When the stressor is gone, the brain signals an "all clear" sign to the body, which stops producing the chemicals that caused the physical reaction. The body then returns to normal.

Problems with stress occur when the brain fails to give the "all clear" signal. If the alarm state lasts too long, you begin to suffer from the consequences of constant stress. Unrelieved stress can lead to many health problems, such as headaches, sleep problems, fatigue, heartburn, colds, and heart disease.

Recognizing Stress

Sometimes it's difficult to recognize or admit that stress is affecting your health. If you can learn to watch for its effects and take corrective action quickly, you will be able to cope with your stress.

The signs of stress are classic. You may get a headache, stiff neck, nagging backache, rapid breathing, sweaty palms, or an upset stomach. You may become irritable and intolerant of even minor disturbances. You may lose your temper more often and yell at your family for no good reason. Your pulse rate may increase and you may feel jumpy or exhausted all the time. You may find it hard to concentrate. Everyone responds to stress differently.

When these symptoms appear, recognize them as possible signs of stress and find a way to deal with them. Just knowing why you're crabby may be the first step in coping with the problem. It is your attitude toward stress, not the stress itself, that affects your health the most.

Managing Stress

When people are under stress, their good health habits often fall by the wayside. Some people try to relieve stress by smoking, drinking, overeating, or taking pills. There is a better way. Avoid the dangerous side effects of tobacco, alcohol, and drugs by learning to control your stress level. You can do this by using your body to soothe your mind and by using your mind to relax your body.

Stress and tension affect our emotions and feelings. By expressing those feelings to others, we are able to better understand and cope with them. Talking about a problem with a spouse or good friend is a valuable way to reduce tension and stress.

Crying can also relieve tension. It's part of our emotional healing process. Expressing yourself through writing, crafts, or art may also be a good tension reliever.

Exercise is a natural response to stress. It is the normal reaction to the fight-or-flight urge. Walking briskly will take advantage of the rapid pulse and tensed muscles caused by stress and relieve your pent-up energy. After a walk, you usually feel better and your stress level is more manageable.

Relaxation Skills

Whatever you do to manage stress, you can benefit from the regular use of relaxation skills. When learning relaxation skills, remove yourself from all outside distractions. It may take some practice to become comfortable with these techniques. Once you've trained your body and mind to relax (after two to three weeks), you'll be able to produce the same relaxed state whenever you want.

This chapter is devoted to skills and techniques to relax your body. In addition to exercise, deep breathing, muscle relaxation, mental relaxation, and imagery are good ways to relieve tension.

Deep Breathing

The way we breathe is also a sign of stress levels. Breath-holding and hyperventilation (the feeling of not being able to catch your breath) are symptoms of tension. Whenever you find yourself doing either, use it as a cue to take time out to relax.

Roll Breathing

The object of roll breathing is to develop full use of your lungs. It can be practiced in any position, but it is best to learn it lying on your back, with your knees bent.

1. Place your left hand on your abdomen and your right hand on your chest. Notice how your hands move as you breathe in and out.

2. Practice filling your lower lungs by breathing so your left hand goes up and down while your right hand remains still. Always inhale through your nose and exhale through your mouth.

3. When you have filled and emptied your lower lungs 8 to 10 times, add the second step to your breathing. Inhale first into your lower lungs as before, and then continue inhaling into your upper chest. As you do so, your right hand will rise and your left hand will fall a little as your stomach draws in.

4. As you exhale slowly through your mouth, make a quiet, whooshing sound as first your left hand and then your right hand falls. As you exhale, feel the tension leaving your body as you become more and more relaxed.

5. Practice breathing in and out in this manner for three to five minutes. Notice that the movement of your abdomen and chest is like the rolling motion of waves rising and falling.

Practice roll breathing daily for several weeks until you can do it almost anywhere, giving you an instant relaxation tool anytime you need one.

Caution: Some people get dizzy the first few times they try roll breathing. If you begin to hyperventilate or become lightheaded, slow your breathing. Get up slowly and with support.

The Relaxing Sigh

During the day you may catch yourself sighing or yawning. A sigh or yawn releases a bit of tension.

1. Sit or stand up straight.

2. Sigh deeply, letting out a sound of deep relief as the air rushes out of your lungs.

3. Don't think about inhaling. Just let the air come in naturally.

4. Each time you breathe out, shake your hands away from your body as if you were throwing your tension away.

5. Repeat this 8 to 12 times whenever needed. Feel the relaxation.

Muscle Relaxation

Stress and tension can lead to tight, sore muscles, especially in the neck and upper back. It may also contribute to headaches and fatigue. Techniques to relax your muscles can relieve tension and lead to relaxation.

Head, Neck, and Shoulder Massage

Massage helps relieve tight shoulder, neck, and back muscles and may work on headaches. It is best to have someone do the massage for you. However, many of the following steps (2, 5, 6, 7) can be done on your own.

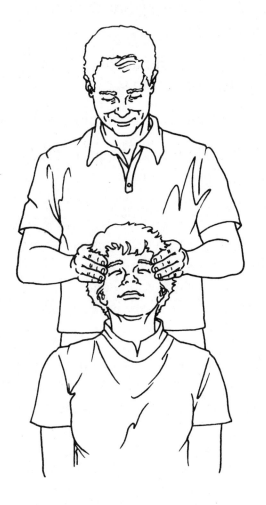

1. Have your partner sit comfortably upright in a chair with her feet flat on the floor. Stand behind her.

2. Using both hands, gently massage across the top of the shoulders with a kneading motion.

3. Apply gentle but firm and even pressure with your thumbs across the top of the shoulders. Work your way toward the neck and then back across to the ends of the shoulders.

4. Locate the vertebrae at the base of the neck. Place your thumbs on either side of the vertebrae and apply gentle but firm pressure away from the spine. Continue down the back. Do *not* press on the spine itself.

5. Locate the indentations at the base of the skull on either side of the spine at the back of the head. Apply gentle rotating pressure with your thumbs.

6. Use three fingers on each hand to massage the jaw muscles. Have your partner clench her jaw. You will easily find the muscles that need to be rubbed. Make sure your partner's jaw is unclenched before you massage the muscles.

7. Gently massage the temples using your fingertips. Work across the forehead and back to the temples.

8. Bring your hands back to the shoulders and allow your hands to say "goodbye" with a few soft, calming strokes.

Progressive Muscle Relaxation

In response to stressful thoughts or situations, the body reacts with muscle tension. Deep muscle relaxation can calm the mind as well as ease muscle tension.

Procedure and Muscle Groups

Choose a place where you can lie down on your back and stretch out comfortably, such as a carpeted floor or firm bed.

You can use a prerecorded tape to help you go through all the muscle groups, or you can just tense and relax each muscle group as described below.

Tense each muscle group for 4 to 10 seconds (hard, but not to the point of cramping); then give yourself 10 to 20 seconds to release it and relax.

Hands: Clench them.

Wrists and forearms: Extend them and bend the hands back at the wrist.

Biceps and upper arms: Clench your hands into fists, bend your arms at the elbows, and flex your biceps.

Shoulders: Shrug them.

Forehead: Wrinkle it into a deep frown.

Around the eyes and bridge of nose: Close your eyes as tightly as possible (remove contact lenses before beginning the exercise).

Cheeks and jaws: Grin from ear to ear.

Around the mouth: Press the lips together tightly.

Back of the neck: Press your head back firmly.

Front of the neck: Try to touch the chin to the chest.

Chest: Take a deep breath, hold it, then exhale.

Back: Arch your back up and away from the supporting surface.

Stomach: Suck it into a tight knot.

Hips and buttocks: Squeeze the buttocks together tightly.

Thighs: Clench them hard.

Lower legs: Point your toes toward your face, as if trying to bring the toes up to touch your head. Then point your toes away and curl them downward at the same time.

When you are finished, arouse yourself thoroughly by slowly counting backwards from five to one.

Mental Relaxation

A lot of stress is the result of worried thoughts or negative "self-talk." By learning to quiet your mind, you can calm and relax your body. You will need a stretch of uninterrupted time and a quiet place for the following mind-relaxing techniques.

Relaxation Response

The relaxation response is the exact opposite of a stress response. It slows the heart rate and breathing, decreases blood pressure, and helps relieve muscle tension.

Exercise: The Natural Way to Relax

A regular fitness program is a natural way to relieve stress and relax. Try walking, swimming, dancing, biking, and stretching your way to relaxation. Exercise strengthens the body's ability to deal with stress, lowering susceptibility to both mental and physical illness.

Vigorous exercise also stimulates the body's production of endorphins. These chemical messengers from the brain produce feelings of well-being. Exercise will help you tap into your brain's own natural tranquilizers.

Technique (adapted from Herbert Benson, MD); also see Resource 53 on page 422.

1. Sit quietly in a comfortable position with your eyes closed.

2. Begin progressive muscle relaxation. See page 368.

3. Become aware of your breathing. As you exhale, say the word "one" (or any other word or phrase) silently or aloud. Instead of focusing on a repeated word, you can also fix your gaze on a stationary object. Concentrate on breathing from your abdomen and not your chest.

   Continue this for 10 to 20 minutes. As distracting thoughts enter your mind, don't dwell on them; just allow them to drift away.

4. Sit quietly for several minutes, until you are ready to open your eyes. Notice the difference in your breathing and your pulse rate.

Don't worry whether you are becoming deeply relaxed. The key to this exercise is to remain passive, to let distracting thoughts slip away like waves on the beach.

Practice 10 to 20 minutes a day, but not within two hours after a meal. When you have set up a routine, the relaxation response should come with little effort.

Imagery

Imagery is a relaxation skill that requires some imagination. In your mind's eye, create a mental picture of a relaxing scene, such as basking in warm sun or strolling through a beautiful garden. Let yourself experience the peace of your mental scene. Your body will respond with lowered pulse rate, controlled breathing, and muscle relaxation.

1. Begin with your choice of a relaxation technique (progressive muscle relaxation, stretching, deep breathing).

2. Use the relaxation response to calm your mind and focus your attention. Then, vividly create within your mind the picture of a peaceful scene. It can be a sunny beach, a mountain meadow, or whatever works for you. Concentrate on the sights, sounds, and smells of your special place, letting the tranquility of the setting permeate your being. Stay as long as you like.

3. Continuing with your deep breathing, slowly come back to reality. Remember, this is your special place to relax. Come here any time you wish.

Color Imagery

1. Close your eyes and scan your body for any points of tension. Associate the color red with this tension.

2. Take a deep breath and change the color from red to blue. Let all the tension go. Experience the relaxation associated with the color blue.

3. Imagine the color blue becoming darker and darker. Relax further with each deepening shade.

4. Practice changing from red to blue with each daily hassle you confront. Use the color blue as your cue to relax.

Eye Relaxation (Palming)

1. Put your palms over your closed eyes. Block out all light without putting too much pressure on your eyelids.

2. Visualize the color black. You may see other colors or images, but focus on black.

3. Continue with this for two to three minutes, thinking and focusing on black. Slowly open your eyes, gradually getting accustomed to the light. Feel the relaxation in the muscles around your eyes.

You've got to accentuate the positive
Eliminate the negative
Latch on to the affirmative
Don't mess with Mr. In-between
From a song by Johnny Mercer

23
Mind-Body Wellness

The Mind-Body Connection

Medical science is making remarkable discoveries about how our expectations, emotions, and thoughts affect our health. One part of this science is called **psychoneuroimmunology**, or PNI. It is the study how the brain communicates with the rest of the body by sending chemical messengers in the blood and how this affects our immune system.

Your brain can trigger your body to make gamma-globulin for fortifying your immune system and interferon for fighting infections, viruses, and even cancer. These and other naturally occurring substances can be combined in the blood to create a defense system for fighting illness and speeding healing. Your brain can also create natural painkillers called endorphins.

The substances that your brain helps your body produce depend in part on your thoughts and feelings. In other words, your body's ability to heal itself is linked to your state of mind and your state of mental wellness.

If you'd like to know more about how you can enlist your mind to boost your immune system and help you manage chronic illness, read on.

Positive Thinking

Your level of optimism and your expectations of what can happen affect what goes on inside your body. People with positive attitudes generally enjoy life more. Aside from that, are they any healthier? The answer is often yes.

Optimism is a resource for healing. Optimists are more likely to overcome pain and adversity in their efforts to improve their outcomes.

For example, optimistic coronary bypass patients generally recover more quickly and have fewer post-operative complications than people who are less hopeful.

Conversely, pessimism seems to aggravate ill health. One long-term study showed that people who were pessimistic in college have significantly higher rates of illness through age 60.

People seem to develop a tendency toward either optimism or pessimism at an early age. However, even if your general outlook on life tends to be gloomy, there are steps you can take to enjoy psychosomatic wellness by using your brain to support your immune system.

The Hardy Personality

Some people have more innate protection from disease than others. Their immune systems appear to be naturally more efficient. Researchers have identified three factors that stand out in the personalities of hardy people.

1. Hardy people show a strong commitment to self, work, family, and other values.

2. Hardy people have a sense of control over their lives.

3. Hardy people generally see change in their lives as a challenge rather than as a threat.

Boosting Your Immune System

Your body's immune system responds to your thoughts, emotions, and actions. In addition to staying fit, eating right, and managing stress, the following three strategies will help your immune system function well:

1. Create positive expectations for health and healing.

2. Open yourself to humor, friendship, and love.

3. Appeal to the Spirit.

1. Create positive expectations for health and healing.

Mental and emotional expectations can influence medical outcomes. The effectiveness of any medical treatment depends in part on how useful you *expect* it to be.

The "placebo effect" proves that expectations affect health. A placebo is a drug or treatment that provides no medical benefit except for the patient's belief that it will help. On the average, 35 percent of patients who receive placebos report satisfactory relief from their medical problems, even though they received no actual medication.

Changing your expectations from negative to positive may give your immune system a boost. Here's how:

- Stop all negative self-talk. Make positive statements that promote your recovery.

- Write your illness a letter. Tell it that you don't need it anymore and that your immune system is now ready to finish it off.

- Send yourself a steady stream of affirmations. An affirmation is a phrase or sentence that sends strong, positive statements to you about yourself, such as "I am a capable person," or "My joints are strong and flexible."

- Visualize health and healing. Add mental pictures that support your positive affirmations.

- Become a cheerleader for your immune system. Talk to it and encourage it to be strong and keep fighting.

2. Open yourself to humor, friendship, and love.

Positive emotions strengthen the immune system. Fortunately, almost anything that makes you feel good about yourself helps you stay healthy.

- Laugh. A little humor makes life richer and healthier. Laughter increases creativity, reduces pain, and speeds healing. Keep an emergency laughter kit of funny videotapes, jokes, cartoons, and photographs. Put it with your first aid supplies and keep it well stocked.

- Seek out friends. Friendships are vital to good health. Close social ties help you recover more quickly from illness and reduce your risk of developing diseases such as arthritis and depression.

- Volunteer. People who volunteer live longer and enjoy life more than those who do not. By helping others, we help ourselves.

- Plant a plant and pet a pet. Plants and pets can be highly therapeutic. When you stroke an animal, your blood pressure goes down and your heart rate slows. Animals and plants help us feel needed.

3. Appeal to the Spirit.

If you believe in a higher power, ask for support in your pursuit of healing and health. Faith, prayer, and spiritual beliefs can play an important role in recovering from an illness.

Your sense of spiritual wellness can help you overcome personal trials and things you cannot change. If it suits you, use spiritual images in visualizations, affirmations, and expectations about your health and life.

Positive Affirmations

An affirmation is a phrase or statement that sends strong, positive messages to you about yourself. Affirmations can raise both conscious and subconscious expectations about your future. They allow you to improve the reality you create for yourself.

An affirmation can be any positive statement. It can be very general: "I am a capable person." Affirmations can also help you with a specific problem: "My memory serves me well."

To create an affirmation:

- Express the statement in positive terms. Instead of "My joints hurt less today," say "My joints are strong and flexible."

- Keep it simple and put it in the present. Instead of saying "I am going to be more relaxed," say "I am completely and deeply relaxed."

- Phrase affirmations with "I" or "my." Try "I am a supportive husband," rather than "Mary appreciates the help I provide."

To practice your affirmation:

- Write it down 10 to 20 times. Then read and reread what you wrote.

- Repeat your affirmation silently or aloud at any time during the day (after waking, during housework, while walking, just before bed, etc.). Repeat it slowly and with conviction.

- If negative self-talk comes up, develop affirmations to counteract these contrary thoughts.

Affirmations help build a more optimistic attitude. However, they are not meant to contradict your true feelings. For problems with depression, anger, anxiety, and emotions, see Chapter 19.

Mentally Managing a Chronic Illness

Many of the health problems discussed in this book, such as headaches, flu, and colds, get better with good home care or medical treatment. These **acute** illnesses tend not to hang on and usually don't do any long-term harm to your body.

As people get older, they tend to get **chronic** problems such as arthritis, high blood pressure, heart disease, or diabetes. Unlike acute illnesses, chronic conditions don't go away. Generally, they can be managed, but not cured completely.

Your frame of mind can make a big difference in how much your chronic illness affects your life and how well you respond to treatment. People who decide not to let their health problems dominate their lives tend to be less bothered by the health problems than people who are overcome by fear and worry about their health.

Living with a chronic condition is not easy. In addition to its symptoms, chronic illnesses are often accompanied by tension, depression, and fatigue. It's difficult to feel positive when it seems like so much is going wrong. However, what you think can determine how good you feel and how "in control" you feel. Negative feelings can inhibit your immune system and limit your body's ability to heal itself and fight disease. On the other hand, positive thoughts and expectations can boost your immune system to help you cope with the disease.

Dealing With Chronic Pain

Chronic pain is a common problem in many chronic diseases. Chronic pain often has a mental as well as a physical component. Pain is not "all in your head," but your thoughts and feelings about the pain often affect how much pain you feel. Feeling anxious, angry, frustrated, or out of control about your pain may make it worse. Your mind and body are important allies in your efforts to manage pain. Your brain can release natural substances called endorphins, which can block pain. Their release depends on how you are thinking and feeling about your pain.

You can train yourself to think and feel differently about chronic pain. These ideas are not a substitute for treatments or advice from your doctor, but they may be a helpful addition to your regular medical care.

- Take control of the pain. This may mean accepting that the pain is not going away while you decide to take active steps toward managing it and keeping it from affecting your life too much.

- Track how your moods, thoughts, and feelings affect your pain. Make a record of your pain level, activities, moods, thoughts, and feelings several times a day for several days. You may find that your pain is worse during or after certain activities or when you are feeling a certain emotion.

- Recognize negative self-talk. Your thoughts can affect your perception of pain. Try to recognize any negative or self-defeating thoughts you have about your pain, such as "This pain will never get better," or "I'll never be able to play with the grandkids with this pain."

- Practice positive self-talk. When you catch yourself in a negative thought, actively replace it with a positive statement, such as "I can manage this pain," or "I will relax before the kids get here."

- Try a relaxation technique. Chronic pain causes stress and tension, which in turn may increase pain. See pages 365 to 370 for relaxation techniques. Gentle exercise, such as walking, also helps relieve tension.

- Change the way you do daily activities so that you can do them with less pain. Try assistive devices (see page 414).

If you can put your mind to work against the pain, you may find that you can manage it better and that it interferes less with your life. Also see "Dealing With Chronic Pain" on page 61 and Resources 48 and 49 on page 422.

Winning Over Serious Illness

A feeling of hopelessness and despair often arrives hand-in-hand with a diagnosis of chronic or life-threatening illness. The best way to triumph over cancer, heart disease, diabetes, or any other serious illness is to shake that feeling of hopelessness and stay in control of your life.

- Remember who you really are. Who you are does not change because of your diagnosis.

- Keep communication open with family and friends. Talking openly about your illness will help them as well as you.

- Gather your support network around you. Forget any notion about being a burden. Letting people help you helps them to feel good about themselves.

- Join a support group of other people coping with the same problem. Finding even one person who has overcome a problem similar to yours can raise your spirits and add to your confidence.

- Avoid guilt. While there is a lot you can do to reduce your risk of illness and improve your chances of recovery, some illnesses develop and persist no matter what you do. Let go of guilt and don't blame yourself. Some things just are.

Lots of people win their struggles over serious illness, either by being cured or by not letting illness control their lives. While there are no guarantees, taking charge of your life will give both your body and your mind the best opportunity to be victorious.

Growing Wiser: Mental Wellness in Later Life

Although some people complain about their age, few would trade age for youth. It would mean giving up wisdom.

Wisdom is one of life's greatest gifts. Cultures the world over recognize the wisdom of their elders. However, although growing wiser is part of the natural aging process, it doesn't happen automatically.

Two Voices

There are two competing voices within each person. One voice is the "Naysayer," the doubter. This voice mutters, "You're too old. You're not useful. You're not wanted. You're getting dependent." The Naysayer tries to limit what we can do and what we can enjoy.

The second voice within us is the voice of the "Sage." This is the voice of experience that tells us, "You have lots to offer. You are needed. You can make it." The ability to hear and listen to the Sage within us is essential to mental wellness.

Visualization

Visualization adds mental pictures to your affirmations. Focus on your affirmation and start thinking of mental images that support it.

- Select one specific affirmation, for example, "My hands are flexible and pain-free."

- Develop a mental image of your affirmation. For example, for pain-free hands, imagine that a cool, soothing fluid is pouring over your hands, making them more and more flexible. Be as creative as you like, but keep it simple.

- Repeat the mental picture over and over. Combine several longer sessions with short replays of the visual picture throughout the day.

- Add positive self-talk and affirmations to the mental picture. If any doubts arise, dismiss them until after the exercise. This time is for positive thoughts only.

- Practice makes perfect. With daily visualizations, you will soon be creating mental pictures that help you meet your goals.

Unfortunately, for many people, the Naysayer dominates the Sage. Myths and negative expectations about aging stifle the Sage while they strengthen the voice of the Naysayer.

Refuse to be limited by negative stereotypes! The secret to developing your wisdom is simply to recognize the Sage within you. The Growing Wiser Formula will encourage the voice of your Sage. Use the formula to help structure your thinking about any problems that may otherwise place limits on you.

Growing Wiser Formula

Step One: Understand the Facts

Wisdom needs information with which to work. Learn all you can about yourself and your problem. Focus not just on the negative consequences, but also on the positive potential within you.

Step Two: Reject Unnecessary Limitations

Carefully probe any uncertainties identified in Step One. If you cannot prove a negative assumption that threatens to limit your life, reject it. You can, for example, accept the fact that you have arthritis while rejecting the idea that it will restrict you unduly.

Step Three: Create Positive Expectations

The most important factor in overcoming a problem is whether you expect to overcome it. Positive expectations can be built around affirmations and visualizations of your goal. When you have a clear vision of what you would like to happen, it is easier to take control of the problem.

Positive expectations also trigger the release of healing substances within your body. The brain releases chemical messengers that affect the healing process. Once you replace unnecessary limitations with positive expectations, your problem is often half-solved.

Step Four: Develop an Action Plan

The other half of problem solving is being ready to act. An action plan will put you in control. It will help you get what you want and expect out of life.

An effective action plan includes these elements:

- It addresses a goal.

- It considers all available options.

- It is something you can visualize.

- It is easy to start.

- It recognizes barriers.

- It includes rewards.

- It encourages support.

- It can be accomplished one step at a time.

For more on mental wellness for older adults, see Resource 36 on page 421.

A great oak is only a little
nut that held its ground.
Anonymous

24
Declaring Independence

You are the captain of your own ship, the chief executive of your own corporation, and the president of your own sovereign state.

As a human being, your most basic right is to independently control your own life and make your own decisions. This means choosing where you will live, how you will spend your money, what health services you will accept, and what, if any, type of help you need and when.

Sometimes, others who care about you may try to make decisions for you. Certainly, you may wish to listen to the suggestions of your loved ones; they can be great sources of information. Listen carefully to the suggestions and options offered you, think them over, and then decide for yourself. Being assertive will help you stay in charge.

You have the right to retain control over the basic decisions of your life for as long as you are able or willing to do so. (By writing down your wishes on a statement called an advance directive, you can retain some control over health care decisions even if you are no longer competent. See page 382.)

Assertiveness

Assertiveness is the art of speaking up for yourself and getting what you want without infringing on the rights of others. As an assertive person, you can exercise your rights without denying or violating the rights and feelings of others. You can learn to state your preferences in a way that others will take seriously.

Assertiveness is the middle ground between aggressiveness and passivity. If you choose aggressiveness, you may get what you want, but the price may be very high. If you get your way by offending others, you could lose friendship and respect.

Passivity, on the other hand, rarely gets you what you want. If you are overly passive, you will not make your needs or wishes known. As a result, others may make decisions for you that you would rather make for yourself.

Passivity may cause you to lose confidence and respect for yourself. You may feel helpless, controlled, and bitter because you rarely get what you really want.

Assertiveness Basics

- Think carefully about what you want and what you need.

- Arrange for a time to discuss the subject.

- Write down what you want and then talk about your problem.

- Describe your feelings about the subject using "I" messages. Say "I feel upset" instead of "You upset me."

- Be very specific about what you want.

- Listen and respond to the other person's concerns. This will improve your chances for agreement.

Being assertive doesn't mean being hard, cruel, or impolite. It simply means being clear about what you want and saying what you mean. It often means negotiating and reaching a compromise. However, the compromise isn't one you're forced into. You agree to it on the basis of what you want.

Your Assertiveness Rights

You have the right to express your feelings.

You have the right to be treated fairly.

You have the right to live your life as you see fit.

You have the right to decide not to assert yourself.

Independence at Home

At some point, you may need to decide whether or not to leave your family home. There are a number of reasons why you might decide to leave: to be closer to children and grandchildren; to move to a place where the climate is better, where it's less expensive or where it's easier to do house and yard chores; or because of health problems, etc.

On the other hand, you may enjoy your current home very much. You may have friends and neighbors whom you would miss if you moved. And there is help available to deal with housecleaning, maintenance, and other tasks that may be becoming more difficult for you. If you prefer not to move, make it clear to everyone that *you* will decide if and when you will move. If you decide to move, consider waiting to see how your new living arrangement works out before selling your home.

However, even with help, it may not be possible for you to stay in your own home. You still have options in addition to moving in with family members or moving to a retirement home. Home-sharing or cooperative living and live-in companions are just a few other possibilities. Take some time to explore all of the options.

Services for Independent Living

The best way to remain independent is to know when to ask for help and where to find it. The following services are available in many communities. You can find out more about services available in your area by calling your local senior center or Area Agency on Aging. Ask for their "Information and Referral" person.

Chore services: help with major housecleaning, yard work, and minor household repairs.

Homemaker services: non-medical care in the home, such as housekeeping, cooking, shopping, and laundry.

Friendly visitors: non-medical attendants who provide companionship and some supervision for a few hours. They do not usually provide any housekeeping or personal care services.

Home health aides or **personal care assistants**: provide personal care (bathing, dressing, help in using the toilet) and basic health care. Home health aides can be very helpful during post-hospital recovery, or to help with caregiving. This service can be provided round-the-clock or for a few hours a week.

Personal Emergency Response System (PERS): a transmitter, generally worn around the neck or on the wrist. When activated, the PERS automatically places a call for help to an emergency response center.

Congregate meals: hot meals served at a central location, usually a senior center. Social activities are sometimes offered too.

Home-delivered meals (also called "Meals on Wheels"): hot, nutritious meals delivered to the home, usually at lunch. Some groups also provide meals that can be warmed for dinner.

Senior centers: sites where older people gather for meals, social activities, and educational programs. Some may offer services such as transportation to and from the site or to doctor visits.

Residential care or retirement homes: special apartment complexes or private homes that provide supportive environments but allow residents to remain somewhat independent. Residents have their own apartments or rooms. Some facilities provide meals in a central location and offer a variety of services, such as laundry, housekeeping, and help with bathing, dressing, and taking medications.

Skilled home care: professional nursing care provided in the home for more serious medical problems. Skilled home care can usually be provided as often as needed and is often supplemented with personal care provided by home health aides. Physical, respiratory, speech, and occupational therapy services are also available in the home.

Advance Directives: Control Over Health Care Decisions

You can make decisions about your health care for as long as you are able to make and communicate them. If you plan ahead, you can maintain some control over health care decisions even if you become unable to make or communicate decisions. An advance directive is a legal document that expresses your personal wishes for future decisions. Three types of advance directives are discussed here.

A **Living Will** is a document that states your wishes regarding life-sustaining measures or other medical treatment should you become unable to speak for yourself. Be very specific about the conditions under which you would or would not want certain kinds of treatment or life-support measures. Some states have a basic form to which you can add your own personal instructions.

A Living Will can be changed or revoked at any time and will not take effect until you are no longer able to make or communicate decisions for yourself. Give your doctor a copy. You do not need an attorney to write a Living Will, but legal advice may be helpful if your state's statutes are unclear or your state does not recognize Living Wills. Many hospitals and nursing homes provide living will forms that comply with state-specific requirements.

A **Durable Power of Attorney for Health Care** is a legal document that gives another person (called a surrogate) the authority to make health care decisions on your behalf if you are unable to do so. The person you choose should understand and respect your wishes about medical treatment. You may specify in the document how

Long-Term Care Insurance

Medicare and private health insurance do not cover nursing home services or extended periods of home health care. Long-term care insurance is designed to protect families from the high costs of custodial care. When shopping for a policy of this kind, look for:

- Allowance of benefits without requiring a prior hospital stay

- Premiums that do not increase because of age or health status

- Benefits for in-home care

- Guaranteed lifetime renewability

- Comprehensive coverage of all levels of long-term care

- Specific coverage for Parkinson's, Alzheimer's, and any other illness involving dementia

- A waiver of premiums while receiving benefits in a long-term care facility

- No waiting period for coverage of preexisting conditions

you would like such decisions to be made. A Durable Power of Attorney may also give another person the authority to make financial and other decisions, if you choose.

You must be mentally competent to draw up a Durable Power of Attorney. For this reason, if you or a spouse or other family member has a progressive brain disorder such as Alzheimer's disease that is still in the early stages, consider drawing up this document as early as possible to avoid later difficulties as judgment becomes impaired.

A **Conservatorship** or **Guardianship** is used if a person has already become incapacitated. It may be the only way for someone else to assume legal control over that person's affairs. A conservator may make decisions in a particular area, such as health or finances, or may have broader responsibility for the person's well-being. A third party may petition the court to ask that a conservator be appointed.

Each state has its own set of laws regarding advance directives. You may wish to consult with an attorney or your local hospital. Hospitals and long-term care facilities that receive Medicare or Medicaid are required to notify all patients of their rights to draw up advance directives stating their wishes about medical or surgical treatment.

Who's In Charge?

For some decisions, you may choose to let someone else take charge. The important thing is that *you* decide what areas of your life you will permit someone else to make decisions about. Do not allow other people to talk you into making decisions that you are not comfortable with, even if you think their intentions are good.

Independence has no age limit. You have the right to make decisions for yourself for as long as you live and are able and willing to do so. There are many options available to help you keep your freedom and independence.

It is up to *you* to make decisions and seek out services that will help you stay independent as long as you wish. Just as you need to exercise your mind and body to keep them strong, you need to exercise your right to make your own decisions.

You *can* control your own life. You *are* in charge.

*One of the deep secrets of life is that all that is
really worth the doing is what we do for others.*
Lewis Carroll

25
Caregiver Secrets

Many older people are caring for a chronically ill or disabled spouse, parent, or other family member. Caregiving can be an enjoyable and rewarding experience, especially when you know that your care has made a positive difference. However, it is difficult. There are three secrets to being a good caregiver:

• Take care of yourself first.

• Don't help too much.

• Don't do it alone.

This chapter will tell you more about these secrets and how they can help both you and the person you care for.

Caregiver Secret #1:
Take Care of Yourself First

If you want to give good care, you have to take care of yourself first.

Caregivers tend to deny their own needs. This strategy may work fine for short-term caregiving. However, for long-term caregiving commitments, it inevitably leads to problems.

Three things happen when caregivers don't take good care of themselves:

1.   They become ill.

2.   They become depressed.

3.   They "burn out" and stop providing care altogether.

These three things are bad for both the caregiver and the person receiving the care.

On the other hand, when caregivers take time to care for themselves, three good things happen:

1. They avoid health problems.

2. They feel better about themselves.

3. They have more energy and enthusiasm for helping others and can continue giving care.

All You Have Is Time

Time is your most important resource. The problem is, you only have 24 hours of it in a day, and after you subtract the time you need to do your basic work and chores, there may be only a few hours left over. That is the time you have to spend on hobbies and exercise, preparing healthy meals, being with friends, and doing other things that you enjoy.

---

10 Ways to Make Extra Time for Yourself

5 Ways That Don't Cost Money

- Trade a morning or an afternoon a week with another caregiver.

- Ask several relatives, friends, church members, or neighbors if each would relieve you for two to four hours per week on a regular schedule.

- Sign up for respite services. Some are available for no cost or for a voluntary donation.

- Barter for services: a loaf of bread, casserole, or errands in exchange for an hour of care.

- Plan some time each day to be alone, perhaps during a time when the person you care for doesn't need your attention (during naps, while reading, or other quiet activities).

5 Ways That Can Cost Money

- Hire a teenager or older adult to stay with the person for a few hours each day.

- Sign up for homemaker or chore services. By saving a few hours of housekeeping, you might have more time (and energy) for more important caregiving tasks.

- Sign up for a home-delivered meal service.

- Enroll the person in adult day care. Even a part-time placement for several hours per week can be helpful to both you and the person for whom you care.

- Hire a home health aide or personal care assistant.

Caregiving requires a large time commitment, perhaps all of the extra time you have for yourself. If that happens, problems can develop.

The best way to prevent the depression, frustration, and resentment that cause caregiver burnout is to hold back some time for yourself.

If you wait until all of your chores and caregiving tasks are done before doing things for yourself, you will wait a very long time. Instead, decide on the minimum amount of time necessary to meet your basic personal needs. Carve that time out of your schedule. Then figure out how the chores and caregiving will get done.

How to Take Care of Yourself

When you are caring for someone else, it's easy to forget to take care of yourself. But if you don't, nobody else will.

- Watch for signs of depression. Depression is very common in caregivers. Maintaining a positive self-image is the most important thing that a caregiver can do to care for herself. Use self-care, extra support, and professional help as appropriate when the earliest signs of depression appear. See page 306 for suggestions.

- Get regular exercise, even just a few minutes several times a day. Exercise can be a good energizer for both physical and emotional health. The guidelines in Chapter 20 can lead you on a path to fitness, one small step at a time.

- Maintain a healthy diet. When you are busy giving care, it may seem easier to eat fast food than to prepare healthy, low-fat meals. However, healthy meals are easy to prepare, and a good diet will give you more energy to carry you through each day. Tips in Chapter 21 can help you reduce fat and increase fiber and carbohydrates in your diet. Don't feel you have to change too much at once. One small diet improvement at a time can make a big difference over a year's time.

- Recognize stress and take steps to manage it. Your need for relaxation increases during periods of caregiving. Chapter 22 can get you started on quick, easy-to-learn relaxation techniques that will help you deal with frustration and stress.

Take heart. You don't need to change everything at once. Just select any area of your health that you would like to improve. This book can help you move closer to your goal, one step at a time.

Caregiver Guilt

The people who provide the most care to others often feel the most guilt. There is an old saying, "Scratch guilt and you will find resentment." When caregiving uses up all of your extra time, you may begin to feel frustrated and angry. Then you may feel guilty because you feel angry, which can cause you to spend even more time on caregiving. This cycle of anger, guilt, and overwork then repeats itself over and over.

The best way to let go of guilt is to accept the fact that you just can't be everything to everyone all of the time.

- Acknowledge your limitations. If you try to do too much, frustration is inevitable.

- Prioritize your caregiving. Decide to do only what is most important. Refuse to feel guilty about unmade beds or dusty windows.

- Allow yourself to be less than perfect. Tell yourself that you are doing a good job at a very difficult task. Pat yourself on the back for your caregiving. Reward yourself.

- Ask for help. Feeling guilty is often a sign that you need a break from your caregiving schedule. If your "guilt-o-meter" starts to increase, explore other options or ask friends and family to pitch in.

Planning for Caregiving

Planning ahead is an important part of caregiving. If you have a plan for what to do if problems come up, you and the person you care for will be better prepared to handle them.

- Talk openly about the person's situation. Identify and discuss any problems. Find out what resources are available to help, and develop a plan.

- Make a plan for what will be done if the person's situation changes for the worse. What types of problems might come up, and what services might be needed? Make sure you both have the names, phone numbers, and addresses of those services.

- Identify friends, neighbors, and other relatives who are currently helping out. Find out what they do now. Be sure you have their names and phone numbers. Contact them, explain the situation, and ask them to call you if they see any problems.

- Consider using a private geriatric care manager. These individuals charge a fee to locate and coordinate caregiving services, often on behalf of an out-of-town caregiver.

Caregiver Secret #2: Don't Help Too Much

The biggest mistake most caregivers make is providing too much care. Even if they don't admit it, people like to help themselves. Every time you provide care that could have been done by the one you are caring for, there is a double loss. First, your effort may have been wasted. Second, the person has missed an opportunity to help himself.

Help Them to Help Themselves

The caregiver's highest goal is to give the person the power and the permission to control as much of his life as possible. Every act your loved one makes toward maintaining independence is a victory for you as a caregiver.

Too often we get trapped in the role of a rescuer. We come to the person's rescue and expect to be rewarded with thanks and praise. Often, the thanks never come.

Too much rescuing teaches the one receiving care to be helpless. Eventually he will lose both the skills and the desire to do things for himself. Instead of rescuing, try to empower.

10 Ways to Empower the Person You Care For

1. Expect more. People respond to expectations. If you expect someone to dress himself, care for his plants, or prepare simple meals, he often will.

2. Limit your availability to help. If you are not always there to help, the person will be forced to do more for himself.

3. Simplify. If you are caring for someone with mild dementia, divide complex tasks into simpler parts: First, get out the cereal box; next get out the milk and the bowl, etc.

4. Make it easy. One of the most productive things a caregiver can do is to find tools that help the person to help himself. See Resource 12 on page 419.

5. Allow for less-than-perfect results or mistakes. The hardest thing about letting someone do something for himself is knowing that you could do it better or faster. Mistakes are okay.

6. Reward both effort and results. Help the person feel good about doing things for herself.

7. Let her make as many decisions as she can, such as what to wear, what to eat, or when to go to bed. Help her retain as much control over her life as possible.

8. Give him responsibility to care for something. Studies show that nursing home patients who are asked to care for pets or plants live longer and become more independent.

9. Match tasks with abilities. Actively identify the person's skills and try to match them with ways she can help herself.

10. Take acceptable risks. A few broken dishes or a few bruises are a small price to pay for letting someone explore what he can do for himself. You can't eliminate all risks without eliminating all opportunities. See pages 266 to 268 for tips to create a safe environment and reduce the risk of accidents.

Caring for a Person With Dementia

Most people who have dementia or Alzheimer's disease are cared for at home by relatives and friends. Also see page 167 for more tips on caring for someone who has dementia.

- If your loved one has been diagnosed as having Alzheimer's disease or another form of progressive dementia, discuss important matters like a will, a living will, and a durable power of attorney early in the course of the disease when his judgment is more clear. See page 382.

- Be aware that confusion often increases around sundown. Don't plan any complicated activities for that time.

- Arrange for respite care. The primary caregiver's need for rest increases as dementia worsens. Regular breaks from caregiving will help give you the stamina you need to care for the person as long as possible. Family and friends can help, but explore other options too. See page 391.

- Recognize when placement in a residential care or nursing home becomes appropriate. When home care can no longer be provided safely or without harm to others, consider placement away from home. Ask if the staff is particularly knowledgeable about dementia. Some facilities have special units designed for people who have dementing illnesses.

- See Resources 8 and 9 on page 419 for information on caring for a person with dementia. Also, contact the Alzheimer's Association at 1-800-272-3900 for the chapter nearest you.

Caregiver Secret #3: Don't Do It Alone

Some caregivers live under the mistaken impression that they are the only available source of help. However, there are often other sources of assistance available that can make your caregiving easier. If you want to be a good caregiver, know where to find help when you need it.

See page 381 for a list and description of services that can help with a variety of needs from shopping to personal care. Other types of services that may be useful to caregivers include:

Respite care may be the most important service for caregivers. Respite services provide someone to stay with the person for a short time while you get out of the house for a few hours. You may also arrange for a short stay in a hospital or nursing home for someone who needs medical care.

Adult day care centers are "drop-off" sites where a person who does not need individual supervision may stay during the day. This service is usually offered during working hours and may or may not be available on weekends. It provides meals, personal care services, and social activities.

Adult foster care or **board-and-care homes** are private homes where older adults receive round-the-clock personal care, supervision, and meals. Some states require that board-and-care homes be licensed.

Caregiver Needs for Respite

If you can answer "yes" to one or more of the following questions, it's time to get more help.

- Do I feel overworked and exhausted?

- Do I feel dissatisfied with myself?

- Do I feel isolated?

- Do I feel depressed, resentful, angry, or worried?

- Do I feel that I have no time for myself?

- Do I have no time to exercise and rest?

- Do I have no time for fun with people outside of my family?

A Caregiver's Bill of Rights

I have the right to take care of myself. This is not an act of selfishness. It will give me the capability of taking better care of my relative.

I have the right to seek help from others even though my relative may object. I recognize the limits of my own endurance and strength.

I have the right to maintain facets of my own life that do not include the person I care for, just as I would if he or she were healthy. I know that I do everything that I reasonably can for this person, and I have the right to do some things just for myself.

I have the right to get angry, be depressed, and express other difficult feelings occasionally.

I have the right to reject any attempt by my relative (either conscious or unconscious) to manipulate me through guilt, anger, or depression.

I have the right to receive consideration, affection, forgiveness, and acceptance for what I do from my loved one for as long as I offer these qualities in return.

I have the right to take pride in what I am accomplishing and to applaud the courage it has sometimes taken to meet the needs of my relative.

I have the right to protect my individuality and my right to make a life for myself that will sustain me in the time when my relative no longer needs my full-time help.

I have the right to expect and demand that as new strides are made in finding resources to aid physically and mentally impaired older persons in our country, similar strides will be made toward aiding and supporting caregivers.

I have the right to:

_____

_____

_____

_____

_____

_____

Nursing homes generally have two levels of care. Intermediate care includes assistance with toileting, dressing, and personal care for people without serious medical conditions. Skilled nursing care is usually for people who have just come from the hospital or others with medical conditions that require more intensive nursing care. Some facilities have special units for people with dementia.

Hospice programs provide social, personal, and medical services to terminally ill patients who wish to spend their remaining time at home or in a less formal environment instead of a hospital or nursing home.

Support groups give you an opportunity to discuss problems or concerns about caregiving with other caregivers.

To learn whether these services are available in your community, look under "Senior Citizen Services" in your Yellow Pages. Your community or county office on aging should be listed.

Take Pride

Now that you know the three secrets of caregiving, you can see that they really aren't secrets at all. There is nothing magical or mysterious about being a good caregiver.

- Care for your own needs first—both your physical and mental health depend on it. Give yourself as much special attention as you give the person you care for.

- Help the person you care for to help himself—this is a gift both to you and to him.

- Recognize when you need extra help, and know where you can get it. A helping hand at the right time can make all the difference.

Take pride in being a caregiver. It is not easy, and those who do it are special people. The three secrets of caregiving can help you feel good about yourself and the care you give.

Paying for Caregiving Services

Long-term nursing home and caregiver services are generally not covered by Medicare or private health insurance. However, if the need is related to a medical problem, short-term services may be covered.

To learn what help is available to you, call your state office on aging. Many of these agencies have a toll-free number.

A merry heart doeth good like a medicine.
Proverbs 17:22

26
Medication Management

What ever happened to "laughter is the best medicine"? Although a positive attitude is more important to our health than we may realize, it alone can't cure everything. Medicines now help to control many diseases that once were crippling or fatal. Arthritis, diabetes, high blood pressure, heart disease, infections, and many other conditions now can be treated successfully with medications. However, medications also have risks. When they are used improperly, they can do more harm than good.

Medications and Older Adults

Medications have special importance for older adults. As a group, people over age 50 receive more prescriptions than people of other ages. Because of changes in many body processes, your body absorbs and uses medications differently as you age. So managing your medications is even more important as you get older.

- You may weigh less, and your body composition changes in ways that affect the amount of medication you may need and how long it stays in your body.

- Your circulation system, liver, and kidneys may work more slowly, which changes how quickly medications are used and disposed of by the body.

- You may take several different medications, which increases the risk of drug interactions.

Good medication management begins in your doctor's office, when a prescription is written, but it doesn't stop there. This chapter includes tips on how to organize and take medications. It also presents useful information on some common over-the-counter and prescription drugs. Guidelines for recognizing and avoiding problems caused by medications are also included.

Be Smart About Pills

- Keep a medication record with:

  o The name of each medication

  o The dose

  o Why you are taking it

  o Who prescribed it

- Include prescription and over-the-counter medications, as well as eyedrops, vitamins, and skin ointments. See page 397 for a form that you can copy for your own use. Take the record to every doctor visit.

- Discuss all medication decisions with your doctor. See page 9 for questions to ask when medications are prescribed. Periodically ask your doctor if there are any medications you can safely stop taking.

- Ask about other treatment options besides medication. Exercise, diet changes, and stress management can provide many of the benefits of medications for some problems.

- Start low; go slow. Ask your doctor if you can begin new medications at a low dose and increase only as needed. Many drugs are tested on young adults. Older adults may need a lower dose.

- Learn about each medication you take. Resource 2 on page 418 will help you learn the side effects and possible interactions of each of your medications.

- Reevaluate your medications regularly. Check for outdated prescriptions and possible inter-actions. If you prefer, clinics, hospitals, and senior centers often offer "brown-bag" medication days. You can put all of your medications in a brown bag and have a doctor or pharmacist review them with you to check for outdated prescriptions, possible interactions, and other problems.

- Don't make any change in the number, kind, or amount of medications you take without consulting your doctor first.

- Remember that your pharmacist is part of your health care team. Pharmacists can answer your questions about prescription and over-the-counter medications.

Organize Your Pills

Good medication management also means organizing your bottles and pills. Taking three or four different drugs at different times each day can

Medication Record			Name _____		
Medica-tion and Dose	Doctor/ Date Prescribed	Color, Size, Shape	Purpose	Times Taken	Notes
(Example) Procardia, 10mg	Jacoby 4-15-96	Blue and gray capsule	Treat angina	1 pill 3 times a day	Take on an empty stomach.

be confusing, but taking your medications exactly as prescribed helps them work better. Develop a system to keep track of when and how you take each medication.

- Show your doctor a complete list of the drugs you take and the times you now take them. Ask if other medications or doses can be used to reduce the number of times you take pills each day.

- List your medication schedule on a daily planner that has spaces for hourly notations. Post it in a prominent place near your medicine cabinet. Take it with you when you travel.

- Use a pillbox designed to hold a week's worth of pills. You can also label empty egg cartons and use them to organize a day's or week's worth of medications.

- Ask if your pharmacist can help you with color-coded containers, easy-open caps, and large-print labels.

- Post reminders near clocks or on the bathroom mirror to help keep you on schedule. Set an alarm clock or kitchen timer to remind you to take your medication.

- Keep medications in a cool, dry place. Hot, steamy bathrooms cause medications to lose their strength. Some drugs need refrigeration. Ask your pharmacist.

- Store drugs in their original containers. Clearly label any drugs that you put in different bottles.

- Inspect your medications at least once a year. Dispose of expired, unused, unlabeled, or discolored drugs by flushing them down the toilet.

Spend Less Money on Pills

Medications are expensive and the costs of several prescriptions add up quickly. Successful medication management will not only prevent adverse health effects, but may save money as well. Besides avoiding unneeded drugs, you can cut your medication costs in these ways:

- Ask your doctor if generic forms of your medications are available and appropriate for you. Generics often may work as well as brand-name drugs but are usually cheaper.

- Compare prices between several pharmacies. It may be worth paying a little more if you are comfortable with the pharmacist, but do shop around. Prices can vary.

- Ask your doctor for samples of newly prescribed medications, or ask your pharmacist to fill only the first week's worth of pills. If the medication has to be changed later, you won't have wasted the price of the full prescription.

• If you can choose where to buy your pills, consider buying regularly used, expensive medications from mail-order pharmacies (see box at right). If your medication has a long shelf-life, you may be able to buy larger quantities at a lower price.

Over-the-Counter (OTC) Medications

An over-the-counter (OTC) medication is any drug that you can buy without a doctor's prescription. However, don't assume that all OTC drugs are safe for you. These drugs can interact with other medications and can sometimes cause serious health problems.

Carefully read the label of any over-the-counter drug you use, especially if you also take prescription medications for other health problems. Ask your pharmacist for help in finding the one best suited to your needs.

Some common OTCs include:

• Antacids and acid controllers

• Antidiarrheals

• Cold and allergy remedies

• Bulking agents and laxatives

• Pain relievers

Mail-Order or the Local Pharmacy?

If you regularly take the same medications, buying them through a mail-order pharmacy may save money. However, before you place your order, talk with your local pharmacist. Most pharmacies offer a senior citizen discount and many compete well with mail-order prices. Your local pharmacy also offers a number of valuable services:

• Convenience and immediate availability

• The pharmacist's professional advice and personal service

• The ability to monitor all of your prescriptions for possible interactions

Before you switch to a mail-order drug company, be sure that the savings are worth the other services that you may be giving up. Your insurance coverage may also limit your choices of where to buy medications.

These drugs can be very helpful when used properly but can also create serious problems if used incorrectly. The following tips will help you use these common OTC drugs wisely and safely. In some cases, you may find that you don't need to take them at all.

Antacids and Acid Controllers

Antacids and acid controllers both treat heartburn, but they work in different ways. Heartburn is often caused by stomach acid backing up into the tube (esophagus) that leads from the mouth to the stomach.

Antacids work by neutralizing excess stomach acid. Acid controllers work by reducing the amount of acid the stomach produces. If you have minor heartburn just a few times a month, an antacid is probably all you need. If you have more severe heartburn, or if it occurs more often, an acid controller may be helpful. In either case, home treatment is also important. See page 125.

Antacids are safe if used occasionally, but can cause problems if taken regularly. There are several kinds of antacids. Get to know what ingredients are in each type so that you can avoid any adverse effects.

- Sodium bicarbonate antacids (Alka-Seltzer and Bromo Seltzer) contain baking soda, which contains a lot of sodium. If you have high blood pressure, or if you are on a salt-restricted diet, avoid these antacids. If used too frequently, they may interfere with kidney or heart function.

- Calcium carbonate antacids (Alka-2, TUMS) are sometimes used as calcium supplements (see page 358). They may cause constipation, so drink plenty of water when taking them.

- Aluminum-based antacids (Amphojel) are less potent and work more slowly than other antacids. Some may cause calcium depletion and should not be taken by women after menopause. Check with your doctor before using aluminum antacids if you have kidney problems.

- Aluminum-magnesium antacids (Di-Gel, Maalox, Mylanta, Riopan) are generally less likely to cause constipation or diarrhea than aluminum-only antacids.

Over-the-counter **acid controllers** such as famotidine (Pepcid AC), cimetidine (Tagamet HB), and ranitidine (Zantac 75) contain a lower dose of some common prescription medications. Each works by reducing the production of stomach acid.

Antacid and Acid Controller Precautions

- Try to eliminate the cause of frequent heartburn instead of taking antacids or acid controllers regularly. See Heartburn on page 125.

- Consult your doctor or pharmacist before taking an antacid or acid controller if you take other medications. Antacids may interfere with the absorption and action of some drugs, such as antibiotics, heart medication (digitalis), and blood thinners (anticoagulants). Also consult your doctor if you have ulcers or kidney problems. Some acid controllers interact with other medications, such as anticoagulants and certain sedatives, heart medications, and asthma medications.

- Acid controllers increase the rate at which your body absorbs alcohol. Avoid alcohol while taking these medications (also good advice to help reduce heartburn).

- Be sure your problem is really heartburn. Heartburn is often confused with other causes of chest pain. If you are not sure about the cause of chest pain, or if antacids or acid controllers don't help, see page 74.

Antidiarrheals

There are two types of drugs for diarrhea (antidiarrheals): those that thicken the stool and those that slow intestinal spasms.

The thickening mixtures (Kaopectate) contain clay or fruit pectin and absorb the bacteria and toxins in the intestine. Although they are relatively safe because they do not go into the system, these products do absorb normal bacteria needed for digestion. Long-term use is not advised.

Antispasmodic antidiarrheal products stop the spasm of the intestine. Loperamide (Imodium A-D, Pepto Diarrhea Control) is an example. Donnagel and Parepectolin contain both thickening and antispasmodic ingredients.

Antidiarrheal Precautions

Diarrhea often helps rid your body of an infection, so try to avoid using antidiarrheal medications for the first six hours. After that, use them only if there are no other signs of illness, such as fever, and if cramping and pain continues.

- Take a dose large enough to be effective. Take antidiarrheal preparations until the stool thickens; then stop immediately to avoid constipation.

- Do not take any antidiarrheal product if you have glaucoma, kidney or liver disease, or prostate problems.

- Replace depleted body fluids. Dehydration can develop when you have diarrhea. See page 120 for information about rehydration drinks.

Cold and Allergy Remedies

In general, if you take drugs for your cold, you'll get better in about a week. If you take nothing, you'll get better in about seven days. Rest and liquids are probably the best treatment for a cold (see page 76). Antibiotics will not help. However, medications help relieve some cold symptoms, such as nasal congestion and cough.

Allergy symptoms, especially runny nose, respond to antihistamines and decongestants. Antihistamines are found in many cold medications, often together with decongestants. The usefulness of antihistamines in treating cold symptoms is under debate. They may worsen cold symptoms by thickening nasal discharge.

It is usually best to take only single-ingredient preparations if you have a cold. For example, if your most troublesome cold symptom is a runny nose, you may want to take a decongestant and avoid medications that also contain an antihistamine.

Decongestants

Decongestants make breathing easier by shrinking swollen mucous membranes in the nose, allowing air to pass through. They also help relieve runny nose and postnasal drip, which can cause a sore throat.

Decongestants can be taken orally or used as nose drops or sprays. Oral decongestants (pills) are probably more effective and provide longer relief, but they cause more side effects. Pseudoephedrine (Sudafed) is an oral decongestant.

Sprays and drops provide rapid but temporary relief. Phenylephrine (Neo-Synephrine) is an effective nasal spray for temporary relief. Sprays and drops are less likely than oral decongestants to interact with other drugs.

Saline Nose Drops

The safest nasal drop for a stuffy nose is homemade saline solution. Saline nose drops will not cause a rebound effect. They keep nasal tissues moist so they can filter the air.

Mix ¼ teaspoon salt in 1 cup distilled water (too much salt will dry nasal membranes).

Place the solution in a clean bottle with a dropper (available at drugstores). Use as necessary. Discard and make a fresh solution weekly.

To insert drops, lie down with your head hanging over the side of the bed. This helps the drops get farther back. Try to prevent the dropper from touching your nose.

Decongestant Precautions

• Do not use decongestant nasal sprays or drops more than three times a day or for more than three days. Continued use will cause a "rebound effect": the mucous membranes swell up more than before using the spray.

• Drink extra fluids when taking cold medications.

• If you have heart disease, high blood pressure, glaucoma, diabetes, or overactive thyroid, use decongestants only under your doctor's advice. Decongestants may also interact with certain antidepressants and some high blood pressure medications. Read the package carefully and ask your doctor or pharmacist to help you choose one.

• Decongestants can cause drowsiness or increased activity in some people. Some brands also interfere with sleep.

• Too much decongestant can cause hallucinations and convulsions and may depress central nervous system functions in older people. Use long-acting formulas only as directed.

Cough Preparations

Coughing is your body's way of getting phlegm and mucus out of your respiratory tract. Coughs are often useful and you usually don't want to eliminate them. However, when a cough is severe enough to interfere with breathing or rest, you may want to relieve it.

Water and other liquids, such as fruit juices, are probably the best cough syrups. They help soothe the throat and also moisten and thin mucus so that it can be coughed up more easily.

You can make a simple cough syrup at home by mixing one part lemon juice with two parts honey. Use as often as needed.

There are two kinds of cough preparations. **Expectorants** help thin the mucus, making it easier to "bring up" when you have a productive cough. Look for expectorants containing guaifenesin, such as Robitussin and Vicks Formula 44E. Plain water is another good expectorant.

Suppressants control or suppress the cough reflex and work best for the dry, hacking cough that keeps you awake. Look for suppressant medications containing dextromethorphan, such as Robitussin-DM and Vicks Formula 44.

Cough Preparation Precautions

• Don't suppress a productive cough so much that you are no longer bringing up mucus, unless it is keeping you from getting enough rest.

- Use cough suppressants with caution if you have chronic respiratory problems. Use care when giving cough suppressants to someone who is very old or frail.

- Cough medicines can cause problems for people with certain health problems, such as asthma, heart disease, high blood pressure, and enlarged prostate. They may also interact with some drugs, such as sedatives and certain antidepressants. Read the package carefully.

- Read the label so you know what ingredients you are taking. Some cough preparations contain a large percentage of alcohol; others contain codeine. Some contain decongestants or antihistamines, which do not treat coughs. There are many choices. Ask your doctor or pharmacist to advise you.

Antihistamines

Antihistamines dry mucous membranes and are commonly used to treat allergy symptoms and itching.

If your runny nose is due to allergies, an antihistamine will help. For cold symptoms, home treatment and a decongestant may be more helpful.

Chlorpheniramine (Chlor-Trimeton) and diphenhydramine (Benadryl) are single-ingredient antihistamine products. Coricidin, Dristan, and Triaminic contain both decongestants and antihistamines.

Antihistamine Precautions

- Drink extra fluids when taking allergy medications.

- Don't drive or operate machinery when taking antihistamines. Antihistamines may cause dizziness, drowsiness, and abnormally low blood pressure in older adults. They may also cause increased activity in some people.

- Antihistamines can cause problems for people with certain health problems, such as glaucoma, epilepsy, and enlarged prostate. They may also interact with some medications, such as certain antidepressants, sedatives, and tranquilizers. Read the package carefully and ask your doctor or pharmacist to help you choose one that will not cause problems.

Bulking Agents and Laxatives

Bulking agents and laxatives are used to prevent or treat constipation.

Bulking agents, such as bran or psyllium (Citrucel, Metamucil), relieve and prevent constipation by increasing the volume of the stool and making it easier to pass. Regular use of bulking agents is generally safe and helps make them more effective. Drink plenty of water and other liquids when using a bulking agent.

Laxatives (Correctol, Dulcolax, Ex-Lax, Senokot) speed up the passage of stool by irritating the intestines. Regular laxative use is not recommended.

There are many other ways to prevent and treat constipation, such as drinking more water. See page 118.

Laxative Precautions

- Do not take laxatives regularly. Overuse of laxatives decreases the efficiency of the large intestine, causing laxative dependence.

- Regular use of some laxatives (Correctol, Ex-Lax, Feen-A-Mint) may interfere with your body's absorption of vitamin D and calcium, which can weaken your bones.

- Do not use mineral oil as a laxative for more than a few days. It interferes with the body's absorption of vitamins and may leak from the anus.

Pain Relievers

There are dozens of over-the-counter pain relievers.

Aspirin, ibuprofen, naproxen sodium, and ketoprofen belong to a class of drugs called **nonsteroidal anti-inflammatory drugs**, or NSAIDs. They relieve pain, inflammation, and fever.

Acetaminophen relieves pain and reduces fever. It does not relieve inflammation.

Generic forms of aspirin, ibuprofen, and acetaminophen will generally work just as well as brand-name products and are often less expensive.

Aspirin is widely used for relieving pain and reducing fever in adults. It also relieves minor itching and reduces swelling and inflammation. Although it seems familiar and safe, aspirin is a very powerful medicine.

Aspirin Precautions

- Keep all aspirin out of children's reach. Do not give aspirin to children and teens younger than 20. It has been linked to a rare but serious condition called Reye's syndrome, which can be fatal.

- Aspirin can irritate the stomach lining, causing bleeding or ulcers. If aspirin upsets your stomach, try a coated brand, such as Ecotrin. Talk with your doctor or pharmacist to determine what will work best for you.

- Some people are allergic to aspirin. (They may also be allergic to ibuprofen.)

- Do not take aspirin if you have gout, and do not take it without your doctor's supervision if you also take blood thinners (anticoagulants).

- Do not take aspirin for a hangover. Aspirin used with alcohol increases the risk of stomach irritation.

- Ringing in the ears is a common side effect of high doses of aspirin. If it develops, reduce the dose. If the ringing persists, call your doctor.

- High doses of aspirin may result in aspirin poisoning (salicylism). Stop taking aspirin and call a health professional if any of these symptoms occur:

  ○ Visual disturbances

  ○ Dizziness

  ○ Rapid, deep breathing

  ○ Persistent ringing in the ears

Ibuprofen (Advil, Motrin IB, Nuprin), **naproxen sodium** (Aleve) and **ketoprofen** (Orudis KT) are other nonsteroidal anti-inflammatory drugs (NSAIDs). Like aspirin, they relieve pain and reduce fever and inflammation. Also like aspirin, they can cause stomach irritation, nausea, and heartburn. All NSAIDs should be taken with caution by people who also take blood thinners (anticoagulants).

NSAID Precautions

- Do not take more than one type of anti-inflammatory medication (aspirin, ibuprofen, naproxen, ketoprofen) at a time. Do not take these medications without your doctor's advice if you are taking a prescription anti-inflammatory. Taking these medications together increases the risk of severe irritation to the stomach lining.

- Long-term use of anti-inflammatory medications can occasionally impair kidney or liver function.

- In some cases, ibuprofen may cause water retention, which can interfere with treatment for high blood pressure.

- If you are taking any anti-inflammatory medication regularly, discuss it with your doctor. He or she may want to do blood tests to check if the medication is affecting your kidneys or liver.

Acetaminophen (Tylenol) reduces fever and relieves pain. It does not have the anti-inflammatory effect of aspirin, ibuprofen, or naproxen, but it also does not cause stomach irritation and other side effects. It is commonly recommended to treat osteoarthritis pain. Acetaminophen is also useful to relieve cold and flu symptoms such as muscle aches and fever.

Prescription Medications

There are thousands of different prescription medications, used to treat hundreds of different medical conditions. Your doctor and your pharmacist are your best sources of information about your prescription medications. Good books are available that contain information on many different prescription drugs. See Resource 2 on page 418.

Information about every kind of prescription medication could fill several books. Common types covered here include antibiotics, minor tranquilizers, and sleeping pills.

Antibiotics

Antibiotics are prescription drugs that kill bacteria (you can also buy antibiotic ointment for skin injuries without a prescription). They help to treat many bacterial infections, such as pneumonia, sinus infections, and skin infections. They are effective only against bacteria and have no effect on viruses. Antibiotics will not cure the common cold, flu, or any other viral illness. Unless you have a bacterial infection, it's best to avoid the possible adverse effects of antibiotics, which may include:

- **Side effects**, including **allergic reactions**. Common side effects of antibiotics include nausea, diarrhea, and increased sensitivity to sunlight. Most side effects are mild, but some, especially allergic reactions, can be life-threatening. If you have any unexpected reaction to an antibiotic, tell your health professional before another antibiotic is prescribed.

- **Secondary infections**. Antibiotics kill most of the bacteria in your body that are sensitive to them, including those that help your body. They may destroy the balance of bacteria in your body, leading to stomach upset, diarrhea, vaginal infections, or other problems.

- **Bacterial resistance**. If you do not take the full dose of a prescription, the stronger bacteria often survive and multiply. This is one way that bacteria build resistance to antibiotics. Many common bacteria have antibiotic-resistant strains, which are very difficult to treat.

When you and your doctor have decided that an antibiotic is necessary, follow the instructions with the prescription carefully.

- Take the whole dose for as many days as prescribed, unless you have severe unexpected side effects. Antibiotics kill off many bacteria quite quickly, so you may feel better in a few days. If you stop taking the antibiotic, the weaker bacteria will have been eliminated, but the stronger bacteria may survive and the infection may persist.

- Be sure you understand any special instructions about taking the medication. They should be printed on the label, but double-check with your doctor and pharmacist.

- Store antibiotics in a dry, cool place. They will usually keep their potency for about a year. However, most antibiotics are prescribed for a specific illness in the amount needed to cure it. Liquid antibiotics are always dated. Check carefully to see if they need refrigeration.

- Do not take an antibiotic prescribed for another illness without a health professional's approval.

- Never give an antibiotic prescribed for one person to someone else.

Minor Tranquilizers and Sleeping Pills

Minor tranquilizers include medications such as chlordiazepoxide (Librium), clorazepate (Tranxene), diazepam (Valium), and alprazolam (Xanax). Examples of sleeping pills include flurazepam (Dalmane), triazolam (Halcion), and temazepam (Restoril). These medications are widely prescribed and used. However, these drugs can cause problems, including memory loss, dizziness, and balance problems that can lead to falls and injuries.

Minor tranquilizers can be effective for short periods of time. However, long-term use may be of limited value and introduces the risk of memory problems, confusion, and addiction.

Sleeping pills may help for a few days or a few weeks. Using them for more than a month generally causes more sleep problems than it solves. For other approaches, see page 315.

If you have been taking minor tranquilizers or sleeping pills for a while, talk with your doctor about whether the medication is still needed or if it may be appropriate to reduce the dose. If you have experienced any dizziness, unsteadiness, memory problems, or any other symptom, tell your doctor. These adverse effects of medications are often mistaken for "normal" signs of aging.

Medication Problems

As the body ages, it becomes more susceptible to medication-related problems. One in five older adults has experienced an adverse drug reaction to a prescription medication.

Aging brings on changes in the stomach, circulatory system, kidneys, and body composition. These changes affect the body's absorption, use, and excretion of medications.

Several different kinds of adverse medication reactions can occur:

Side effects: Predictable, but unpleasant reactions to a drug. They are not usually serious but can be inconvenient. In some people, they are severe and dangerous.

Drug-drug interactions: Two or more prescription or over-the-counter drugs mixing in the body and causing an adverse reaction. The symptoms can be severe and may be misdiagnosed as a new illness.

Drug-food interactions: Medications reacting with food. Some drugs work best when taken with food, but others should be taken on an empty stomach. Some drug-food reactions can cause serious symptoms.

Over-medication: Sometimes the full adult dose of a medication is too high for people over age 60. This may cause severe reactions soon after the drug is taken or after it has been taken for a while and has built up in the body.

Addiction: Use of some medications over time leads to dependence on them and severe reactions if they are withdrawn suddenly. Narcotics, tranquilizers, and barbiturates should all be used with care to avoid addiction. See page 308.

Prevention

- Take a list of all your medications (prescription and over-the-counter) to every doctor visit. See page 397 for a sample medication record. Don't forget eyedrops, skin ointments or patches, and vitamins.

- When a new medication is prescribed, ask your doctor whether it may interact with other medications you are already taking.

- Tell your doctor and pharmacist if you have any medication allergies.

- Never take a prescription that was written for another person. Don't share your medications with anyone. A drug that works wonders for you might harm someone else.

- Do not ignore symptoms that you suspect are related to a medication. Even mild symptoms can sometimes cause serious problems, and if any symptom is bothersome, your doctor should know about it. Sometimes the dose or medication can be adjusted to reduce the symptoms.

- Keep a record of any symptom or side effect you have, even if it is minor. Show it to your doctor.

When to Call a Health Professional

- If any symptom, such as vomiting, breathing difficulties, headache, confusion, or drowsiness, is severe or persistent.

- If symptoms develop soon after you have started taking a new medication, changed the dose of a medication, or eaten a certain food.

- If symptoms such as forgetfulness, depression, confusion, or fatigue develop slowly over a period of weeks or months. Some adverse drug effects take a while to show up.

- If you suspect that a symptom is related to an adverse drug reaction.

- If any side effect, such as dry mouth or constipation, interferes with your enjoyment of life or makes it hard for you to keep taking the medication as directed.

Adverse Drug Reactions

Side effects, drug-drug and food-drug interactions, over-medication, and addiction may cause:

- Nausea, indigestion, vomiting

- Constipation or diarrhea

- Incontinence or difficulty urinating

- Dry mouth

- Headache, dizziness, ringing in the ears, or blurred vision

- Confusion, forgetfulness, disorientation, drowsiness, or depression

- Difficulty sleeping, irritability, or nervousness

- Difficulty breathing

- Rashes, bruising, and bleeding problems

Don't assume any symptom is a normal side effect or "just part of getting older." Call your doctor or pharmacist anytime you think your medicines are making you sick.

Be prepared.
Boy Scout Motto

27
Your Home Health Center

Who provides most of the care for your health problems? Chances are, it's you. If you have the right tools, medicines, supplies, and information on hand, you can do a good job.

Store all your self-care resources in one central location, such as a large drawer in the bedroom or family room. Use the charts on tools and supplies and the list of resources in this chapter as checklists for keeping your home health center well stocked.

Note: If small children are around or visit, keep your supplies out of reach or protected by childproof safety latches.

Be familiar with the disaster preparation and response plan for your area. Keep the appropriate supplies on hand.

Self-Care Tools

Self-care tools are the basic equipment of your home health center.

Cold Pack

A cold pack is a plastic envelope filled with gel that remains flexible at very cold temperatures. Buy two cold packs and keep them in the freezer. Use them for bumps, bruises, back sprains, turned ankles, sore joints, or any other health problem that calls for ice. A cold pack is more convenient than ice and may become the self-care tool you use the most. See page 294 for guidelines.

You can make your own cold pack:

- Put one pint of rubbing alcohol and three pints of water in a one-gallon heavy-duty plastic freezer bag.

- Seal the bag and then seal it in a second bag. Mark it "Cold pack: Do not eat," and place it in the freezer.

A bag of frozen vegetables will also work as a cold pack.

Heating Pad

Heating pads are a convenient way to apply heat to sore joints (do not apply heat to a swollen joint) or to minor sprains and bruises after a day or so of cold pack treatment.

However, heating pads can cause serious burns. Do not fall asleep with a heating pad on. Use them with care if you have diabetes, peripheral vascular disease, or other conditions that impair circulation or make it hard for you to notice if the pad is getting too hot. Do not allow a person who is confused or who has dementia to use a heating pad without supervision.

Humidifier and Vaporizer

Humidifiers and vaporizers add moisture to the air, making it less drying to your mouth, throat, and nose. A humidifier produces a cool mist and a vaporizer may put out hot or cool mist.

However, humidifiers are noisy, produce particles that may be irritating to some people, and need to be cleaned and disinfected regularly. This is especially important for people who are allergic to mold.

Self-Care Tools

Keep these on hand:
- Blood pressure cuff*
- Cold pack*
- Dental mirror
- Eyedropper
- Heating pad*
- Humidifier or vaporizer*
- Medicine spoon*
- Nail clippers
- Penlight*
- Scissors
- Stethoscope*
- Thermometer*
- Tweezers

*Described in text

A vaporizer's hot steam does not contain any irritating particles, and you can add medications such as Vicks VapoRub to ease breathing. However, the hot water can burn anyone who overturns it or gets too close.

Humidity in the air can help to soothe a scratchy throat, ease a dry, hacking cough, and make it easier for someone with a stuffy nose to breathe. Added humidity will make your home more comfortable, especially in the winter when dry air is a problem.

Medicine Spoon

Medicine spoons are transparent tubes with marks for typical dosage amounts. A medicine spoon makes it easy to give the right dose of liquid medicine. Medicine spoons are convenient if you frequently take liquid medications. Buy one at your local pharmacy.

Penlight

A penlight has a small intense light that can be easily directed. It is useful for examining the throat or ears and is easier to handle than a flashlight.

Stethoscope and Blood Pressure Cuff

If you have high blood pressure, it's a good idea to have a blood pressure cuff (sphygmomanometer), either an electronic model or the type that requires a stethoscope, to monitor your blood pressure regularly.

Blood pressure cuffs come in many models. If you have difficulty reading the gauge on a regular cuff, look for an electronic digital model. (If you use an electronic digital model, or one attached to an upright mercury column, you will not need a stethoscope.) Ask your pharmacist to recommend a blood pressure kit and show you how to use it. If you use a blood pressure cuff, take it to a doctor visit and compare the reading to the one in your doctor's office.

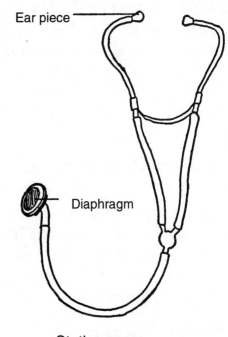

Ear piece

Diaphragm

Stethoscope

Purchase a flat diaphragm model stethoscope rather than a bell-shaped one. The flat surface makes it easier for you to hear.

Thermometer

Buy a thermometer with easy-to-read markings. Digital electronic thermometers are accurate and easy to read. Temperature strips are very convenient and safe but are not as accurate as mercury or electronic thermometers and should only be used to measure armpit (axillary) temperature. Thermometers that measure the temperature in the ear are fast, easy to use, and quite accurate, but they are expensive.

Rectal thermometers with enlarged bulbs are helpful for anyone who cannot hold an oral thermometer in his mouth. Do not use a rectal thermometer if the person is confused or uncooperative.

Self-Care Supplies

See the Self-Care Supplies box at right for a list of supplies that are useful to keep on hand in your home health center. These products are inexpensive, easy to use, and generally available at any drugstore or pharmacy.

Assistive Devices

If your hands and other body parts aren't as nimble as they used to be, consider assistive devices such as large-handled tools and kitchen utensils, appliances with large buttons and large-print displays, devices that allow you to reach, lift, or carry items more easily, etc. They can help you with meal preparation, personal care, housekeeping, hobbies, and other activities. See Resource 12 on page 419 for a catalog of assistive devices.

Over-the-Counter (OTC) Products

The chart on page 415 lists some common health problems, suggests over-the-counter (OTC) products to treat them, and refers you elsewhere in this book for more information. For more information about some of these products, see Chapter 26, Medication Management:

Self-Care Supplies

Keep these on hand:

- Adhesive strips ("Band-Aids") in assorted sizes
- Adhesive tape, one inch wide
- Butterfly bandages
- Sterile gauze pads, two inches square
- Elastic ("Ace") bandage, three inches wide
- Roll of gauze bandage, two inches wide
- Cotton balls
- Safety pins
- Tweezers
- Dental disclosing tablets and dental floss

- Antacids and acid controllers, page 400.
- Antidiarrheals, page 401.
- Cold and allergy remedies, page 402.
- Bulking agents and laxatives, page 404.
- Pain relievers, page 405.

OTC Products for Home Use

Problem	OTC Product (example)	Comments
Allergies	Antihistamine (Benadryl, Chlor-Trimeton)	Useful for allergies and itching. See page 404.
Colds	Decongestant	See page 403 for precautions.
Constipation	Bulking agent (Metamucil) or laxative	Avoid long-term or regular use of laxatives. See page 404.
Cough, non-productive	Suppressant (Vicks Formula 44)	Ease a dry, hacking cough. See page 403.
Cough, productive	Expectorant (Vicks Formula 44E)	Thin and help clear the mucus. See page 403 for precautions.
Diarrhea	Antidiarrheal (Pepto Diarrhea Control)	Avoid long-term use. See page 401.
Dry skin	Lubricating cream (Vaseline Intensive Care)	Also see page 215.
Heartburn	Antacid (Maalox, TUMS) or acid controller (Pepcid AC, Tagamet HB)	Avoid long-term use unless your doctor recommends it. See page 400.
Itching	Hydrocortisone cream (Cortaid)	Antihistamines are also helpful. See page 215.
Pain, fever, inflammation	Aspirin, ibuprofen, naproxen, ketoprofen	Help relieve swelling and pain. May cause stomach upset or ulcers. See page 406.
Pain, fever	Acetaminophen (Tylenol)	Less stomach irritation. Safe for children. See page 406.
Scrapes, skin infections	Antibiotic ointment (Bacitracin, Polysporin)	May cause local allergic reaction. Keep creams cool and dry. Discard if out of date.

Home Medical Tests

Many common medical tests are now available in home kits. Combined with regular visits to your health professional, home tests can help you monitor your health and, in some cases, detect problems early.

Some medical tests must be very accurate (over 95 percent) to be approved by the Food and Drug Administration. However, they must be used correctly to give such accurate results. Follow the package directions exactly. If you have questions, ask your pharmacist or check the label for the company's toll-free phone number to call.

Home medical tests are especially helpful if you have a chronic condition that requires frequent monitoring, such as diabetes, asthma, or high blood pressure. Ask your doctor which home medical tests would be appropriate for you. Some common tests are described below.

Blood Cholesterol

These tests allow you to test your cholesterol level at home using a few drops of blood from a finger prick. They are fast and easy. However, most people don't need to check their cholesterol frequently.

The results may also not give you all the information you need. Some types measure only total cholesterol and do not measure HDL and LDL cholesterol levels. If your cholesterol is high, it is important to know your total, HDL, and LDL levels. If a home cholesterol test indicates that your cholesterol is high, report it to your doctor. Also see page 352.

Blood Glucose Monitoring

If you have diabetes, you may already monitor your blood sugar (glucose) levels using a finger prick and a test strip or an electronic monitor.

This test should always be used under a doctor's supervision. Never adjust your insulin dose based on a single abnormal test, unless your doctor has specifically instructed you to do so.

Check with your doctor if you have symptoms of abnormal blood sugar levels, even if the test is normal. See page 150.

Blood Pressure Monitoring

If you have high blood pressure, it is important to monitor your blood pressure frequently. With a little instruction, you can easily monitor your blood pressure at home.

By checking your blood pressure at home, when you are relaxed, you will be able to track changes due to your home treatment and medications.

- Do not make any changes to your medications based on your home blood pressure readings without consulting your doctor.

- Check your blood pressure at different times of day to see how rest and activities affect it. For regular readings, check it at the same time of day. Blood pressure is usually lowest in the morning and rises during the day.

- For the most accurate reading, sit still for five minutes before taking your blood pressure.

- Check the accuracy of (calibrate) the blood pressure device yearly.

Peak Flow Meter

If you have asthma, your doctor may recommend that you monitor your lung capacity regularly. A peak flow meter is a device with a mouthpiece attached to a meter. When you exhale forcefully into the mouthpiece, the meter records the amount of air you blow out. This is your peak airflow. Record the highest of three measurements.

A decrease in peak airflow can be the first symptom of an asthma attack. Monitoring your peak airflow may allow you to prevent an asthma attack or treat it before it becomes severe. Ask your doctor for a treatment plan that you can follow if your peak airflow decreases. Call your doctor if your peak airflow is less than 50 percent of your normal.

Tests for Blood in Stool

The fecal occult blood test can detect hidden blood in the stool, which may indicate colon cancer or other problems. However, this test has a very high rate of false positive and false negative results.

The test for blood in the stool is very sensitive to blood from other sources, such as bleeding gums, ulcers, or red meat in your diet. Follow the package instructions exactly, and report any positive results to your doctor, even if some tests are negative.

Your doctor may also recommend a more accurate screening test for colon cancer called a flexible sigmoidoscopy. See page 117.

Urinalysis

Some of the more common medical lab tests on urine can be done at home. Home urinalysis can help you monitor diabetes, although it is not often used for this anymore. It is also useful if you have frequent bladder infections.

Home Medical Records

Your home health center is a good place to keep your family's medical records. A three-ring binder or wire-bound notebook with dividers for each member of the family is helpful. Each person should have a cover sheet listing:

- Diagnosed chronic conditions: arthritis, asthma, diabetes, high blood pressure, etc.

- Any known allergies to drugs, foods, or insects.

- Information that would be vital in an emergency, such as a pacemaker, a hearing aid, diabetes, epilepsy, or if someone is deaf or blind.

- Name and phone number of primary doctor.

Other important information that should be included:

- An up-to-date list of medications. Include name of drug, purpose, dose, instructions, doctor, and date prescribed. A sample chart is included on page 397.

- Immunization records: Tetanus, influenza, pneumonia.

- Health screening results: Blood pressure, cholesterol, vision, hearing.

- Records of major illnesses and injuries, such as pneumonia, bronchitis, broken bones, or major infections.

- Records of any major surgical procedures and hospitalizations.

- Records listing major diseases in members of your family: heart disease, stroke, cancer, diabetes.

Your Home Health Library: Self-Care Resources

Good information is the most important self-care resource for the home. Many of the resources listed below are available at your local bookstore or public library. If not, ask the bookstore to order the ones you want.

Other sources of health information may be available in your community or from your health plan. Check the phone book for your local chapter of the American Cancer Society, American Heart Association, Arthritis Foundation, American Diabetes Association, American Lung Association, and other organizations.

If you subscribe to an on-line service such as America On-Line, CompuServe, or Prodigy, check for health databases, electronic bulletin boards and discussion groups, and other services. You may be able to access medical journal articles, textbooks, and other publications on-line.

Two Books Every Home Should Have

1. D. W. Kemper et al., *Healthwise for Life* (2nd ed.), Healthwise, 1996. Available from Healthwise, Inc., P.O. Box 1989, Boise, ID 83701, (208) 345-1161.

2. J.J. Rybacki, Pharm. D, and J. W. Long, MD, *The Essential Guide to Prescription Drugs,* Harper Collins, 1996.

General Purpose Resources

3. D. Vickery, MD, and J. Fries, MD, *Take Care of Yourself* (5th ed.), Addison-Wesley, 1993.

4. D. E. Larson, MD, ed. *Mayo Clinic Family Health Book,* William Morrow, 1990.

5. S. Margolis, MD, PhD, and J. Moses III, MD, eds. *The Johns Hopkins Medical Handbook: 100 Major Medical Disorders of People Over the Age of 50*, Random House, 1992.

6. M.E. Williams, MD, *The American Geriatric Society's Complete Guide to Aging and Health*, Harmony Books, 1995.

Special Concerns Resources

Alcohol Problems

7. *Alcoholics Anonymous: The Story of How Thousands of Men and Women Have Recovered From Alcoholism* (3rd ed.), Alcoholics Anonymous World Services, Inc., 1986.

Alzheimer's Disease

8. N. L. Mace and P. V. Rabins, MD, *The 36-Hour Day: A Family Guide to Caring for Persons with Alzheimer's Disease, Related Dementing Illnesses, and Memory Loss in Late Life,* The John Hopkins University Press, 1991. Also available from the Alzheimer's Association, 1-800-272-3900.

9. M. Larkin, *When Someone You Love Has Alzheimer's*, Dell, 1995.

Arthritis

10. K. Lorig and J. Fries, MD, *The Arthritis Helpbook,* Addison-Wesley, 1995.

11. J.F. Fries, MD, *Arthritis*: *A Comprehensive Guide to Understanding Your Arthritis* (3rd ed.), Addison-Wesley, 1990.

Also see Resource 19.

Assistive Devices

12. A.I. Abrams and M.A. Abrams, *The First Whole Rehab Catalog: A Comprehensive Guide to Products and Services for the Physically Disadvantaged,* Betterway Publications, Inc., 1990.

Asthma

13. The American Lung Association, *Help Yourself to Better Breathing,* 1991. Available from your local chapter of the American Lung Association.

14. A. Weinstein, MD, *Asthma: The Complete Guide to Self-Management of Asthma for Patients and Their Families,* McGraw-Hill, 1987.

Also see Resource 19.

Back and Neck Pain

15. R. McKenzie, *Treat Your Own Back,* Spinal Publications, 1989.

16. R. McKenzie, *Treat Your Own Neck,* Spinal Publications, 1989.

Cancer

17. M. Dollinger, E. H. Rosenbaum, G. Cable, *Everyone's Guide to Cancer Therapy*, Somerville House Books, 1991.

18. B. Siegel, MD, *How to Live Between Office Visits*, HarperCollins, 1993.

Also see Resource 19.

Chronic Illnesses

19. K. Lorig, H. Holman, D. Sobel et al., *Living a Healthy Life With Chronic Conditions: Self-Management of Heart Disease, Arthritis, Stroke, Diabetes, Asthma, Bronchitis, Emphysema, and Others*, Bull Publishing, 1993.

20. D. Spiegel, *Living Beyond Limits: New Hope and Help for Facing Life-Threatening Illness*, Ballantine, 1994.

Diabetes

21. L. Jovanovic-Peterson, MD, C. M. Peterson, MD, and M. B. Stone, *A Touch of Diabetes: A Guide for People Who Have Type II, Non-Insulin Dependent Diabetes,* Chronimed Publishing, 1991.

22. D.W. Guthrie, RN, PhD, and R.A. Guthrie, MD, *The Diabetes Sourcebook*, Lowell House, 1995.

Also see Resource 19.

Elder Care

23. D. W. Kemper et al., *Growing Wiser: The Older Person's Guide to Mental Wellness,* Healthwise, Inc., 1986. Available from Healthwise, P.O. Box 1989, Boise, ID, 83701, (208) 345-1161.

Fitness

24. J. Clarke, *Full Life Fitness*, Human Kinetics Publishers, 1992.

25. B. Anderson, *Stretching,* Shelter Publications, 1992.

Grief

26. H. Fitzgerald, *The Mourning Handbook*, Simon and Schuster, 1994.

27. C. Staudacher, *A Time to Grieve*, HarperCollins, 1994.

Heart Disease

28. D. Ornish, MD, *Dean Ornish's Program for Reversing Heart Disease,* Ballantine, 1992.

29. M.D. McGoon, MD, ed., *Mayo Clinic Heart Book*, William Morrow and Company, 1993.

30. G.C. Griffin, MD, and W.P. Castelli MD, *How to Lower Your Cholesterol and Beat the Odds of a Heart Attack*, Fisher Books, 1993.

Also see Resource 19.

Medical Consumerism

31. D. W. Kemper et al., *It's About Time: Better Health Care in a Minute (or two),* Healthwise, Inc., 1993. Available from Healthwise, P.O. Box 1989, Boise, ID 83701, (208) 345-1161.

32. R. Arnot, MD, *The Best Medicine,* Addison-Wesley, 1992.

33. C. B. Inlander, *Good Operations, Bad Operations: The People's Medical Society's Guide to Surgery,* Penguin Books, 1993.

Medications

34. *Consumer Reports Books Complete Drug Reference*, Consumer Reports, 1996.

35. *Physician's Desk Reference*. Available at most hospital and public libraries.

Also see Resource 2.

Mental Self-Care

36. D.W. Kemper, et al. *Growing Wiser: The Older Person's Guide to Mental Wellness*, Healthwise, Inc., 1990. Available from Healthwise, P.O. Box 1989, Boise, ID 83701, (208) 345-1161.

37. D. Burns, MD, *The Feeling Good Handbook,* New American Library/Dutton, 1990.

38. D. Sobel, MD, *The Healthy Mind, Healthy Body Handbook,* DRx, 1996.

39. B. Moyers, *Healing and the Mind,* Doubleday, 1993.

40. M. Seligman, *Learned Optimism,* Random House, 1991.

Men's Health

41. *Staying Strong for Men Over 50: A Common Sense Health Guide.* Available from AARP, Stock no. D15296, 601 E Street NW, Washington, DC 20049.

42. P.C. Walsh, MD, and J.F. Worthington, *The Prostate: A Guide for Men and the Women Who Love Them*, The Johns Hopkins University Press, 1995.

Newsletters

43. *University of California at Berkeley Wellness Letter.* Available from Health Letter Associates, P.O. Box 420148, Palm Coast, FL 32142.

44. *Mental Medicine Update*, The Center for Health Sciences, P.O. Box 381069, Cambridge, MA 02238-1069. Phone 1-800-222-4745.

45. *Harvard Health Letter,* P.O. Box 420285, 11 Commerce Blvd., Palm Coast, FL 32142.

Nutrition

46. *Health Counts.* John Wiley and Sons, Inc., 1991.

47. E. R. Blonz, *The Really Simple, No-Nonsense Nutrition Guide,* Conari Press, 1993.

Pain

48. E. Mohr-Catalano, *The Chronic Pain Control Workbook: A Step-by-Step Guide for Coping With and Overcoming Your Pain,* New Harbinger Publications, 1987.

49. M. Caudill, *Managing Chronic Pain: A Behavioral Medicine Program Workbook*, Guilford, 1994.

Safety and First Aid

50. *American Red Cross First Aid and Safety Handbook*, Little, Brown, and Company, 1992.

Self-Help Groups

51. *The Self-Help Sourcebook* (4th ed.), American Self-Help Clearinghouse, 1992. Saint Clares-Riverside Medical Center, 25 Pocono Road, Denville, NJ 07834.

Smoking

52. T. Ferguson, MD, *The No-Nag, No-Guilt, Do-It-Your-Own-Way Guide to Quitting Smoking,* Putnam, 1988.

Stress

53. H. Benson and M. Klipper, *The Relaxation Response,* Avon Books, 1976.

54. M. Davis et al., *The Relaxation and Stress Reduction Workbook*, New Harbinger, 1994.

Stroke

55. *American Heart Association Family Guide to Stroke*, Random House, 1994.

Wellness

56. H. Benson and E. M. Stuart, *The Wellness Book,* S&S Trade, 1993.

57. D. W. Kemper et al., *Pathways: A Success Guide for a Healthy Life,* Healthwise, Inc., 1985. Available from Healthwise, P.O. Box 1989, Boise, ID 83701, (208) 345-1161.

58. R. Ornstein and D. Sobel, MD, *Healthy Pleasures,* Addison-Wesley, 1989.

Women's Health

59. P.B. Doress-Worters and D.L. Siegal, *Ourselves, Growing Older*, Simon and Schuster, 1994.

60. B.D. Shephard, MD, and C.A. Shephard, *The Complete Guide to Women's Health*, Penguin Books, 1990.

Index

A

Abdominal pain, 115, 116, 117, 123, 124, 129, 132, 135
    in lower left abdomen, with constipation and fever, 123
    in upper right abdomen, with fever and vomiting, 124
    ulcers and, 135
    with diarrhea, 122
    with fever, 123, 124
    with gas and bloating, 129
    with vomiting, 132
    with vomiting and diarrhea, 132
Abdominal problems, see Digestive problems
Abscess, skin, see Boils, 214
Accidents, preventing, 266
Acetaminophen, 406
Achilles tendinitis, 58
Acid controllers, 400
    heartburn and, 126
    ulcers and, 136
Acquired immune deficiency syndrome (AIDS), 263
Actinic keratoses, 227
Addiction
    alcohol, 299
    drug, 308
    sleeping pills or tranquilizers and, 408
    to medications, symptoms of, 410
Adult day care, 391
Adult foster care, 391
Advance directives, 382
Advice nurse, 12

Advil, 406
Age spots, 211
Al-Anon, 302
Alcohol
    memory loss and, 299, 313
    moderate use of, 300
    problems, 299
    screening test for problems, 301
Alcoholics Anonymous, 300
Alcoholism, 299
Aleve, 406
Alka-2, 400
Alka-Seltzer, 400
Allergic reaction, 65
    anaphylaxis, 65, 66
    antibiotics and, 407
    hives and, 219
    insect bites and, 286, 288
Allergies, 63
    antihistamines, 404
    immunotherapy, 66
    severe, see anaphylaxis, 65, 66
    shots, 66
Aluminum, Alzheimer's disease and, 164
Alzheimer's disease, 163
    caregiver tips for,167, 390
    durable power of attorney and, 383
    mental status exam, 169
Ambulance services, wise use of, 15
Ampho-jel, 400
Amsler grid, 187
Anal itching, 127
Anaphylaxis, signs of, 66

Anger, 302
  grief and, 310
Angina, 97
  change in pattern of, 100
Angiomas, cherry, 226
Ankles, swelling in, 101
Antacids, 400
  heartburn and, 126
  ulcers and, 136
Anti-inflammatory drugs, 405, 406
  heartburn and, 126, 127
  high blood pressure and, 104
  nausea and vomiting and, 132
  ulcers and, 135
Antibiotics, 407
  nausea and vomiting and, 132
Antidiarrheals, 401
Antifungals, 218
Antihistamines, 404
  hives and, 219
Anus
  itching, 127
  lump on, 127, 128
  pain in, with bowel movements,
  127
Anxiety, 303
  hyperthyroid and, 152
Apnea, 316
Arm pain, 42
  with chest pain, 74
Arrhythmias, see Irregular heartbeats,
  105
Arthritis, 43, 44
  ice and cold packs for, 294
  types of, chart, 44
Artificial tears, for dry eyes, 184
Aspirin, 405
  bruises and, 269
  nosebleeds and, 289
  stroke and, 110

Assistive devices, 414
Asthma, 67
Atherosclerosis, 95
  cholesterol and, 352
  coronary artery disease and, 96
  peripheral vascular disease and,
  107
Athlete's foot, 217
Atrial fibrillation, 105
Atrophic vaginitis, 236, 240
Audiologist, 196
Automobile safety checklist, 266

B
Back pain, 27
  exercises to prevent, 32
  first aid for, 28
  osteoporosis and, 57
  posture and, 30
  ruptured disc and, 29
  sudden and unexplained, 57
  surgery, 38
  with fever (men), 255
  with leg or buttock pain (sciatica),
  29
  with leg weakness, 37
  with painful urination, fever, chills
  (men), 254, 255
  with painful urination, fever, chills
  (women), 141
Bacteria, ulcers and, 135
Bacterial infections, 70
  compared to viral, 71
Bacterial vaginosis, 240
Bad breath, 202
  gingivitis and, 204